psychiatry

The National Medical Series for Independent Study

psychiatry

EDITOR

James H. Scully, M.D., F.A.P.A.

*Associate Professor of Psychiatry
Director, Medical Student Education
  in Psychiatry
Director, Psychiatric Residency
  Training Program
University of Colorado School of
  Medicine
Director, Psychiatric Liaison Division
Veterans Administration Medical
  Center
Denver, Colorado*

A WILEY MEDICAL PUBLICATION
JOHN WILEY & SONS
New York • Chichester • Brisbane • Toronto • Singapore

Harwal Publishing Company, Media, Pennsylvania

Library of Congress Cataloging in Publication Data
Main entry under title:

Psychiatry.

(The National medical series for independent study)
(A Wiley medical publication)
   Includes index.
   1. Psychiatry—Examinations, questions, etc.
I. Scully, James H. II. Series. III. Series: Wiley med-
ical publication. [DNLM: 1. Psychiatry—examination
questions. 2. Psychiatry—outlines. WM 18 P9765]
RC457.P77   1985   616.89′0076   85-7679
ISBN 0-471-82345-7

©1985 by Harwal Publishing Company, Media, Pennsylvania

10 9 8 7 6

Contents

Contributors

Jon A. Bell, M.D.
Assistant Professor of Psychiatry
University of Colorado School of Medicine
Medical Director, Psychiatric Emergency
  Service
Veterans Administration Medical Center
Denver, Colorado

Steven L. Dubovsky, M.D., F.A.P.A.
Associate Professor of Psychiatry and
  Medicine
Associate Dean
University of Colorado School of Medicine
Attending Physician, Colorado Psychiatric
  Hospital and University Hospital
Denver, Colorado

Eugene V. Friedrich, M.D.
formerly, Assistant Professor
  of Psychiatry
University of Colorado School of Medicine
Ward Chief
Veterans Administration Medical Center
Denver, Colorado

William V. Good, M.D.
formerly, Assistant Professor
  of Psychiatry and Pediatrics
University of Colorado School of Medicine
Denver, Colorado

James H. Scully, M.D., F.A.P.A.
Associate Professor of Psychiatry
Director, Medical Student Education in
  Psychiatry
Director, Psychiatric Residency Training
  Program
University of Colorado School of Medicine
Director, Psychiatric Liaison Division
Veterans Administration Medical Center
Denver, Colorado

Preface

This book is designed to outline the major clinical areas of psychiatry, and the current understanding of the diagnosis and treatment of psychiatric illness is presented in outline form. While only a few physicians specialize in the area of mental illness, almost every physician sees patients with psychiatric disorders in his or her clinical practice. Many surveys of practice patterns reveal that nearly one-half of the patients with psychiatric illness receive most, if not all, of their care from nonpsychiatric physicians. It is clearly necessary then for all physicians to know something about the diagnosis and treatment of psychiatric illness.

A recent major advance in our ability to diagnose mental illness has been achieved by a publication of the American Psychiatric Association, the *Diagnostic and Statistical Manual of Mental Disorders,* third edition, which is known as the *DSM III.* Although psychiatric illnesses have been described for thousands of years, particular mental disorders have been subject to interpretation. The *DSM III* attempts to bring descriptive and observable criteria to the diagnosis of psychiatric illness.

A great deal of research is under way in our attempt to understand the brain and behavior. Research in psychiatry is now at a point comparable to where it was in general medicine about 20 years ago. The future looks promising for better understanding the basic mechanisms of mental illness as well as for improving the treatment of those who suffer.

James H. Scully

Acknowledgments

We would like to express our deep appreciation to Jim Harris of Harwal Publishing Company, who developed the concept for this series, and to Jane Velker, Project Editor, for her support, guidance, and patience over the months. Special thanks are also due Naomi Miller for her tireless efforts in preparing the manuscript in addition to all of her other duties as Staff Assistant for Medical Student Education in the Department of Psychiatry at the University of Colorado School of Medicine.

Publisher's Note

The objective of the *National Medical Series* is to present an extraordinarily large amount of information in an easily retrievable form. The outline format was selected for this purpose of reducing to the essentials the medical information needed by today's student and practitioner.

While the concept of an outline format was well received by the authors and publisher, the difficulties inherent in working with this style were not initially apparent. That the series has been published and received enthusiastically is a tribute to the authors who worked long and diligently to produce books that are stylistically consistent and comprehensive in content.

The task of producing the *National Medical Series* required more than the efforts of the authors, however, and the missing elements have been supplied by highly competent and dedicated developmental editors and support staff. Editors, compositors, proofreaders, and layout and design staff have all polished the outline to a fine form. It is with deep appreciation that I thank all who have participated, in particular, the staff at Harwal—Debra L. Dreger, Jane Edwards, Gloria Hamilton, Jeanine Kosteski, Wieslawa B. Langenfeld, Keith LaSala, June A. Sangiorgio, Mary Ann C. Sheldon, and Jane Velker.

The Publisher

Introduction

Psychiatry is one of six clinical science review books in a series entitled *The National Medical Series for Independent Study*. This series has been designed to provide students and house officers, as well as physicians, with a concise but comprehensive instrument for self-evaluation and review within the clinical sciences. Although *Psychiatry* would be most useful for students preparing for the National Board of Medical Examiners examinations (Part II, Part III, FLEX, and FMGEMS), it should also be useful for students studying for course examinations. These books are not intended to replace the standard clinical science texts but, rather, to complement them.

The books in this series present the core content of each clinical science area, using an outline format and featuring a total of 300 study questions. The questions are distributed throughout the book at the end of each chapter and in a pretest and post-test. In addition, each question is accompanied by the correct answer, a paragraph-length explanation of the correct answer, and specific reference to the outline points under which the information necessary to answer the question can be found.

We have chosen an outline format to allow maximal ease in retrieving information, assuming that the time available to the reader is limited. Considerable editorial time has been spent to ensure that the information required by all medical school curricula has been included and that each question parallels the format of the questions on the National Board examinations. We feel that the combination of the outline format and board-type study questions provides a unique teaching device.

We hope you will find this series interesting, relevant, and challenging. The authors, as well as the John Wiley and Harwal staffs, welcome your comments and suggestions.

Pretest

QUESTIONS

Directions: Each question below contains five suggested answers. Choose the **one best** response to each question.

1. What is the most important feature of addiction?

(A) Overwhelming involvement in seeking and using a drug
(B) Physical dependence on a drug
(C) Use of narcotics
(D) Antisocial behavior
(E) Tolerance, withdrawal, and abstinence syndromes

2. Almost all theories about the etiology of the borderline personality disorder postulate

(A) problems in neurotransmitter function
(B) problems in separation-individuation
(C) cognitive disorganization
(D) low levels of monoamine oxidase (MAO) activity in platelets
(E) oedipal conflicts

3. A man is found to have injected himself with a foreign matter for no apparent reason, but he denies this. The most likely diagnosis is

(A) hypochondriasis
(B) malingering
(C) somatization disorder
(D) conversion disorder
(E) factitious disorder

4. Night terrors are most likely to occur at what time during the night?

(A) Between 9:00 P.M. and 1:00 A.M.
(B) Between midnight and 3:00 A.M.
(C) Between 2:00 A.M. and 5:00 A.M.
(D) Between 5:00 A.M. and 6:30 A.M.
(E) At any time

5. What percentage of patients who die by suicide have sought medical help within 6 months of their deaths?

(A) 20%
(B) 30%
(C) 40%
(D) 50%
(E) 60%

6. A 58-year-old man complains of moodiness and disinterest in his normal activities. At times he is confused and forgetful. His gait is unsteady. Deep-tendon reflexes are diminished. He frequently experiences tingling in his legs. What is the most likely diagnosis?

(A) Hypothyroidism
(B) A cerebellar neoplasm
(C) Multiple sclerosis (MS)
(D) Vitamin B_{12} deficiency
(E) Manganese intoxication

7. An example of a simple phobia is fear of

(A) horses
(B) public transportation
(C) bridges
(D) social situations
(E) crowds

8. All of the following statements about the epidemiology of affective disorders are true EXCEPT

(A) the lifelong risk for bipolar disorder is about 1%
(B) depression may occur at any age
(C) dysthymic disorder is frequently associated with chronic medical and psychiatric illnesses
(D) men are diagnosed as depressed more often than women
(E) the risk for major affective illness is greater in family members of those afflicted than in the population as a whole

9. The dramatic decrease in the number of hospitalized schizophrenic patients since 1955 is due to

(A) successful primary prevention, resulting in a decreased incidence of the disorder
(B) increased social acceptance, resulting in decreased stigmatization
(C) successful symptomatic treatment with neuroleptics, permitting an earlier return to the community
(D) successful curative treatment, resulting in a decreased prevalence of the disorder
(E) increased social mobility, with an increased population in urban areas

10. All of the following statements about normal sexual response are true EXCEPT

(A) physical stimulation of the bladder may produce an involuntary sexual response
(B) erection and lubrication depend upon arousal of the parasympathetic nervous system
(C) arousal of the sympathetic nervous system inhibits sexual response
(D) stages of sexual response include excitement, plateau, and resolution
(E) psychic stimuli are mediated through the prefrontal cortex and the anterior spinal cord

11. A young woman with anorexia nervosa steadfastly refuses to eat. She is not yet in imminent medical danger from starvation, and she remains an outpatient. A logical approach at this point would be to

(A) break off treatment with the patient, refusing to treat her unless she agrees to eat
(B) set a critical weight for the patient below which she will be hospitalized if necessary and forced to gain weight
(C) insist that the patient must increase her caloric intake or she will be hospitalized
(D) try to curtail her physical activities (e.g., running and dancing)
(E) none of the above

12. A 22-year-old woman has just delivered a healthy boy by caesarean section under general anesthesia. When she awakens she is frantic because she has not bonded to her child. The physician should

(A) reassure the patient that bonding is a lengthy process
(B) suggest that the mother breast-feed to offset the effects of poor postnatal bonding
(C) return in 1 day to see if the patient's concerns have dissipated
(D) recommend psychiatric counseling aimed at helping the patient attach to her child
(E) none of the above

13. Effects of amphetamine intoxication include all of the following EXCEPT

(A) tachycardia
(B) depression
(C) suspiciousness
(D) anorexia
(E) insomnia

14. Which of the following disorders is most likely to present as violent behavior?

(A) Bipolar disorder, manic
(B) Anxiety disorder
(C) Major depressive episode
(D) Somatoform disorder
(E) Obsessive-compulsive personality disorder

15. Which of the following personality types is most commonly associated with anorexia nervosa?

(A) Schizophrenic
(B) Borderline
(C) Sociopathic
(D) Hysterical
(E) None of the above

16. All of the following statements about major depression are true EXCEPT

(A) some patients are treated with increased exposure to light
(B) 50% of patients suffer a recurrence
(C) levels of dopamine and its metabolites are decreased
(D) symptoms of dysphoria are unaltering during the episode
(E) medication can shorten the depressive episode in many cases

17. Anxiety may be a symptom of all of the following illnesses EXCEPT

(A) hypoglycemia
(B) hypothyroidism
(C) pheochromocytoma
(D) porphyria
(E) hypocalcemia

18. A 26-year-old woman presents with a history of emotional lability and anxiety punctuated by episodes of confusion and abdominal pain. She takes birth control pills but uses no other drugs or medications. Which of the following diagnoses is most likely?

(A) Acute intermittent porphyria
(B) Toxic vapor exposure
(C) Premenstrual syndrome
(D) Petit mal seizures
(E) Presenile dementia

19. What is the most common reason for cessation of sexual activity in married couples?

(A) Aging
(B) Marital discord
(C) Physical illness
(D) Cultural prohibitions
(E) Depression

20. All of the following statements about child abuse are true EXCEPT

(A) children are often reluctant to admit to abuse
(B) physicians may be hesitant to intervene in family matters
(C) abuse is more prevalent in families of lower socioeconomic level
(D) any unexplained trauma should raise the question of abuse
(E) abusive parents may appear overly concerned about the child's welfare

21. Which of the following conditions is pathognomonic of schizophrenia?

(A) A progressive deteriorating course
(B) Auditory hallucinations of a derogatory nature
(C) Bizarre delusions of influence by an outside force
(D) Loose associations with overinclusive ideas
(E) None of the above

22. Which of the following personality types is most likely to respond to a placebo?

(A) Obsessive-compulsive
(B) Histrionic
(C) Narcissistic
(D) Paranoid
(E) None of the above

Directions: Each question below contains four suggested answers of which **one or more** is correct. Choose the answer

    A if **1, 2, and 3** are correct
    B if **1 and 3** are correct
    C if **2 and 4** are correct
    D if **4** is correct
    E if **1, 2, 3, and 4** are correct

23. The classic psychosomatic disorders include

(1) hypothyroidism
(2) multiple sclerosis (MS)
(3) hyperventilation
(4) peptic ulcer

24. The developmental history of a patient with anorexia nervosa is likely to reveal which of the following factors?

(1) Little or no negativism at the age of 2 years
(2) A very compliant personality style
(3) High achievement
(4) An obsessive-compulsive personality type

25. Factors associated with a poor prognosis for schizophrenia include

(1) acute onset with agitation
(2) absence of affective symptoms
(3) verbal aggressiveness
(4) unmarried status

26. Premature ejaculation can be described as

(1) the most common form of sexual dysfunction reported by men
(2) occasioned by hostile feelings towards the sexual partner
(3) usually caused by psychological factors such as anxiety
(4) psychologically mediated by arousal of the parasympathetic nervous system

27. True statements about sexual abuse include

(1) father- (or stepfather-) daughter incest is most common
(2) sexual abuse often precipitates running away from home
(3) sexual abuse may present as vaginal trauma
(4) children are often ashamed of their incestuous activity

28. Cocaine abuse can manifest as

(1) sexual dysfunction in men
(2) an increased need for sleep
(3) severe anxiety and paranoid ideation
(4) hallucinations

29. Which of the following conditions can cause encopresis?

(1) Night terrors
(2) Crohn's disease
(3) Rheumatoid arthritis
(4) Hirschsprung's disease

30. True statements concerning narcotic abuse include which of the following?

(1) Narcotic abuse does not increase mortality significantly
(2) Most addicts are introduced to opioids by drug pushers
(3) Narcotic abuse is common in young adults
(4) Narcotic abuse tends to occur in an epidemic fashion

31. A 37-year-old man is brought to the emergency room by the police. He was apprehended while driving 100 mph on the highway at night without his headlights on. He is agitated and belligerent. He warns the physician that he has spoken to God and that God will punish those who have incarcerated him. Diagnostic possibilities include

(1) hyperthyroidism
(2) arsenic intoxication
(3) amphetamine intoxication
(4) Addison's disease

Questions 32–34

A 17-year-old boy was brought to the emergency room by his father after admitting that he had taken three of his father's sleeping pills [30 mg of Dalmane (flurazepam)] in a suicide attempt. He was medically cleared, with the physicians and nurses making jokes about "a three-Dalmane overdose." The patient appeared depressed, but he minimized the episode, saying that he was just upset about school. The father was angry about "running up a bill for nothing" and was impatient to take his son back home. Both were resistant to a psychiatric evaluation.

32. Since neither the patient nor his father wanted to stay and since the overdose was not life-threatening, the most appropriate treatment at this time would include

(1) calling other family members to come to the hospital
(2) referring the boy to the school counselor to discuss his academic problems
(3) insisting that the father and son stay to be interviewed individually
(4) encouraging the father to watch out for his son

33. Additional treatment approaches at this point would include

(1) beginning antidepressant therapy since the medication takes 10 to 14 days to be effective
(2) encouraging the father to hide his sleeping pills and other medications
(3) giving the son an excuse from school for a couple of days so that he may rest
(4) suggesting family counseling to help to relieve tensions

The boy remained silent, and the father continued to insist on going home. The decision was made to send the boy home with his father. He was brought in the following morning dead of a self-inflicted gunshot wound to the head. The father had left his loaded revolver in his dresser before going to work.

34. This case represents errors in suicide evaluation, including

(1) not adequately evaluating the son's feelings about being alive
(2) not appreciating the meaning of the suicide attempt for both the son and the father
(3) not assessing adequately the father's capacity to be a resource and support
(4) not immediately hospitalizing the patient against his will

Directions: The groups of questions below consist of lettered choices followed by several numbered items. For each numbered item select the **one** lettered choice with which it is **most** closely associated. Each lettered choice may be used once, more than once, or not at all.

Questions 35–39

Match each statement below with the type of medication that it describes.

(A) Benzodiazepines
(B) Antihistamines
(C) Barbiturates
(D) Neuroleptics
(E) Tricyclic and tetracyclic antidepressant drugs

35. These drugs may cause tardive dyskinesia if taken chronically

36. There is low incidence of toxicity, but these drugs are not always effective

37. Addiction rarely occurs with these drugs

38. These drugs are indicated for endogenous anxiety and phobias

39. There is high danger of tolerance, abstinence syndromes, and addiction

Questions 40–45

Match each statement below with the sex-related condition it best describes.

(A) Transsexualism
(B) Transvestism
(C) Exhibitionism
(D) Impotence
(E) Homosexuality

40. It often occurs for the first time after overindulgence in alcohol

41. Most men with this disorder have a history of dressing in female clothing before the age of 4 years

42. Psychologically immature young men with hostile feelings towards their "victims" need this behavior to achieve sexual gratification

43. Anxiety about sexual performance is the most common psychological cause

44. Incidence and prevalence of mental illness in this condition is about the same as in the general population

45. Men with this disorder have excessively close physical and emotional ties to their mothers and have fathers who were absent during their childhoods

Questions 46–50

Match each substance listed below with the characteristic sign of intoxication.

(A) Suggestibility
(B) Insomnia
(C) Decreased pain sensitivity
(D) Violence
(E) Postural hypotension

46. Phencyclidine (PCP)

47. Marijuana

48. Stimulants

49. Barbiturates

50. Alcohol

Questions 51–55

Match each disorder listed below with the appropriate clinical presentation.

(A) Binging followed by purging
(B) Unusual regurgitation and vomiting
(C) Fluctuating weight loss and weight gain
(D) Encephalopathy
(E) Weight loss

51. Failure to thrive

52. Anorexia nervosa

53. Bulimia

54. Pica

55. Rumination

Questions 56–60

Match each condition listed below with its appropriate corollary.

(A) It probably begins at birth
(B) It can be treated with tricyclic antidepressants
(C) It can be a side effect of phenobarbital treatment
(D) It occurs in anxiety-producing situations
(E) It is associated with lower socioeconomic status

56. Infantile autism

57. Mental retardation

58. Enuresis

59. Hyperactivity

60. Thumb sucking

ANSWERS AND EXPLANATIONS

1. The answer is A. (*Chapter 4 I C*) Although addiction is defined differently by different clinicians, the most agreed-upon definition is overwhelming involvement and preoccupation with obtaining and using any type of drug. Addicts often are physically dependent, but it is possible to become preoccupied with drug use even if one is not dependent on the substance. Any drug, including alcohol, that acts upon the central nervous system can be addictive. Although antisocial behavior often develops as a result of attempting to obtain drugs, it is not the defining feature of addiction.

2. The answer is B. (*Chapter 11 III A 4*) Borderline personality is thought to be caused by problems in early development, which usually include the mother not allowing the infant to separate and keeping him or her too close or, alternatively, abandoning and pushing away the infant so that there is no smooth separation. This leads to a persistance of the symbiotic relationship with the parent. Cognitive disorganization may occur under high stress situations, but this is secondary rather than etiologic. Low levels of monoamine oxidase (MAO) activity in platelets occur in patients with schizotypal disorder, not borderline disorder. All of these problems precede issues of oedipal struggles in the young child, which occur later in development.

3. The answer is E. (*Chapter 6 III A*) Factitious disorder is the most likely diagnosis because, although the patient must be aware that he has caused his illness, he probably is not aware of his motivation for doing so. Hypochondriasis is a preoccupation with the sick role but does not usually involve the patient causing harm to him- or herself. Malingering is closer in nature to this case, but the goals of malingering behavior must be apparent. Diagnosis of somatization disorder requires multiple symptoms, and that of conversion disorder requires a psychoneurologic loss of function.

4. The answer is A. (*Chapter 10 VI A 2*) Night terrors occur during the deep stages (stages 3 and 4) of sleep, which are early in the sleep cycle. Therefore, night terrors would be most likely to occur between 9:00 P.M. and 1:00 A.M. The physiology of night terrors is only partly understood. Apparently, arousal from these deep stages of sleep triggers night terrors in some children. Since so many children (30%) experience night terrors, delayed central nervous system maturation is hypothesized as a cause.

5. The answer is D. (*Chapter 9 III A 5*) ''Medical help'' does not mean psychiatric help; rather, most patients go to their family physicians looking for help but in a covert fashion. As many as 70% of patients who commit suicide have some active medical illness that keeps them in contact with their physicians. They may not reveal feelings of depression or suicidal ideation unless directly asked. Furthermore, many depressed patients initially present to nonpsychiatric physicians with various somatic complaints, fatigue, and insomnia; again they may not describe depression or suicidal ideation unless asked. If the diagnosis is missed, these patients may attempt suicide with the prescriptions that they are given for anxiety or sleeplessness.

6. The answer is D. (*Chapter 3 IV H 4*) The patient has presented with psychiatric symptoms of apathy and moodiness. Memory impairment is suggested by his forgetfulness. There is evidence of neurologic impairment. Destruction of the myelin sheaths could explain all of these symptoms, phenomena that are seen in both multiple sclerosis (MS) and vitamin B_{12} deficiency. Without a relapsing, remitting course, vitamin B_{12} deficiency is the more likely diagnosis.

7. The answer is A. (*Chapter 5 I B 5 a*) Irrational fear of a situation in which help might not be immediately available or from which escape might be difficult, such as being in crowds, on public transportation, and crossing bridges, are types of agoraphobia. Fear that one will humiliate oneself in certain social situations indicates a social phobia. Simple phobias, such as fear of horses, include fears that are not primarily associated with being alone, in public places, or in certain social situations.

8. The answer is D. (*Chapter 2 III A 2*) Depression is diagnosed in women about two times as often as in men, possibly because women get depressed more readily than men. The signs of depression (e.g., tearfulness and hopelessness) may be more easily recognized in women because societal norms allow such expressions from women. Examiners may overlook depressive symptoms in men for similar societal reasons.

9. The answer is C. (*Chapter 1 V D; VII H*) The development and widespread use of neuroleptics since 1954 has permitted successful treatment of positive symptoms of schizophrenia. While not curative (and, in this regard, there has not been any decrease in the prevalence of the disorder), successful symptomatic treatment dovetailed with the community mental health movement to allow the deinstitutionalization of even chronic patients. While there may be somewhat increased societal acceptance of mental illness, having schizophrenia continues to be a significant stigma. In the absence of a specific etiology or etiologies, no successful primary prevention is possible, and thus the incidence of the disorder has remained between 0.043% and 0.069% of the population in the United States over the past 25 years. Not only does an increase in social mobility not effect a decrease in hospitalized patients, schizophrenics tend to drift into the lower socioeconomic classes of larger cities, creating an increased incidence in these particular areas.

10. The answer is E. (*Chapter 7 I*) Psychic stimuli are mediated through the limbic system, the hypothalamus, and the lateral spinal cord. Physical stimulation of the bladder and the bowel as well as the genitals may produce an involuntary sexual response through the spinal cord. The parasympathetic nervous system is responsible for erection and lubrication; sympathetic arousal inhibits this response. Among the stages of sexual response are excitement, plateau, orgasm, and resolution.

11. The answer is B. (*Chapter 8 I F 3 a, c*) The weight of a patient with anorexia nervosa should be followed closely, and limits should be reinforced; that is, weight that is too low should result in hospitalization or curtailment of privileges if the patient is already hospitalized. Although increasing caloric intake would normally result in some weight gain, anorectic patients have learned that they can compensate for ingested calories by vomiting, exercising, or abusing laxatives. Likewise, decreased exercise would be met with vomiting, laxatives, or decreased caloric intake. It is too difficult to eradicate all of the weight-losing maneuvers; therefore, weight should be monitored.

12. The answer is A. (*Chapter 10 II A, B*) Bonding and attachment are processes that occur over a lengthy period of time. Although many parents worry that a caesarean section interferes with this process, simple reassurance usually is helpful to them. Breast-feeding would not necessarily offset any sort of aberration in bonding and attachment. At first, many new mothers feel that their babies do not belong to them. This feeling can last several days. Returning to see the patient is a good idea but should be done 3 to 4 days later; however, conditions can warrant returning sooner. When the mother is severely depressed, anxious, or psychotic, she should be evaluated for psychiatric treatment and follow-up.

13. The answer is B. (*Chapter 4 II C*) Amphetamine intoxication produces tachycardia, hypertension, a paranoid psychosis, loss of appetite, and sleeplessness. Depression is caused by withdrawal from amphetamines. Amphetamine psychosis may be indistinguishable from schizophrenia; it is treated with haloperidol. Withdrawal depression, which may result in a high risk of suicide, is treated with a noradrenergic antidepressant such as imipramine.

14. The answer is A. (*Chapter 9 IV C*) Bipolar patients in the midst of a manic episode are frequently extremely irritable and have a low frustration tolerance in conjunction with great pressure in their thinking and activity. They may quickly become aggressive if they are slighted or frustrated in their plans. Patients with the other diagnoses mentioned may present with considerable psychomotor agitation (e.g., those with anxiety disorder or major depressive episodes) or dramatic demands (e.g., those with somatoform disorder) but are far less likely to strike out at others. An individual with an obsessive-compulsive personality disorder tends to be overly controlled and avoids direct expression or acknowledgment of anger.

15. The answer is D. (*Chapter 8 I E 11*) The hysterical personality is one of three personality types that have been associated with anorexia nervosa. The other two are obsessive-compulsive and schizoid. Hysterics sexualize their relationships. Since sexual concerns can be at the root of anorexia nervosa, hysterics may be at greater risk for developing this illness. Individuals with obsessive-compulsive personality styles can become preoccupied with the details of eating and calorie counts. Schizoid individuals may have had bizarre mannerisms or behavior prior to the onset of anorexia, placing them at risk for this disorder, too.

16. The answer is C. (*Chapter 2 IV A 2; V A 2, 3; VIII A 3 b*) Alterations in norepinephrine and serotonin metabolism have been found in depressed individuals. Levels of both norepinephrine and serotonin have been found to be decreased, although levels may also be normal. To date, dopamine has not been shown to play a role in depression. A group of individuals who are depressed only during months with fewer hours of sunlight have been recently identified. Bodily rhythms change in response to sunlight, and increased exposure to light has proved to be successful treatment in some cases. Symptoms of dysphoria are prominent and unaltering in depressive episodes, which have been shortened in many individuals by medication.

17. The answer is B. (*Chapter 5 III C, D*) Hypothyroidism is more likely to cause depression than anxiety. Hypocalcemia may produce anxiety accompanied by increased neuromuscular irritability. Anxiety due to hypoglycemia and pheochromocytoma may be accompanied by signs of increased adrenergic activity such as sweating and tachycardia. Porphyria may produce a variety of psychiatric complaints, including psychosis and anxiety.

18. The answer is A. (*Chapter 3 IV I 2*) Key elements in this history are the episodic nature of the disturbance, the age of onset, the association between abdominal pain and confusion, and the use of birth control pills. Acute intermittent porphyria is an episodic disorder that first gains expression in young adults in the age group of 20 to 40 years. Anxiety and emotional lability may be chronic. Abdominal pain accompanies exacerbations. The use of estrogens may precipitate episodes of disturbance.

19. The answer is B. (*Chapter 7 V B 2*) Many factors can affect the sexual activity of couples, including aging, physical illness, and psychiatric illness such as depression. However, more commonly than not, the reason that sexual activity ceases is discord in the marital relationship. Cultural prohibitions may play a role but usually not as frequently as discord.

20. The answer is C. (*Chapter 9 V A*) Child abuse is as prevalent in upper- and middle-class families as it is in lower-class families, but the physician may find that he or she has a more difficult time addressing the issue in the former groups, particularly if they seem similar to his or her own socioeconomic group. In addition, the physician may feel reluctant to raise questions about the severity of family discipline and make a judgment as to what is too severe. He or she may mistakenly interpret the parents' overly concerned attitude or the child's reluctance to talk as evidence of a close, happy family. Vague or evasive answers from either children or parents about the cause of the trauma should never be accepted at face value but always should be investigated further.

21. The answer is E. (*Chapter 1 IV B*) Auditory hallucinations, bizarre delusions, and loose associations all are common symptoms of schizophrenia. Evidence of a deteriorating course is also necessary for the diagnosis. However, no single feature is pathognomonic of schizophrenia. While they may be more commonly observed in schizophrenia, all of the above features can be seen in affective disorders with psychotic features. In these cases, the psychotic symptoms are preceded by a mood disturbance and do not persist after resolution of the mood disturbance.

22. The answer is E. (*Chapter 6 V*) Placebo response is unrelated to personality type. It is often incorrectly thought that patients who respond to placebos must have a psychiatric disorder or at least have a hysterical or histrionic personality. The reaction to a placebo does not help determine if the symptoms are organic in nature, and placebo response should not be used as a test for proving that patient symptoms are psychogenic in nature.

23. The answer is D (4). (*Chapter 6 I A 1*) Hyperthyroidism or thyrotoxicosis rather than hypothyroidism was initially felt to be a psychosomatic disorder. Multiple sclerosis (MS), while often misdiagnosed in the early stages as a psychiatric illness, has generally not been thought to be caused by psychological factors. Hyperventilation is clearly a phenomenon with strong psychological components, but it is not generally classified as a disease. Peptic ulcer is the only one of these conditions that was originally studied as a psychosomatic disorder.

24. The answer is E (all). (*Chapter 9 I E 11*) Children with anorexia nervosa are often described as having been model 2 year olds. They comply with parental requests and feel a need for achievement in school and at home. They are not independent. Although they seem to follow no recommendations about eating, they usually remain dependent and easily persuaded in other areas.

25. The answer is C (2, 4). (*Chapter 1 V D 2; Table 1–1*) There are a number of factors that are consistently associated with a good prognosis or a poor prognosis for schizophrenia. Florid psychiatric symptoms with agitation and verbal aggressiveness are associated with a good prognosis, particularly when they arise acutely after a significant stress in an individual with good premorbid functioning. The factors associated with a poor prognosis, including an absence of affective symptoms and an unmarried status, predict future functioning more accurately than do those associated with a good prognosis. Poor performance on neuropsychological tests and abnormalities demonstrated by computed tomographic (CT) scans are more likely to be found in patients with symptoms indicative of a poor prognosis.

26. The answer is A (1, 2, 3). (*Chapter 7 V H*) The most common form of sexual dysfunction reported by men is premature ejaculation, in which the patient ejaculates within a few strokes of or even before insertion. It is almost always caused by psychological factors rather than by physical ones. The most common cause is anxiety, which leads to arousal of the sympathetic nervous system, which then causes premature ejaculation. Occasionally it is caused by hostile feelings towards the sexual partner, but this is unusual. In general, the parasympathetic nervous system is not aroused but is overridden by the sympathetic nervous system in the physiology of this disorder.

27. The answer is E (all). (*Chapter 9 V B 1, 2*) Sexual abuse includes all forms of sexual contact, including intercourse. Although intercourse is more common with teenaged girls, grade-school–aged girls may also be affected, with a higher incidence of vaginal trauma. Any perineal or vaginal trauma in young girls, and even infants, should indicate the need for an evaluation of sexual abuse. Sexual abuse is most common between father and daughter, and, regardless of how close their relationship is in other respects, the daughter usually experiences some shame and guilt. The feeling of shame and guilt may be increased by the father's threats or pressures to keep their behavior secret. Over one-half of female runaways give sexual abuse as the reason for leaving home.

28. The answer is E (all). (*Chapter 3 IV F 2 y*) Users of cocaine often feel that they perform better in many areas when intoxicated. This misperception probably results from the overriding effects of euphoria and stimulation caused by the drug. Chronic cocaine use can lead to erectile and ejaculatory dysfunction in men as well as hypersomnia. Acutely, cocaine can cause severe anxiety with paranoia and hallucinations.

29. The answer is D (4). (*Chapter 10 VIII B 1, C 1*) The main illness in the differential diagnosis of encopresis is Hirschsprung's disease. Crohn's disease could conceivably cause encopresis, but the child would be so symptomatic in other ways that the diagnosis would be easily known. An empty rectal vault on physical examination can indicate Hirschsprung's disease. In encopresis the vault is usually full of stool. A fecal impaction can cause overflow encopresis, necessitating disimpaction before beginning psychiatric treatment.

30. The answer is D (4). (*Chapter 4 V A, B*) The combined mortality rate for narcotic abuse, suicide, and murder is approximately 10 per 1000. Although many adolescents and young adults experiment with a variety of drugs, hallucinogens, stimulants, and central nervous system depressants are more popular than narcotics. Two to three percent of this group have tried heroin, and a smaller percentage are addicted to opioids. Most addicts are introduced to the drug by their friends rather than by pushers. Heroin abuse tends to occur in epidemics in which individuals become addicted and then ''infect'' their friends.

31. The answer is B (1, 3). (*Chapter 3 IV F 2 e, G 3 e, K 3 a, 5 a*) Hyperthyroidism can lead to an agitated, excited state characterized by pressured, erratic behavior. Although delusions and hallucinations may occur in hyperthyroidism, as they do in this case, the mechanism is unknown. Amphetamines have potent effects on the central nervous system. With chronic use, an organic delusional syndrome may develop, which resembles paranoid schizophrenia. The individual becomes suspicious and paranoid; he or she experiences hallucinations. Unpredictable and dangerous behavior is predicated upon irrational fears and beliefs. Acute arsenic intoxication, if severe, leads to serious medical symptomatology. Chronic intoxication typically leads to apathy and lethargy, and the individual would appear to be depressed, ill, or both. Addison's disease results from chronic adrenal insufficiency. In a state of chronic corticosteroid depletion, an individual becomes depressed, lethargic, and easily fatigued: The energetic and psychotic behavior that is seen in this case is highly unlikely.

32. The answer is B (1, 3). (*Chapter 9 III D, E, F*) Any suicide attempt must be taken very seriously because the lack of success may reflect ambivalence or a miscalculation, not the lack of a serious intent to die. The suicide rate climbs dramatically for males over 15 years of age. Since this boy has probably not studied pharmacology, one can assume that he did not know that three flurazepam would not be lethal. Rather, his expectations and fantasies about what would happen are more important than the actual pharmacologic toxicity. Both the boy and his father minimized the event based on the outcome, but what of the initial intent? Also, some tension between them and anger on the father's part raises questions about the home situation in general and the father as a support in particular. Given the father's response it would be important to call other family members and see them in person both to evaluate the family completely and to emphasize the severity of the situation. Both the boy and the father might provide more information individually; the boy in particular will be unlikely to talk about his depression and suicidal feelings in the presence of his angry father. Referring the boy to a school counselor is not adequate treatment following an attempted suicide; it does not address the need for evaluation and treatment of depression and assessment of the home situation. Similarly, encouraging the father to watch out for the son is a treatment intervention without adequate evaluation. It assumes that the son must be watched, but without an assessment of ongoing suicidal intent or of the father's interest and ability to be a reliable support.

33. The answer is D (4). (*Chapter 9 III D, E, F*) Suggesting family counseling assumes that family conflict contributed to the boy's suicide attempt; the counseling must start on the spot with as complete an evaluation of the family as possible if the boy is to go home. Beginning antidepressant therapy immediately in the emergency department suggests first that a complete evaluation for depression in the boy has been done and second that there is a symptomatic depression apparent. There is no evidence that such an evaluation has been done, and if the boy is that depressed, hospitalization should be considered. Encouraging the father to hide the sleeping pills and giving the son an excuse from school suggest that a serious and continuing problem is perceived but is not directly addressed and evaluated.

Both interventions reflect an acknowledgment of the boy's depression and suggest an awareness of continuing suicidal ideation. More active intervention is required (i.e., more extensive evaluation of the boy and his support system or hospitalization).

34. The answer is A (1, 2, 3). (*Chapter 9 III D, E, F*) Outpatient treatment following a suicide attempt is a reasonable option. Not every suicide attempt requires hospitalization, and hospitalization should not be automatic as this may ultimately interfere with an ongoing treatment alliance if it is used prematurely or unnecessarily. However, if the protective environment of the hospital is not used, there should be some crisis resolution, evidence of mild concurrent psychopathology, a mobilization of environmental resources, and a therapeutic response to the interview. There is no evidence from the data that any of these criteria were present. There was neither an adequate evaluation of the son's depression and continuing wish to die nor of the father's understanding of the seriousness of the situation and willingness to be supportive of and responsible for his son. In fact, the father's continuing anger at his son and denial about the suicidal intent was apparent when he left a loaded weapon in the house and in his reluctance to have his son completely evaluated. Eight out of ten eventual suicides give prior warning. The boy had given his, and it was unheeded by the emergency room staff and his father.

35–39. The answers are: 35-D, 36-B, 37-A, 38-E, 39-C. (*Chapter 5 VII C*) Recent evidence indicates that few medical patients become addicted to benzodiazepines when the drugs are prescribed appropriately. Barbiturates, on the other hand, tend to cause tolerance, abstinence syndromes, and addiction. Antihistamines can be particularly useful as antianxiety drugs or hypnotics in the elderly, but they are not as predictably effective as other medications and may cause anticholinergic side effects. In low doses, nonsedating neuroleptics (antipsychotic drugs) may help to relieve anxiety in patients who fear sedation, but the danger of tardive dyskinesia must not be ignored. Antidepressants may be very effective in the treatment of endogenous anxiety and phobias.

40–45. The answers are: 40-D, 41-A, 42-C, 43-D, 44-E, 45-A. (*Chapter 7 III A; IV C 2, 5; VI A 1*) An overindulgence in alcohol is often the initial cause of failure of erection; this event leads to anxiety about performance. Other sexual disorders, such as transvestism and exhibitionism, may also occur when a lack of impulse control is exacerbated by alcohol; however, paraphilias are not usually precipitated for the first time by drinking.

Although anxiety is an issue in many of the sexual disorders, it is a primary cause of secondary erectile failure or impotence. Sympathetic nervous system arousal decreases the ability to have an erection, which is mediated by the parasympathetic nervous system. A man must relax in order to achieve erection, and anxiety interferes with this reaction.

The etiology of transsexualism in males is thought to be associated with an excessively close physical and emotional relationship with the mother and with the absence of the father during childhood. Over 75% of transsexual males have a history of being crossdressed by their mothers in girls' clothing before the age of 4 years. Transvestites also dress in women's clothes; however, they do not have a history of doing so as early in life. Although these associations have also been postulated as causes of homosexuality, homosexuality is no longer considered to be a disorder.

The incidence and prevalence of mental illness in homosexuals is about the same as it is in heterosexuals, which is one of the reasons that homosexuality is no longer considered to be a mental illness. Exhibitionists may have concurrent and more pervasive personality disorders, including one that encompasses pedophilia. Transvestites, transsexuals, and patients with failure of erection may suffer other mental illnesses to varying degrees, but actual statistics are unknown.

Men who expose themselves (usually to women and girls) in order to achieve sexual gratification often feel hostile towards their "victims" and wish to frighten them. They often do not take further action. Transsexuals wish to change their sex and are not necessarily hostile towards anyone. Transvestites are more concerned about wearing women's clothing to achieve sexual gratification than scaring women by this behavior.

46–50. The answers are: 46-D, 47-A, 48-B, 49-E, 50-C. (*Chapter 4 II A, B, C, D*) Phencyclidine (PCP) intoxication causes violent behavior much more frequently than other hallucinogens; on the other hand, marijuana is associated with suggestibility, but intoxication rarely produces hallucinations. Stimulants disrupt sleep. Alcohol intoxication, in contrast to that caused by barbiturates, increases the pain threshold. Postural hypotension is commonly a result of barbiturate intoxication.

51–55. The answers are: 51-E, 52-C, 53-A, 54-D, 55-B. (*Chapter 9 I A 1–7; II A; III A, B, C; IV D 2; V A*) Failure to thrive presents as weight loss. As the illness progresses, short stature can develop. Failure of head growth is a very late and ominous sign because it implies that the brain has stopped growing. Psychological factors most commonly cause failure to thrive. However, the workup should include a search for organic etiologies (e.g., diabetes mellitus and chronic infection).

Anorexia nervosa causes weight loss also. Frequently there is a history of mild-to-moderate obesity. Many girls fluctuate between starvation and obesity.

Bulimia consists of binging followed by guilt and purging. Frequent weight fluctuations occur, but profound weight loss does not. Purging can consist of self-induced vomiting.

Pica is defined as eating nonfood products. When it occurs in adults, it frequently is due to iron deficiency anemia. It can be normal in children. However, eating lead-based paint chips (e.g., from old houses) leads to lead poisoning. If severe, lead poisoning presents as encephalopathy. Milder cases present as intellectual deterioration or behavior change.

Rumination is a syndrome of regurgitation and vomiting. It is a rare disorder of infancy. Rumination usually indicates parent-child difficulties. Parents may be immature and distant. Treatment should focus on the parents' relationship with the child. Because rumination can lead to nutritional problems, a careful medical workup is indicated.

56–60. The answers are: 56-A, 57-E, 58-B, 59-C, 60-D. (*Chapter 10 III A 1; VII C 3; X; XI B*) Infantile autism probably begins at birth, although it can be diagnosed up to the age of 30 months. It is a syndrome of abnormal social responsiveness, altered responses to the environment, and language abnormalities. It occurs in all socioeconomic groups. There is no medication that treats this condition.

Mental retardation is more common in lower socioeconomic groups, in which poor nutrition and environmental understimulation are prevalent. Mental retardation can be caused by a variety of medical conditions (e.g., hypothyroidism and congenital infection). Treatment is aimed at improving any underlying condition, improving nutrition, which sometimes plays a role in this condition, and providing social and environmental stimulation.

Enuresis can be treated with imipramine. This drug has anticholinergic properties that cause increased bladder capacity. It also affects the central nervous system, which may be a pathway for its effectiveness. Other forms of treatment for enuresis include behavior modification and psychotherapy. Because enuresis is self-limited, no treatment may be indicated. Organic causes of the condition should be sought.

Hyperactivity is best considered as a symptom. The differential diagnosis includes depression, severe central nervous system disease, anxiety, constitutional factors, vulnerable child syndrome, adjustment reactions, learning disabilities, as well as sedative (e.g., phenobarbital) effects. Many children with seizures are started on phenobarbital; subsequently, they may develop hyperactivity.

Thumb sucking occurs in some children when they are anxious. It can cause problems with dentition after the age of 3 years. Treatment consists of behavior modification.

1
Schizophrenic Disorders
Eugene V. Friedrich

I. DEFINITION. Schizophrenia is best considered as a group of several, if not many, disorders, which are heterogeneous with respect to etiology, pathogenesis, response to treatment, and prognosis. The various subgroups are considered to be a syndrome by virtue of characteristic presenting symptoms. These **presenting symptoms include alterations in thinking, perception, affect, and behavior**, which reach psychotic proportions at some point during the course of the illness. On a more general and abstract level, schizophrenia has been regarded in essence as a **disorder of multiple ego functions**, which results in the inability of the affected individual to discriminate accurately and reliably between inner and outer reality and to maintain a stable and cohesive internal representation of him- or herself and the outside world.

II. DIAGNOSIS. There have been many approaches to the diagnosis of schizophrenia over the years. However, at the present time, there has been no reliable identification of any of the subgroups of the schizophrenic disorders, whether this identification is based upon particular symptom clusters, biologic markers, or etiologic markers.

A. Emil Kraepelin differentiated **dementia praecox** from manic depressive illness on the basis of a progressive, deteriorating course in the former.

B. Eugene Bleuler renamed the disorder schizophrenia, believing that the basic disturbance was a **split or disharmony among various groups of mental functions**. While Bleuler did not accept Kraepelin's idea of the absoluteness of a progressive deteriorating course, neither did he believe that complete recovery to the premorbid state was possible. Bleuler described fundamental symptoms, which have been called "the four A's"; these are disturbances of associations, affect, autism, and ambivalence. He believed that delusions and hallucinations were secondary to the four fundamental symptoms. Bleuler's conceptualization greatly broadened the diagnostic limits of schizophrenia.

C. Kurt Schneider based the diagnosis of schizophrenia on clusters of symptoms, which he considered pathognomonic and designated as "first-rank symptoms." These symptoms include auditory hallucinations, thought insertion, thought withdrawal, thought broadcasting, and experiences of somatic passivity. This diagnostic approach was popular in Europe and considerably narrowed the concept of schizophrenia in comparison to Bleuler's approach. Nevertheless, these pathognomonic symptoms for schizophrenia have been reported recently to be present in 20% to 50% of patients with established manic depressive illness. The more first-rank symptoms that are present in a particular patient, the more likely the diagnosis is schizophrenia; however, a set of these symptoms alone cannot provide a valid diagnosis of schizophrenia. Furthermore, some affective symptoms have been found to be more accurate than schizophrenic symptoms in the differential diagnosis and in prediction of outcome.

D. The *Diagnostic and Statistical Manual of Mental Disorders*, third edition, *(DSM III)* takes elements from each of these diagnostic systems to generate criteria for the diagnosis of a schizophrenic disorder.

1. The essential features of such a diagnosis include the presence of certain psychotic symptoms during the active phase of the illness, characteristic symptoms involving multiple psychological processes, a deterioration from the previous level of functioning, onset before the age of 45 years, and a duration of at least 6 months. An affective disorder or organic mental disorder must be excluded before this diagnosis can be made.

2. The criteria identified by the *DSM III* is valid with respect to the following parameters:
  a. Differential response to somatic therapy
  b. Presence of a familial pattern
  c. A tendency towards onset in early adult life
  d. Recurrence and deterioration in social and occupational functioning

III. EPIDEMIOLOGY.

The **incidence**, that is, the number of new cases of schizophrenia diagnosed in a given year, has been 0.043% to 0.069% of the population in the United States over the past 25 years; the incidence in Asia and Europe has been 0.085%. The **prevalence**, which is that fraction of the population diagnosed as having schizophrenia during a given year, is 0.23% to 0.47% in the United States. The **lifetime prevalence**, that is, the percentage of those now living who have had or who are likely to have schizophrenia in their lifetimes is 1% in the United States, which is over 2 million individuals. The total annual direct and indirect **cost of schizophrenia** to the United States is estimated to be between $10 billion and $20 billion. There has been a dramatic decrease in the number of hospitalized schizophrenic patients since 1955. In fact, between 1965 and 1975, the schizophrenic population of psychiatric hospitals decreased to 40% of previous levels. However, readmission rates have doubled, and one-half of all hospitalized mental patients are schizophrenics.

A. **The sex ratio of schizophrenia** is considered to be equal in women and men, although the syndrome may be more common in women who are divorced or separated. Schizophrenic men are more likely to remain single.

B. **Ethnic and religious subgroups** show differences in the occurrence of schizophrenia, with Jews being slightly less likely to develop schizophrenia than either Protestants or Catholics. Blacks and Puerto Ricans, however, are two to two and one-half times as likely to have schizophrenia as whites. The transition from one culture to another often increases the frequency of psychopathology; however, European Jews who emigrated to Israel show a lower incidence of schizophrenia compared to the indigenous population of Israel. There are isolated towns in northern Sweden that have an incidence of schizophrenia three times that of the European and Asian incidence of 0.085%.

C. **Socioeconomic status.** The incidence of schizophrenia is highest in the lower socioeconomic classes of cities with populations greater than 100,000. The incidence increases with the increasing sizes of the cities. This correlation between incidence and size has not been noted in small towns or rural areas.

D. **Familial pattern.** There is a higher prevalence of this disorder among family members. First-degree relatives have a 10% to 15% risk of developing the disorder in comparison to the risk of the general population, which is 1%. **No definite biologic pattern has been established.** Ninety percent of schizophrenics do not have a first-degree relative with the disorder. Manic-depressive parents may produce schizophrenic children; however, it is rare to observe a manic-depressive psychosis in the children of schizophrenic parents.

E. **Season of birth.** Children who develop schizophrenia tend to be born in the late winter and early spring months. There are differences in this pattern in different parts of the world and even in different regions of the United States. In the United States as a whole, **there is a highly significant rise in schizophrenic births from December to May**, which peaks in March and April. A similar peak in incidence is found in the winter months (i.e., July, August, and September) in the Southern Hemisphere.

IV. CLINICAL FEATURES

A. **Onset.** The onset of schizophrenia usually is apparent in **late adolescence or early adulthood**, and in 50% of cases symptoms are present before the age of 25 years. Symptoms of overt psychosis are obvious. Prodromal symptoms, which may be subtle and insidiously progressive, may be manifested by gradual deterioration in function, social withdrawal, and preoccupation with strange ideas and experiences. Family and friends may feel that the affected individual has changed in some indefinite or unspecified way.

B. **Symptoms.** There are usually several areas of disturbances in different psychological processes. There may be severe impairment in one or several areas, while good function is preserved concurrently in others. Symptoms may change throughout the course of the illness. **No single feature is pathognomonic of schizophrenia.**

  1. **Form of thought** refers to the quantity and quality of cognition and verbal communication. Several types of disturbances are frequently seen.

   a. Loosening of associations results when the logical connections among ideas are obscure or absent; the goal-directedness of speech is impaired or lost. The affected individual shifts from one subject to another without clear transition.

     (1) Word use. Words may be given personalized, idiosyncratic meanings, and speech becomes more self-expressive than communicative.

     (2) Concept formation. The schizophrenic appears unable to exclude irrelevant or competing ideas from consciousness. Boundaries between concepts are blurred. Thinking becomes overinclusive, with unessential details, unrelated items, and personalized material forming the basis of concepts, which then have only private meaning.

     (3) Logic. Schizophrenic logic is similar to that seen in normal dreaming and that used by young children. Subjects are considered identical merely on the basis of common properties. Isolated parts represent the whole; the slightest similarity in appearance and simple proximity in time or space mean that the subjects are identical and causally related.

     (4) Concreteness and abstraction. The thinking of the schizophrenic patient is overly concrete, and the patient's ability to form abstract hypotheses is impaired. Like the brain-damaged patient, the schizophrenic interprets symbols and metaphors literally; however, the schizophrenic patient differs from the brain-damaged patient in that often strange, personalized material intrudes into schizophrenic thinking. The schizophrenic patient who is preoccupied with esoteric ideas such as those of philosophy, religion, and psychology may use overly abstract and misapplied symbolic concepts. Thus schizophrenic thought may be simultaneously very concrete, overly abstract, bizarre, and idiosyncratic.

     (5) Incoherence can result from severe loosening of associations. Although it may occur transiently in the midst of an acute decompensation, it usually occurs only in severely regressed, chronically institutionalized patients. In this extreme thought disorder, the patient may invent new words (**neologisms**), senselessly repeat the same words or phrases (**verbigeration**), or repeat the words of a question in an answer (**echolalia**).

   b. Poverty of content of speech occurs when speech is vague, overly concrete, overly abstract, or perseverative. Although adequate in amount, verbal expressions are empty of meaning; the individual may speak at length but actually convey little information.

   c. Mutism is the inhibition of voluntary speech. It can last for hours or days, and in the past, before the advent of modern treatment methods, it was known to last for years in some catatonic patients. In milder forms, spontaneous speech is limited, with brief, unelaborated answers given to questions.

   d. Thought blocking is an interruption of speech in the middle of a stream of thought. The affected individual appears to be preoccupied and distracted by internal stimuli; he or she may not be able to complete the train of thought. The patient may report the sensation of someone putting thoughts into or taking thoughts out of his or her head.

2. Content of thought. The most frequent disturbances in this area are **delusions**, which are beliefs that lack consensual validation and that are maintained despite evidence that they are false. Delusions may provide a central organizing function for the patient's thoughts and perceptions. They range from overvalued ideas to simple, limited delusions to complex systems that pervade all aspects of the patient's life. All of the delusions described may have elements or themes that involve body function or body parts (**somatic delusions**) and the destruction of the self or the world (**nihilistic delusions**). There is frequently evidence of religious and sexual preoccupations. Some of the ideas may be believable, while others are patently absurd (**bizarre delusions**).

   a. Overvalued ideas are unreasonable beliefs that are persistent but that are less vehemently insisted upon than delusions. If not too bizarre, they may be considered eccentric rather than pathologic. Unlike obsessive thoughts against which an individual struggles, overvalued ideas are comfortable and are not a source of internal conflict.

   b. Delusions of reference attribute personal significance to the behavior of others or to unrelated external events. The significance attributed is often ominous, negative, or at least vaguely threatening. The special meaning may be deduced from an overriding delusional belief (e.g., the patient finds repeated evidence of threats and danger, which confirms his or her other, persecutory, delusion). At other times, self-referential experiences are treated as clues to be assembled by the affected individual and from which a delusional conclusion is drawn. Ideas of reference are similar but are maintained with less intensity.

   c. Delusions of influence and control are quite common in schizophrenia. Thoughts, feelings, behavior, and even will are felt to be manipulated or controlled by outside, often mysterious, forces. If the forces are malevolent, the delusions may also be frankly persecutory. Delusions of influence and control include the belief that thoughts are being removed from (thought withdrawal) or are being put into (thought insertion) the mind or that thoughts are broadcast externally so that others can hear them. The patient may believe that his or her actions, feelings, and impulses are the products of someone else as well as being influenced and directed by someone else.

d. Persecutory and grandiose delusions are common and range from simple to complex. They overlap with the other types of delusions described previously. Persecutory delusions are the belief that others are spying on, making fun of, or plotting to harm the involved individual. There is an implicit grandiosity in that the affected individual is the center of attention, although in a negative way. Grandiose delusions reflect an exaggerated sense of importance, power, or knowledge. They may also involve a relationship or an identity with an omniscient and omnipotent figure. The patient may present himself or herself as persecuted on the basis of these grandiose attributes or relationships.

3. **Perceptual disorders** are disturbances in the patient's experience of him- or herself and the environment. They may involve any sensory modality; they are often accepted as reality and are given delusional explanations as to their origins. The false sensory experiences that occur while dreaming, falling asleep (hypnagogic experiences), or waking up (hypnopompic experiences) are similar but are not considered to be pathologic. Similar perceptual disturbances can be due to the ingestion of drugs and other toxic substances.

   a. Hallucinations are sensory experiences that occur in the absence of any corresponding external stimuli.

     (1) Auditory hallucinations, usually in the form of voices, are the most common. The voices may be single or multiple, muffled or distinct, familiar or unrecognizable. They may offer support and reassurance but are more often critical and insulting. They may speak directly to the affected individual, often maintaining a running commentary of his or her behavior. Frequently two or more voices discuss the individual in the third person. The individual may experience his or her own thoughts spoken aloud.

     (2) Command hallucinations issue an order that the patient may feel obliged to obey or unable to resist. The situation becomes dangerous when the hallucinatory commands involve injury to the patient or others.

     (3) Other hallucinations include tactile, somatic, visual, gustatory, and olfactory. The latter three rarely occur in the absence of auditory hallucinations in schizophrenia. Almost invariably the false sensations are accompanied by a delusional interpretation.

   b. Illusions are misperceptions of identifiable sensory stimuli. They occur in schizophrenia but are more common in organic mental disorders. They may occur in any sensory modality and are often given delusional explanations. Such disturbances include:

     (1) Deja vu, in which there is an unwarranted feeling of familiarity and a new situation is felt to have been experienced previously

     (2) Jamais vu, in which a familiar situation is experienced as novel

     (3) Hypersensitivity to light, sound, or smell

     (4) Distorted perception of the passage of time

     (5) Misperception of movement and perspective

     (6) Changes in the perception of one's face and body or those of other individuals

4. **Affect refers to the observable expression of emotion**, and it is assumed to reflect internal states of feeling. There are several such disturbances in schizophrenia, but they are difficult to judge objectively and are also influenced by neuroleptic medication.

   a. Blunted affect is reduced intensity in emotional responsiveness. The impression that it gives is of a lack of depth of feeling. Severe blunting suggests pervasive personality deterioration. Well-preserved emotional responses are good prognostic signs.

   b. Flat affect is extremely diminished responsiveness. The affected individual may appear totally indifferent and apathetic, with a monotone voice, an immobile face, and no accessory gestures. He or she seems to be wooden or mechanical and may describe him- or herself as having no feelings.

   c. Inappropriate affect is emotional expression that is incongruous with the content of the affected individual's speech. A simple neutral question may evoke a rage response, or the patient may smile broadly when discussing the agonizing death of a loved one. This may have a disconcerting and even eerie effect on an observer.

   d. Unusual emotions are feelings that are rarely experienced under normal circumstances. These include feelings of ineffable pleasure associated with a conviction of an omniscient understanding of life or oceanic oneness with the universe. The terror and panic accompanying the experience of the disintegration of one's body or the destruction of the world are equally indescribable.

5. **Sense of self** is one's individuality and continuity in time and space. A stable sense of self implies clear and enduring boundaries between oneself and others and a developing identity capable of self-direction. This is frequently impaired in the schizophrenic, who feels uncertain about his or her own existence and confused about his or her sexual identity. Other in-

dividuals may be experienced in an equally fragmented and discontinuous way. The schizo-phrenic is excessively responsive to the immediate stimulus and is excessively dependent on external structure to modulate his or her feelings and impulses. This may be reflected in the experience of being influenced or controlled by outside forces.

6. **Volition** is related to a disturbed sense of self and may result in apparent apathy. The individ-ual may be so ambivalent as to be paralyzed, so lacking in interest as to make self-initiated and self-directed activity impossible, or so fearful of imagined disastrous consequences that he or she dares not think, feel, or move. Patients may experience themselves as having no will of their own.

7. **Relationship to the external world.** A schizophrenic individual's experiences with and rela-tionship to the external world are likely to be quite impaired. The external world is perplexing and unpredictable; the individual may markedly withdraw and become preoccupied with egocentric thoughts, fantasies, delusions, and hallucinations. If the thought disorder is severe, communication with others becomes increasingly difficult and frustrating. Extreme preoc-cupation with an internal world and concomitant withdrawal from the external world is called **autism**.

8. **Behavior.** As with thought and affect, the disturbances of behavior may be quantitative or qualitative.
   a. **Quantitative disturbances.** The schizophrenic individual may show agitation and in-creased psychomotor activity, particularly early in an acute psychotic episode. Converse-ly, the schizophrenic may be withdrawn and inactive, evidencing reduced spontaneity and initiative. The extremes of quantitative disturbances in behavior are catatonic stupor and catatonic excitement, both of which are infrequently seen in present practice and are more likely to be associated with affective illness.
      (1) **Catatonic stupor.** The patient shows little or no response to the environment, to the point of requiring tube feedings, catheterizations, and total nursing care. Although ap-pearing unaware as well as unresponsive, on emerging from the stuporous state, it is apparent that the patient may have been acutely perceptive of all going on around him or her.
      (2) **Catatonic excitement.** The patient's activity and speech are frenzied and purposeless, apparently driven by internal stimuli and not responsive to external stimuli. The patient is not only physically dangerous to others but is medically at risk due to dehydration, hyperpyrexia, and complete exhaustion.
   b. **Qualitative changes.** Movement and gait may be awkward, stiff, and stereotyped. Inap-propriate and bizarre gestures and actions may be exhibited. Behavior appears both strange and poorly integrated.
      (1) **Catatonic posturing.** The affected individual may voluntarily assume bizarre postures and hold them for long periods of time.
      (2) **Catatonic rigidity.** The affected individual maintains a rigid posture and resists efforts to be moved.
      (3) **Catatonic waxy flexibility.** The patient's limbs yield in a wax-like fashion when moved and may remain in the position where they are placed for long periods of time, how-ever uncomfortable.
      (4) **Mannerisms and grimacing.** The patient's manner may appear artificial and stilted. Grimacing may range from the subtle to the grotesque.
      (5) **Echopraxia** is analogous to echolalia. The schizophrenic individual imitates the move-ments and gestures of an individual whom he or she is observing.
      (6) **Automatic obedience in robot-like fashion** may immediately follow any command given to the patient. Conversely, the patient may refuse to follow any request, even the simplest; this is **negativism**. When actively negativistic, the patient may do the opposite of what is requested.
      (7) **Stereotyped behavior** may present as the repetitive performance of strange gestures or patterns of walking or moving. The behavior may be purposeless or ritualistic and as-sociated with magical ideas.

9. **Associated features.** The symptoms described previously may appear in any combination and to varying degrees. An individual's symptom picture may change over time. The presen-tation of the syndrome as a whole has changed: Catatonic symptoms are infrequently seen; the content of delusions has broadened to include current aspects of civilization—in addition to be being influenced or controlled by witchcraft or hypnotism, patients feel at the mercy of radiation, lasers, and mind-altering drugs. There is generally some deterioration in personal appearance and hygiene. There may be little regard for expected or acceptable behavior in social situations.

C. **Syndromes.* The diagnosis of a particular type of schizophrenia is based on the predominant symptomatology at the time of the evaluation**; the clinical picture in any individual may vary over time.

1. **Disorganized (hebephrenic) schizophrenia** often has an early and insidious onset and a chronic course without remissions, resulting in severe impairment in social and occupational functioning. The essential features include the following.
   a. Speech is often incoherent.
   b. Delusions that are present are fragmentary and are not organized around a particular theme.
   c. Blunted, inappropriate, or silly affect is more apparent in disorganized schizophrenia than in other types of schizophrenia.
   d. Other symptoms include grimaces, mannerisms, hypochondriacal complaints, and extreme social withdrawal.

2. **Catatonic schizophrenia**, which is now uncommon in Europe and North America, often involves a family history that is positive for affective illness. At the extremes of catatonic stupor and catatonic excitement, the affected individual may be in danger of malnutrition or hyperpyrexia and exhaustion, respectively. Short-acting intravenous (IV) barbiturates dramatically ameliorate the catatonic stupor. This type of schizophrenia is characterized by a predominance of any of the following catatonic symptoms: stupor, mutism, negativism, rigidity, excitement, or posturing.

3. **Paranoid schizophrenia** tends to have a later onset than other types, and the affected individual may be better established socially and occupationally. Thought processes are tightly organized and tend toward overabstraction. Affective response may be maintained, although there may be excessive intensity in certain situations, particularly in those relating to delusions: At such times, the individual may be extremely angry and argumentative and even dangerous. At other times, social interactions may appear to be normal, although the individual tends to have a stilted, condescending manner. The patient is often concerned with homosexual impulses in him- or herself or in others. Paranoid schizophrenia is characterized by delusions, hallucinations with persecutory or grandiose content, or both.

4. **Undifferentiated schizophrenia** has prominent symptoms such as delusions, hallucinations, and disordered thinking, but it does not fit the criteria for classification in any of the other categories.

5. **Residual schizophrenia** is characterized by a history of at least one previous episode of schizophrenia with prominent psychotic symptoms. However, the current clinical picture does not evidence these psychotic symptoms. Residual symptoms, such as eccentric behavior, bizarre ideation, blunted affect, and vague speech are obvious.

V. **PATHOGENESIS.** An **active phase with psychotic symptoms** is always present at some time during the course of schizophrenia. There are also certain characteristic personality traits and nonpsychotic symptoms that may precede or follow the active phase and that accompany the patient's deterioration from a previous level of functioning.

A. **Premorbid personality.** The prepsychotic personality abnormalities that are frequently observed include shyness, withdrawal, social awkwardness, and an inability to form close relationships comfortably. An individual with a prepsychotic personality may also be suspicious, introverted, or eccentric. Despite an apparent distance in interpersonal relationships, the affected individual is often extremely sensitive and vulnerable to rejection by others. A volatile prepsychotic personality has also been described. This individual has a less effective pattern of living than does an individual with a schizoid personality. The individual with a stormy prepsychotic personality has more conscious anxiety, a less distinct self-image, and frequent crises, which are often precipitated by minor incidents. The result is a chaotic, self-destructive life-style. Characteristics of both personality types are recognizable in childhood and become more apparent in adolescence, when the individual is expected to function with greater autonomy and cope with a greater range of situations. The prepsychotic personality may meet diagnostic criteria for paranoid, schizoid, schizotypal, or borderline personality disorders.

B. **The initiating factors** described here are not specific for schizophrenia but frequently are associated with the appearance of symptoms in an individual who is predisposed to the disorder.

---

*The syndromes listed in section IV C are defined according to the diagnostic nomenclature of the *DSM III.*

1. Time of onset
   a. The peak time of onset of schizophrenia is **the end of adolescence**, which is a period of significant stress. An individual leaves home, often for the first time, to work or attend school. He or she must assume greater responsibility for his or her life, whether married or living alone. There is a mixed reaction to the losses and gains with each developmental step. There may be mourning at the loss of childhood dependency and anxiety with the increased responsibilities of adulthood.
   b. There is a second, smaller peak time of illness in the **fourth decade**, particularly for women. It may follow divorce or the death of a parent, child, or spouse.

2. Precipitating events
   a. Signs of the illness can appear following a traumatic incident. The trauma may seem to be relatively minor, such as being rejected by a friend, or it may be severe, such as being assaulted or raped.
   b. A **period of drug** [including lysergic acid diethylamide (LSD), marijuana, and amphetamines] **and alcohol use** may precede the onset of symptoms.

C. Clinical course

1. Onset. The type of onset is variable, and it has prognostic significance.
   a. The onset of schizophrenia may be **acute**, with the appearance of florid psychiatric symptoms following an identifiable stressor. The more confusion, agitation, and affective reaction accompanying the presenting symptoms, the better the prognosis. It is unusual that such a presentation leads to chronic, severe psychosis.
   b. Sometimes there may be a **transient episode of neurotic symptoms**, which may last from 1 to 2 months. Symptoms such as anxiety, phobias, and obsessional preoccupations can occur and may mirror elements of the approaching psychotic decompensation.
   c. Alternatively, there may be a **prodromal phase** of varying severity and duration, which precedes the active psychotic phase. The more insidious the onset and the more progressive the deterioration noted in this phase, the worse the prognosis. The symptoms are, in many cases, milder forms of the pathology seen in the active phase and include:
      (1) Social withdrawal
      (2) Markedly impaired role functioning and deterioration in grooming
      (3) Diminished or inappropriate affect
      (4) Bizarre ideation
      (5) Unusual perceptual experiences
      (6) Vague, overelaborate, or metaphoric speech

2. Active phase. The symptoms of the schizophrenic active phase include delusions, hallucinations, loosening of associations, disturbances of affect, and disorganized behavior (see section IV B). The duration of these symptoms ranges from 1 week to continuous.

3. Residual phase. The symptoms of this phase are the same as those of the prodromal phase. **Increasing impairment of role functioning** is especially apparent, and, together with diminished affective responsiveness, it suggests a poor prognosis. Some of the residual symptoms may be difficult to distinguish from those of a postpsychotic depression, which affects up to 25% of schizophrenics recovering from a psychotic episode. The severity of this depression can range from isolated depressive symptoms to a full-blown major depressive episode.

4. Duration. A **duration of at least 6 months** with continuous signs of the illness is required for the diagnosis of schizophrenia. Evidence of active-phase psychotic symptoms is always necessary; prodromal or residual symptoms may or may not be present. If the same symptoms occur for less than 6 months, other diagnoses are required, depending upon the specific time course of the symptoms and the presence or absence of psychosocial stressors. These alternative diagnoses include schizophreniform disorder, brief reactive psychosis, and atypical psychosis, and in general they have better prognoses.

5. Deterioration from a previous level of functioning in one or, more typically, several areas is a cardinal feature of schizophrenia.
   a. The affected individual may **recompensate** with or without chronic psychotic symptoms and function at an effective but lower level than previously. For example, he or she may have a less stressful job or may be more isolated interpersonally than would have been predicted prior to the illness. There may be no further decline, whether or not there are future episodes of schizophrenia.
   b. More commonly, there is **progressive deterioration**, resulting from increasing residual impairment following repeated acute exacerbations. The exacerbations may follow major stressful events or even seemingly minor events, which have potent intrapsychic meaning

to an individual whose adaptation is already compromised by residual symptoms. The risk of further personality deterioration increases with each relapse.

   c. Silvano Arieti has described four stages of increasing regression in schizophrenic individuals who are untreated or who are unresponsive to treatment. These stages do not imply an inevitable course for all patients but rather a possible course for some.

     (1) Stage 1 consists of three substages, which include the **progressive development of psychotic symptoms** that are seen in the active phase of schizophrenia.

     (2) Stage 2, or the **advanced stage**, is characterized by reduced anxiety and an apparent resignation. The patient's behavior becomes more asocial, routine, and stereotyped. Psychotic symptoms may persist, but the patient does not seem to be bothered by them.

     (3) Stage 3, or the **preterminal stage**, begins 5 to 15 years after the onset of the psychosis. Earlier symptoms are not distinct and appear to have burned out. Primitive behaviors such as hoarding useless objects, bizarre self-decoration, and stereotypy predominate.

     (4) Stage 4, or the **terminal stage**, begins 7 to 40 years after the onset of the psychosis. The patient appears to have moved from a psychological state to a neurologic one. The patient may grab and eat food impulsively; he or she becomes increasingly indiscriminate and ingests inedible small objects. He or she may be intermittently or regularly incontinent of urine and feces. The patient seems insensitive to pain, temperature, and taste but often retains a strong reaction to olfactory stimuli. This terminal stage of deterioration is infrequently observed with the advent of modern pharmacologic and social treatment.

D. Prognosis. Recovery from schizophrenia is possible, but a complete return to premorbid functioning is unusual, even with treatment. It is more realistic to speak in terms of social recovery or the ability to function in the community despite residual symptoms, which limit optimal functioning.

   1. Statistics. Kraepelin reported that 13% of patients recovered from a first episode in 1898. Most of these relapsed later, and only 2.6% had lasting recoveries. Some clinicians feel that the chances for complete remission and full recovery have improved but are probably not significantly better than in Kraepelin's day. At present, however, about 90% of patients achieve some state of recovery with modern treatment and rehabilitation. Only 10% require chronic hospitalization. The range of functioning subsumed under the term "social recovery" is vast, including definite but minimal impairment as well as progressive deterioration with frequent hospitalizations.

     a. After 5 years of illness, about two-thirds (60% to 70%) of patients are socially recovered and are employed 50% of the time.

       (1) Fifty percent of these patients (or thirty-three percent of the total) have had one or two episodes from which they have recovered reasonably well.

       (2) The other 50% (or 33% of the total) have definite impairment and continuing exacerbations but are able to function within society.

     b. The remaining one-third of patients have marked impairment with a chronic downhill course requiring frequent hospitalizations. This group includes the 10% of patients who need chronic institutionalization.

   2. Prognostic variables. A number of predictors of prognosis have been identified; despite different labels, this **bimodal clustering** of certain predictive elements has remained rather constant over time. A related approach has been to classify schizophrenia according to the predominance of **positive symptoms** (hallucinations, delusions, and formal thought disorder) or **negative symptoms** (affective flattening, social withdrawal, apathy, anhedonia, and poverty of speech). These subtypes, positive and negative schizophrenia, have internal consistency and distinctly different prognostic implications. The good and poor prognostic factors are compared in Table 1-1.

     a. Good prognostic variables have been called schizophreniform disorder, reactive schizophrenia, and good-prognosis schizophrenia. Patients show a predominance of positive symptoms, which are likely to respond well to neuroleptic treatment. Some authors do not believe that these symptoms represent schizophrenia at all but rather are consistent with affective illness.

     b. Poor prognostic variables have been called process, nuclear, true, and poor-prognosis schizophrenia. These patients show a predominance of negative symptoms, which respond poorly to neuroleptic treatment and which seem to reflect a defect state (i.e., a state characterized by diminished or absent function in some areas). These prognostic variables predict a poor outcome with 80% to 90% accuracy, which is more reliable than predictors of a good outcome. Associated findings for this group of patients include an increased incidence of abnormal computed tomographic (CT) scans and poor performance on neuropsychological tests of cognitive functioning.

Table 1-1. Prognostic Variables of Schizophrenia

Good Prognosis	Poor Prognosis
Acute onset with obvious precipitating factors	Insidious onset with no precipitating factors
Good premorbid social and work history	Schizoid or asocial premorbid functioning
Depressive symptoms	Withdrawn behavior
Concern over guilt and death	Emotional blunting
Verbal aggression	Little overt hostility
Tension and anxiety	Excessive persecutory delusions and paranoia
Confusion and disorientation	Absence of affective symptoms
Married state	Hebephrenic clinical picture
A family history of an affective disorder	Single state
No family history of schizophrenia	A family history of schizophrenia

   E. Complications

   1. **Impaired educational achievement.** Despite average or high intelligence, the schizophrenic individual frequently is unable to complete college or vocational training successfully.

   2. **Poor work history.** In addition to settling for mundane, low-level jobs, he or she may be unable to work consistently at one job and may make frequent changes.

   3. **Celibacy.** Schizophrenic women marry more frequently than schizophrenic men but still at a lower rate than does the general population.

   4. **Prolonged hospitalizations.** Schizophrenic patients may have frequent or chronic hospitalizations.

   5. **Crime.** Minor crimes such as shoplifting and disturbing the peace are related to the chronically ill patient's attempts to live in the community without adequate structure and support. Although the violent crimes committed by schizophrenics are often bizarre and excessively publicized, it is not known whether they are committed with greater frequency than by the general population.

   6. **Shortened life expectancy.** In addition to a higher suicide rate among schizophrenic individuals, there is shorter life span, resulting from a variety of other causes, including chronic malnutrition and debilitation from deprived environments and inadequate medical evaluation and treatment.

VI. DIFFERENTIAL DIAGNOSIS. Inasmuch as there are no true pathognomonic symptoms of schizophrenia, the mode of onset, clinical course, family history of mental illness, and personal medical history (including medications and drugs that have been taken), in addition to the types of symptoms present, are important in making the diagnosis. Following are the most common diagnoses that may be confused with schizophrenia. A more exhaustive listing is found in Table 1-2.

   A. Organic mental disorders. Any disease or condition that disrupts the normal function of the central nervous system (CNS) may present with symptoms such as hallucinations, delusions, impaired thinking, and changes in affective responsiveness. The dysfunction can result from pathophysiologic processes both inside and outside of the CNS. The etiologies are multiple and usually result in some impairment of memory and concentration, although this impairment may be subtle and may be missed if it is not discovered by a mental status examination.

   1. **Substance-induced organic mental disorders** include states of both intoxication and withdrawal from drugs, which are used both medically and nonmedically. The syndromes generally manifest confusion, disorientation, or fluctuating levels of consciousness in addition to some physical symptoms such as ataxia, nystagmus, sympathetic nervous system hyperactivity, and parasympathetic blockade. Onset is acute, the course is brief with good resolution, and premorbid functioning may be very good. Careful history reveals past and current drug intake; toxicologic evaluation of urine and serum specifies the substances involved. The most common states that mimic schizophrenia include the following.
      a. States of intoxication
         (1) Cocaine and amphetamines cause a state of acute intoxication, with hyperactivity, elation, grandiosity, and evidence of sympathetic nervous system stimulation. An organic delusional syndrome can result from long-term use of moderate to high doses of these drugs. Persecutory delusions predominate in this syndrome and may be accompanied by ideas of reference, hostility, aggressiveness, anxiety, and agitation. There may also

be tactile or visual hallucinations of insects and vermin crawling on or under the skin (i.e., formication). The delusions or hallucinations are usually transient with cocaine intoxication, but they may persist for weeks or months beyond the state of acute intoxication with amphetamines.

(2) **Phencyclidine (PCP)** intoxication causes psychological symptoms that include euphoria, severe agitation, anxiety, a sensation of slowed time, and synesthesia. Hallucinations, paranoid ideation, and bizarre behavior can also occur and appear identical to symptoms occurring in schizophrenia, particularly in the absence of a delirium. Numerous physical symptoms include vertical and horizontal nystagmus, increased blood pressure, diaphoresis, ataxia, and dysarthria.

(3) **Hallucinogen and cannabis** ingestion causes disturbances of perceptions, which include illusions, hallucinations, especially visual hallucinations, depersonalization, and derealization. Additionally there may be anxiety, fear of losing one's mind, panic,

---

Table 1-2. Differential Diagnosis of Schizophrenia

Substance-Induced Disorders

Caused by
  Amphetamines
  Cocaine
  Psychotomimetics
    Lysergic acid diethylamide (LSD)
    Phencyclidine (PCP)
    Cannabis
  Alcohol
  Barbiturates
  Steroids
  Anticholinergics

Infections

Viral
  Herpes simplex encephalitis
  Meningitis
Bacterial
  Meningitis
  Neurosyphilis
  Subacute endocarditis

Endocrine System and Metabolic Disorders

Thyroid disease
  Hyperthyroidism
  Hypothyroidism
Adrenal disease
  Addison's disease
  Cushing's disease
Acute intermittent porphyria
Electrolyte imbalances

Space-Occupying Lesions

Tumors
  Primary
  Metastatic
    Lung
    Breast
Subdural hematomas
Brain abscess

Nutritional Deficiencies

Niacin
  resulting in
    pellagra
Thiamine
  resulting in
    Wernicke-Korsakoff syndrome

Vascular Abnormalities

Collagen disorders
Aneurysms
Intracranial hemorrhage

Cerebral Hypoxia/Hypercapnia

Secondary to
  Anemia
  Decreased cardiac output
  Chronic obstructive pulmonary disease

Miscellaneous

Complex partial seizures (temporal lobe
  epilepsy)
Wilson's disease
Normal-pressure hydrocephalus

Functional Disorders

Paranoid disorders
Affective disorders
  Manic episode
  Major depressive episode
  Postpsychotic depression
Schizoaffective disorder
Schizophreniform disorder
Atypical psychosis
Personality disorders
  Paranoid
  Schizotypal
  Borderline
Pervasive developmental disorders
Obsessive-compulsive disorder
Hypochondriasis
Phobic disorders
Factitious disorder with psychological symptoms
Beliefs of religious and subcultural groups
Mental retardation

ideas of reference, and paranoid ideation. The affected individual may also have a mystical experience of tremendous insight or oneness with the universe. Physical symptoms include sympathetic nervous system overactivity. An organic delusional syndrome persisting beyond the state of acute intoxication can also occur and may appear identical to symptoms of schizophrenia.

    (4) **Anticholinergic** intoxication with drugs such as benztropine or trihexyphenidyl produces an agitated delirium with hallucinations and characteristic signs of cholinergic antagonism, including mydriasis, tachycardia, and diminished bowel sounds. Anticholinergic intoxication is clinically important because schizophrenic patients frequently take anticholinergic medications in conjunction with neuroleptics. These medications may produce a mild euphoria and have abuse potential. It is essential to differentiate between anticholinergic intoxication and an exacerbation of an individual's schizophrenia.

  b. Withdrawal states. Alcohol is most likely to produce withdrawal symptoms that may be confused with schizophrenia.

    (1) **Delirium tremens** (alcohol withdrawal delirium) is usually recognizable on the basis of tremulousness, instability of the autonomic nervous system, hyperpyrexia, gross delirium, and a history of heavy ethanol abuse.

    (2) **Alcohol hallucinosis** is most often confused with schizophrenia. It is manifested by vivid auditory hallucinations, which develop within 48 hours of cessation of ethanol ingestion and without evidence of delirium. This disorder usually lasts less than 1 week but may become chronic. Ideas of reference and persecutory delusions may develop, and at this point the illness becomes clinically indistinguishable from schizophrenia. There is a history of heavy alcohol abuse; however, there is no family history of schizophrenia. The typical age of onset is later than that of schizophrenia.

2. Neurologic disorders may present with behavioral manifestations before cognitive impairment and specific neurologic signs become apparent. The patient usually has a good premorbid social history and may have a family history positive for genetic or neurologic disease.

  a. Infections. Any CNS infectious process can produce aberrant behavior. Infections with subacute or chronic courses are more likely to be mistaken for schizophrenia. In particular, **herpes encephalitis**, which has special affinity for the temporal lobes, may present with a subacute onset of irritability, personality change, psychosis, and bizarre behavior. Some memory impairment and fluctuation in mental status are usually present also.

  b. Vascular disorders. Cerebral vasculitis associated with systemic lupus erythematosus may produce a schizophreniform psychosis with hallucinations and delusions in a clear sensorium. Differentiation from schizophrenia is complicated by the insidious onset and early appearance of psychiatric symptoms before the appearance of fever, anemia, or skin rash.

  c. Complex partial seizures (temporal lobe epilepsy) may have unusual and even bizarre ictal manifestations, including cognitive, psychosensory, and psychomotor disturbances. Although they are often difficult to diagnose as a seizure disorder, these symptoms are usually too transient to be mistaken for schizophrenia. However, an interictal schizophreniform psychosis with paranoid features has been described in association with long-standing temporal lobe epilepsy. Some authors believe that affective responsiveness is better preserved in this psychosis associated with temporal lobe epilepsy than in true schizophrenia.

  d. Degenerative diseases, particularly those beginning in adolescence, may cause diagnostic confusion. Again, personality change, often a deterioration, and psychotic symptoms may precede cognitive impairment or overt neurologic symptoms. **Huntington's chorea**, which is a genetic disease with autosomal dominant transmission, is an excellent example of such an illness. A detailed family history usually establishes the early diagnosis, but often the patient becomes a chronic and terminal resident of a state mental institution. Without identification of the neurologic symptoms, such a patient history could appear consistent with poor-prognosis schizophrenia.

3. Metabolic and endocrine system disturbances produce a multitude of psychiatric symptoms, including anxiety, depression, and sometimes psychosis. **Acute intermittent porphyria (AIP)**, although an uncommon illness, may present with an acute delusional psychosis without disorientation or confusion. Abdominal pain and vomiting are also usually present. AIP is inherited as an autosomal dominant trait and may be precipitated by ingestion of any number of substances, including barbiturates and estrogens.

4. Nutritional disorders. Severe pellagra secondary to niacin deficiency can produce a range of psychiatric symptoms, including those consistent with a schizophrenic disorder.

5. Other disorders. Schizophreniform episodes have also been reported in cases of cerebral trauma, intracranial tumor, narcolepsy, sleep deprivation, presenile cerebral degeneration, and cerebral anoxia. A complete list is presented in Table 1-2.

B. Functional disorders

1. Paranoid disorders, including paranoia, shared paranoid disorder, and acute paranoid disorder, are characterized by persistent persecutory delusions or delusional jealousy, but there is no evidence of thought disorder, bizarre delusions, or hallucinations. Delusional beliefs may be quite complex and elaborate and are usually organized around a central theme. Emotional reactions and behavior are consistent with the delusional ideas and frequently interfere with the patient's interpersonal functioning. Although the course may be chronic, progressive deterioration does not occur; in fact, the affected individual may be able to function very well occupationally. Onset is in middle or late adult life.

2. Affective disorders. If hallucinations and delusions are present in an affective disorder, they develop after the mood disturbance and do not persist beyond the resolution of the mood disturbance. Mood-incongruent psychotic symptoms may be identical to those seen in schizophrenia and may be impossible to distinguish on the basis of clinical observations alone. Age at onset, clinical course, family history, and lack of residual impairment following the psychotic episode are important diagnostic features.

    a. A major depressive episode (including bipolar disorder, depressed) may present with social withdrawal and prominent paranoid symptoms, suggesting schizophrenia. In addition, the slowed thinking, decrease in spontaneous speech, and indecisiveness may be mistaken for the thought blocking, mutism, poverty of speech, and ambivalence that occurs in schizophrenia.

    b. A manic episode, with irritability and paranoid delusions, may be indistinguishable from acute paranoid schizophrenia. This is particularly true in the midst of an acute psychosis, where severe pressure of speech, distractibility, and flight of ideas result in incoherence and disorganized, even bizarre, behavior. The precise diagnosis may not be possible until later in the course of the illness.

    c. Postpsychotic depression. A schizophrenic individual may manifest dysphoric moods during and after psychotic decompensation. There may be other depressive symptoms, sometimes severe enough to warrant a diagnosis of a major depression, after a psychotic episode. It is essential to distinguish depression from oversedation or akinesia secondary to neuroleptic medication.

3. Schizoaffective disorder has no specific criteria but has features of both schizophrenia and an affective disorder, mania or depression; therefore, a differential diagnosis cannot be made with assurance. It is not known whether this disorder represents a distinct diagnostic entity or a variant of an affective disorder. Individuals with schizoaffective disorder have a higher incidence of an affective disorder in relatives and a better prognosis than schizophrenics. Effective treatment may require medication with neuroleptics, lithium, and tricyclic antidepressants.

4. Schizophreniform disorder is diagnosed if the symptoms of schizophrenia are present but the duration of the condition is less than 6 months. Since the duration is shorter, there is less deterioration in function and a better prognosis.

5. Atypical psychosis describes a psychotic illness that does not fit another specific category. There may be several symptoms consistent with schizophrenia, including delusions, hallucinations, loosening of associations, and bizarre behavior, but not enough to meet the criteria for the syndrome.

6. Personality disorders, such as borderline, paranoid, schizoid, and schizotypal, may predispose to the development of schizophrenia. In addition, these disorders may have transient psychotic symptoms, which last for hours to days, usually with a return to the previous level of functioning. Their onset is in adolescence or early adulthood, which may further complicate the diagnosis.

7. Mental retardation. The cognitive, affective, and behavioral disturbances of mental retardation may suggest schizophrenia; however, in retardation alone, there is no progressive deterioration, but constant low-level social and occupational functioning. A concurrent diagnosis of schizophrenia can be made if psychotic symptoms are definitely present.

C. Religious and subcultural groups
may have beliefs and experiences that appear psychotic to outside observers but that should not be so described if they are shared by the group. It should be noted that the schizophrenic may find temporary acceptance in such groups until the symptoms become too florid or bizarre to be tolerated by the group.

VII. ETIOLOGIC THEORIES. The heterogeneity of the schizophrenic disorders with respect to symptoms, course, response to treatment, family history, and prognosis precludes any single etiologic explanation. There are no definite biologic markers that identify specific subtypes of schizophrenia. The theories that are described are best considered as factors that, if present, increase the likelihood of schizophrenia or, in some cases, a specific subtype of schizophrenia.

A. Genetic theories

  1. Theories. Both monogenic and polygenic theories have been proposed in the etiology of schizophrenia.

   a. A single gene with variable penetrance has been suggested as etiologic in petit mal epilepsy, which may be transmitted as an autosomal dominant trait. Whether or not this trait is expressed in the form of petit mal seizures depends upon the age of the individual and some acquired brain damage. Similar factors might operate in schizophrenia.

   b. Polygenic inheritance (as probably occurs in diabetes mellitus, atherosclerotic heart disease, and cleft lip) allows for the transmission of the abnormality by two normal parents, which is the situation for 90% of schizophrenics. According to this theory, the number of affected genes determines the individual's liability and threshold and allows for the influence of environmental factors. If the theory of polygenic inheritance is true, other features would include the following.

     (1) Severity of the condition would range from borderline to severe, depending upon the number of inherited "bad" genes.

     (2) Severely ill probands would be expected to have more affected relatives than mildly ill probands.

     (3) As the number of family members who are affected by the illness increases, the risk to unaffected relatives would increase.

     (4) The risk to relatives would decrease as the number of genes in common decreases (e.g., a monozygotic twin of a schizophrenic has a 40% to 60% risk of illness; a first cousin has a 2% risk).

     (5) The illness would be distributed on both maternal and paternal sides of the family.

  2. Evidence. There are a number of studies that suggest that genetic predisposition is involved in the etiology of schizophrenia.

   a. Family studies compare the prevalence of a given disorder among relatives of the affected individuals to the prevalence of the disorder among the general population. Although suggestive of genetic involvement, the studies cannot separate genetic transmission from familial and other environmental factors. The rate of schizophrenia in the general population is nearly 1%. Among first-degree relatives of a schizophrenic, the average risk for the disorder ranges from 4% to 12%. Siblings, at 8%, and children, at 10% to 12%, have higher risks than do parents, at 4%. Two affected parents increase the risk of schizophrenia to roughly 40%. The fewer genes in common, the more the risk decreases.

   b. Twin studies examine the differences in the concordance rate of schizophrenia between monozygotic and dizygotic twins. **All major twin studies show a higher concordance rate in monozygotic twins (40% to 60%) than in dizygotic twins (10% to 12%).** The dizygotic rate is similar to that in nontwin siblings (8%). If the severity of the schizophrenic illness is considered, the monozygotic concordance rate is 77% for severely ill patients and 27% for mildly ill patients. Even with twin studies, sociocultural and familial factors are not excluded.

   c. Adoption studies examining the frequency of the occurrence of schizophrenia in children of schizophrenic parents who are adopted at birth show that the risk to the child (about 10% to 12%) is the same as if the child is raised by the biologic parents. Identical twins who are reared apart have the same concordance rate as those who are reared together. The adoptive relatives of schizophrenic individuals do not have an increased risk of schizophrenia; biologic relatives of schizophrenic adoptees do. Children of normal parents who are adopted into a home with a schizophrenic parent do **not** have increased rates of the disorder.

  3. Conclusions. Although many of the predictions made by the polygenic theory are observed in schizophrenia, neither this nor the monogenic theory has been consistently substantiated. Nevertheless, whatever the mechanism, the theory that some genetic predisposition is involved in the etiology of schizophrenia is widely accepted.

B. Biochemical theories

  1. The role of neurotransmitters and hallucinogens. These theories suggest that an excess or a deficiency of certain neurotransmitters, an alteration of pre- or postsynaptic receptor sites, or the presence of endogenous psychotogenic amines produce the symptoms of schizophrenia.

a. Dopamine (DA)
   (1) Theory. It is suggested that certain central dopaminergic systems, most likely the mesolimbic and mesocortical systems, are overactive and produce some of the pathologic behavior seen in schizophrenia, particularly the psychotic symptoms.
   (2) Evidence
   (a) Primarily psychopharmacologic research has elucidated the role of central dopaminergic systems in the brain inasmuch as these systems cannot be investigated directly in humans. Methylphenidate and D-amphetamine, which both potentiate release of DA, can, in high doses, produce a florid psychosis in normal volunteers, which is identical to that found in paranoid schizophrenic individuals. Neuroleptics, which are potent dopaminergic antagonists, ameliorate these symptoms. Methylphenidate and D-amphetamine in small doses markedly worsen preexisting psychotic symptoms in acutely ill schizophrenic individuals.
   (b) Some studies have found evidence **against** the theory that a simple dopaminergic excess produces schizophrenic symptoms. First, decreased rather than increased levels of homovanillic acid (HVA), which is the primary metabolite of DA, have been found in the cerebrospinal fluid of schizophrenic patients. Second, L-dopa, which is a DA precursor, worsens positive symptoms but improves negative symptoms when given in moderate doses to schizophrenic patients maintained on neuroleptics. Third, apomorphine, which is a DA receptor agonist, can, in low doses, improve symptoms in chronic schizophrenics. Such findings have led some researchers to study both pre- and postsynaptic DA receptors; however, postmortem studies have been inconclusive as to whether or not there is an increase in specific DA receptors.
   (3) Conclusions. Dopaminergic pathology is important in the etiology of schizophrenia but not in a simple or exclusive way. Neuroleptics also reduce psychotic symptoms in other disorders; not all symptoms of schizophrenia (i.e., negative symptoms) are improved by dopaminergic receptor-blocking drugs. Considerable confusion remains concerning the role played by DA and its receptors and autoreceptors in the varied symptoms of schizophrenia.
b. Norepinephrine (NE)
   (1) Theory. It is hypothesized that overactivity of noradrenergic projections to the brain stem, cortex, and cerebellum causes a sensitization to sensory input and thus the sensory flooding experienced by acutely psychotic patients.
   (2) Evidence. Some patients, especially acutely psychotic patients, may respond to propranolol, which is a β-adrenergic receptor blocker. Neuroleptics themselves are potent noradrenergic receptor blockers. NE release is regulated by presynaptic α_2-receptors, and clonidine, which is an α_2-receptor agonist, has been shown to have antipsychotic properties in neuroleptic-responsive patients. Lastly, increased levels of NE in the mesencephalon and increased levels of 3-methoxy-4-hydroxyphenylglycol (MHPG), a major metabolite of NE, have been found in the nucleus accumbens in paranoid schizophrenics.
   (3) Conclusions. As is suggested by the hypothesis concerning the dopaminergic system, abnormalities in the noradrenergic systems are probably involved in the production of some schizophrenic symptoms.
c. Gamma-aminobutyric acid (GABA) neurons are primarily inhibitory in interaction with other systems. Reduced levels of GABA and glutamic acid decarboxylase, an enzyme involved with its formation, have been found in the nucleus accumbens in postmortem tissue samples; increased levels of DA have been found in the same area. Furthermore, neuroleptics increase GABA turnover, and there is some evidence that diazepam, which is a GABA agonist, has an antipsychotic effect in some schizophrenic patients. Interference with the normal GABA inhibitory effect on dopaminergic neurons has been suggested as a possible mechanism for the role of GABA in schizophrenia; however, evidence is conflicting, and this neurotransmitter appears to have a secondary role compared to those of DA and NE.
d. Serotonin. A disruption in serotonergic systems in schizophrenia was suggested when it was observed that the hallucinogen LSD binds to serotonin receptors; neuroleptics also bind to serotonin receptors. However, the hallucinations produced by the hallucinogenic drugs are different from the usual psychotic symptoms observed in schizophrenia, in contrast to the reaction produced by amphetamines, which exacerbates the usual psychotic symptoms. Other evidence suggests that, in acute schizophrenia, there is a decrease in the plasma level of the serotonin precursor, tryptophan, which then increases with clinical improvement. Also, long-term amphetamine treatment decreases levels of serotonin, suggesting that a deficiency in serotonin, rather than an excess, may have a role in schizophrenia. The role of this neurotransmitter is more confusing than that of the others described.

e. Phenylethylamine (PEA) is not a true neurotransmitter but is an endogenous amine, which is structurally and pharmacologically similar to amphetamine. It is found in the blood, urine, and cerebrospinal fluid, and it is highest in concentration in the limbic areas of the brain. Urinary PEA has been found to be significantly elevated in paranoid chronic schizophrenics when compared to nonparanoid chronic schizophrenics and to normal controls, a fact that is particularly interesting when considering that chronic amphetamine administration can produce a paranoid psychosis. However, urinary PEA levels have also been found to be decreased in unipolar depressed patients and increased in manic patients, although not increased to the extent that they are in paranoid schizophrenics. PEA does not appear to have a specific etiologic role in schizophrenia, but rather increased levels may represent an endogenous vulnerability to psychosis, whether drug-induced, schizophrenic, or affective in origin.

f. Hallucinogens, similar to LSD, do not produce a psychosis that is similar to that seen in schizophrenia. However, **PCP** can produce a long-lasting psychosis similar to that seen in schizophrenia, and **mescaline** is structurally similar to a methylated form of NE. The suggestion was made that some naturally occurring amines might serve as substrates for abnormal methylation, resulting in endogenous hallucinogenic substances. Such an enzyme has been found, and administration of methionine, a methyl donor, has caused an exacerbation of schizophrenic symptoms. However, no difference in the amount of such methylated compounds has been found between normal controls and schizophrenic individuals, and beyond this, administration of methyl donors does not consistently increase the level of methylated compounds. Thus, there is no reliable data that such a mechanism is responsible for even a subtype of schizophrenia.

2. The role of enzymes
   a. Monoamine oxidase (MAO)
   (1) Theory. Deamination by MAO is a major pathway for catabolism of central amine neurotransmitters, especially NE, DA, and serotonin. These neurotransmitters have been hypothesized to be involved in the causation of psychosis. Thus, decreased activity of MAO could increase the availability of these neurotransmitters, resulting in a relative excess or overactivity. The level of MAO activity in platelets has been used as a model for the level of MAO activity in the brain.
   (2) Evidence. Levels of platelet MAO activity have been found to be lower in schizophrenic individuals than in controls. At one time, an association between low levels of MAO activity in platelets and auditory hallucinations and delusions was made. More recently, an association between low levels of platelet MAO activity and paranoid schizophrenia in particular has been suggested. Decreased levels of MAO activity in platelets has also been found in other mental disorders, including bipolar illness and alcoholism.
   (3) Conclusions. Reduced levels of MAO activity in platelets is best thought of as a biologic trait that is associated with severe psychopathology in general and a subtype of schizophrenia in particular.
   b. Dopamine-β-hydroxylase (DBH) is the enzyme that catalyzes the conversion of DA to NE in noradrenergic neurons. Agents that inhibit this enzyme, causing an accumulation of DA, have been demonstrated to increase psychosis in manic and schizophrenic patients. Studies have shown conflicting results about levels of DBH activity in plasma and postmortem brain samples of schizophrenics.
   c. Catechol-O-methyltransferase (COMT) is the principal extraneuronal route for catecholamine metabolism. Although this enzyme could be involved in the production of abnormally methylated substances (see section VII B 1 f), there is no consistent data confirming an elevation or deficit of this enzyme in schizophrenia.
   d. Creatine phosphokinase (CPK) in elevated levels in the serum has been found in significant numbers of newly hospitalized patients with schizophrenic and affective psychoses. Anatomical and neurophysiologic abnormalities in motor innervations to skeletal muscle have been observed in some psychotic patients. The meaning and implications of these findings are not clear; however, rather than being etiologic in themselves, they are probably secondary to other processes, such as central neurotransmitter abnormalities or viral infections, and simply indicate disturbed CNS function.

3. The role of endorphins. Endorphins are a group of opiate-like peptides that are naturally found in the brain. Studies are conflicting as to whether enhancing or diminishing central transmission of endorphins is therapeutic in schizophrenia. One group of researchers has identified a gamma endorphin fragment, des-tyrosine-gamma endorphin (DT-gamma-E), which has neuroleptic-like activity, particularly in the area of the nucleus accumbens; treatment with this fragment has produced a therapeutic effect in some patients. Opiate receptors are probably also involved in the regulation of DA and serotonin synthesis and release. However, at the present time, there is no conclusive data about the role of these neuropeptides in schizophrenia.

4. The role of prostaglandins (PGs). PGs are groups of cyclic fatty acids that have a number of neurophysiologic properties, especially the prostaglandin E (PGE) series. PGE_1 decreases catecholamine release, and catecholamines enhance PG release; neuroleptics inhibit the secretion of PGs. Results are conflicting as to whether a PG excess or deficiency is associated with schizophrenia. Antiprostaglandin drugs have no effect on schizophrenic symptoms. The normal effects of PGE are inhibited by a deficiency in essential fatty acids, especially linoleic acid; symptomatic improvement in some schizophreniform patients has been observed in conjunction with treatment with linseed oil, which is high in linolenic and linoleic acids. Any connection between PGs and schizophrenia remains speculative at present.

5. The role of gluten. Gluten is a component of wheat protein, and an abnormal reaction to gluten has been proposed as a pathogenic factor in schizophrenia. The incidence of schizophrenia was observed to correlate with wheat consumption during World War II. An increased incidence of celiac disease in schizophrenic patients and an increased incidence of psychosis in patients with celiac disease provide further indirect evidence of such a relationship. More direct evidence comes from a study in which patients improved on a gluten- and milk-free diet only to worsen when gluten was added back in a double-blind fashion. Repeat challenge studies have been equivocal; however, there may be a subgroup of schizophrenic patients who are gluten-intolerant. With regard to the pathophysiologic mechanism involved, some gluten-derived polypeptides have been shown to have endorphin properties.

6. The role of immunology
  a. Theory. It has been proposed that schizophrenia is an autoimmune illness in which brain function is altered either by antibodies cytotoxic to neurons or by changes in cellular immunity.
  b. Evidence. Alterations in levels of immunoglobulin M (IgM), IgA, and IgG have been found in the serum and cerebrospinal fluid of various subtypes of schizophrenia, but generally reports are inconsistent with each other. Likewise, studies of human leukocyte antigens (HLAs) have produced inconsistent results.
  c. Conclusions. Although immunologic factors may be involved, the weight of the evidence does not yet support an autoimmune theory for the etiology of schizophrenia. In addition, the long-term use of neuroleptics may alter the immune system.

7. The role of viruses
  a. Theory. A viral hypothesis would suggest that some schizophrenic syndromes are produced by a neurotropic slow virus acting upon a subgroup of genetically predisposed individuals, who develop a chronic illness from the acute infection.
  b. Evidence. Herpes simplex encephalitis has caused syndromes that mimic schizophrenia. Other viruses may cause injury to specific areas of the brain following a slow onset and a long latency period. A virus-like agent in the cerebrospinal fluid and increased levels of serum IgA have been found in some patients with a schizophrenia-like illness and in some patients with chronic neurologic disease. These patients have tended to have poor prognoses and poor responses to drugs.
  c. Conclusions. A slow virus hypothesis is supportable for some schizophrenic patients and is attractive additionally because of its compatibility with multiple other theories, including immunologic, genetic, and developmental theories, as well as with observations about the seasonal patterns of schizophrenic births.

C. Neurophysiologic theories. Psychophysiology involves the study of the central and peripheral nervous systems via bioelectric signals from the surface of the skin and their variation in relation to behavior and psychological states. Such measures are a more direct reflection of brain activity and can be relatively independent of the motivation of the experimental subjects. Some findings seem to be consistent with state-dependent characteristics (i.e., characteristics present only at certain times), and other findings seem to represent enduring traits and could be used as biologic markers to identify populations at risk.

1. Electrodermal activity. Several different components of skin conductance have been studied in multiple experimental situations. **Skin conductance recovery**, which refers to the rate of return to baseline of a phasic skin conductance change in response to some stimulus, appears to predict schizophrenia in high-risk prepsychotic children. Children who showed a fast skin conductance recovery were more likely to become psychotic in later life. **Skin conductance habituation** refers to the process in which skin conductance ceases to change after a repetitive orienting stimulus. It has been found that acute schizophrenic patients who habituate show a positive response to neuroleptic treatment; nonhabituators do not and have a poorer prognosis.

2. Cardiovascular activity. Both tonic (or resting) levels of heart rate and phasic heart rate responses to stimuli have been studied in schizophrenia and seem to have more significance than other parameters of cardiovascular activity.

  a. Tonic heart rate levels are higher in schizophrenic individuals than in normal controls and are not affected by neuroleptic medication. This may reflect a state of hyperarousal, which has been postulated to exist in schizophrenia.

  b. Phasic heart rate response studies have produced more divergent findings than those studies of tonic heart rate levels but do suggest that schizophrenics differ from normal controls in the phasic response to neutral stimuli, although the direction of the response (acceleration versus deceleration) is not consistent.

3. Smooth pursuit eye movements

  a. Findings. Smooth pursuit eye movements are the slow-tracking lateral eye movements seen when an individual watches a swinging pendulum; they occur normally in a smooth sinusoidal pattern. Schizophrenics and other psychotic patients deviate from this normal pattern by having many velocity arrests, in which the eye comes to a complete stop, resulting in an irregular pattern. In addition, this eye-tracking deviance is found in 45% of first-degree relatives of schizophrenics and in only 10% of relatives of nonschizophrenic patients. The concordance rate of this anomaly is significantly higher in monozygotic than in dizygotic twins. Although some nonschizophrenic psychotic patients show this deficit, patients who have evidence of thought disorder in psychological testing show significantly more eye-tracking deviance than other psychotic patients.

  b. Conclusions. The exact significance of these findings is not clear, but this deficit may reflect an impairment of involuntary attention in which the schizophrenic individual is unable to suppress the background stimuli behind the pendulum and is distracted from following its movement. Furthermore, evidence of an increased incidence of eye-tracking deviance in relatives of schizophrenics suggests that this may be a genetic marker for vulnerability to schizophrenia.

4. Electroencephalography

  a. Findings. The electroencephalogram (**EEG**) suggests nonspecific abnormalities in schizophrenics more often than in the general population. Power spectral analysis of the EEG involves a computer-based analysis of the total amount of each wave frequency after artifacts such as eye movements and muscle tension have been filtered out; this approach reveals clear differences between normal and schizophrenic individuals. Schizophrenics have a significant increase in early delta waves (3 Hz to 4 Hz), a significant reduction in late alpha waves (10 Hz to 12 Hz), and a significant increase in fast beta waves (24 Hz to 33 Hz). A very similar pattern has been observed in normal adults using LSD and in some prepsychotic high-risk children. This pattern of high beta waves and low alpha waves also occurs in normal controls when sensory stimulation is presented or tasks are performed. A new technique, brain electrical activity mapping (BEAM), which generates color maps of EEG and evoked potential (EP) data, has demonstrated increased bilateral delta activity, especially in frontal regions, and increased fast beta activity, especially in the left temporal-parietal area, in schizophrenics compared to normal controls. Lastly, schizophrenics with hyperstable EEG records (i.e., more slow wave and less fast wave activity) tend to have limited responses to neuroleptic treatment.

  b. Conclusions. These EEG findings suggest that some schizophrenics may be in a chronic state of hyperarousal and cortical processing, which involves deficient filtering and integration of sensory input. Those schizophrenics with low alpha, high beta wave patterns before treatment respond better to neuroleptics, which enhance alpha wave activity and reduce increased delta and beta wave activity. Thus, the EEG spectra may identify those patients who will be neuroleptic-responsive. Furthermore, this pattern in high-risk children may indicate an electrophysiologic marker for a genetic predisposition to schizophrenia.

5. Evoked potentials (EPs)

  a. Definition. An EP is the reaction of the brain electrical activity to sensory stimuli of any modality (auditory, visual, or somatosensory) measured by EEG. Because of the high level of background EEG activity compared to the small amplitude EP waves following a single stimulus event, a computerized process averaging multiple trials and using various amplifiers and filters is required to obtain readable EP records. Different components of EP recordings have been identified depending upon the time of their appearance as measured from the stimulus presentation and whether they are positive (P) or negative (N) [e.g., P 100 is a positive peak at about 100 msec]. They have been designated as **early** (EP waves within about 50 msec of stimulation), **middle** (EP waves from about 100 msec to 200 msec), and **late** (EP waves occurring from 300 msec and later). These waves may vary in shape, latency, and amplitude, depending upon sensory modality and location. They are believed to reflect different aspects of stimulus registration, attention, and information processing.

b. Findings. This is a relatively new area of study with considerable variation in recording techniques and stimulus paradigms; however, there does appear to be some consensus about the following findings.

(1) Early EPs tend to have shortened latencies in individuals with chronic schizophrenia compared to normal controls. The amplitudes of early EPs may be increased or decreased, depending upon the stimulus modality and intervals. The persistent nonsuppression of an early auditory EP wave (P 50) in chronic schizophrenic patients, regardless of the clinical status or medication level, distinguishes these patients from normal controls and may represent an enduring trait. The peak of early somatosensory EPs (N 60) in the central regions of the brains of chronic schizophrenic patients differentiates them from normal controls, whose peak for these waves is in frontal areas, and parallels observations of differences in regional blood flow (see section VII C 6).

(2) Middle EPs tend to be reduced in amplitude as a whole complex (i.e., P 100, N 140, and P 200) in reaction to most stimulus modalities in schizophrenia. The middle components are sensitive to attention and arousal and are very reactive to medication; neuroleptics reduce the amplitude and increase the latency of these components.

(3) Late components are substantially reduced in amplitude in schizophrenics when compared to normal controls. However, rather than being a primary defect, this characteristic may represent a failure to attend to the task because of internal preoccupation.

(4) Significant heritability is reflected in the observation that identical twins have very similar EPs, which are more alike than those of fraternal twins. In addition, nonsuppression of an early auditory EP wave (P 50) has been observed in nonschizophrenic relatives of schizophrenic patients with five times the frequency found in normal controls, and its presence in relatives is significantly associated with a family history of psychosis.

(5) With increasing levels of stimulus intensity, schizophrenics may show an **augmenting response**, which means that their EPs increase in amplitude as stimulus intensity increases. This response is different from that of normal controls, who have a **reducing response** (i.e., their EPs decrease in amplitude with increasing stimulus intensity).

(6) Strong **inverse relationships** have been observed between EP reduction and augmentation and between high and low levels of MAO activity in platelets and are associated with the degree of psychopathology. Additionally, a low level of MAO activity in platelets has been associated with a stimulus-seeking pattern of behavior, while a high level of MAO activity in platelets has been associated with a stimulus-avoiding pattern of behavior. Patients with chronic schizophrenia tend to have low levels of MAO in platelets as well as an augmenting EP response.

c. Conclusions. EP studies provide exciting data that can be integrated with that from other areas of research, in particular, research areas of cerebral blood flow, biochemistry, genetics, and attention and arousal. One theory suggests that preschizophrenic children with low MAO levels and augmenting EPs seek sensory stimulation but lack sensory protection with increasing stimulus intensity; such a child might be hyperactive and overaroused. In the schizophrenic adult, the elevated early EP components might indicate abnormal amounts of information reaching higher brain centers, especially the postcentral regions, due to inadequate brain stem filtering and resulting in disorganization. The attenuated later components might reflect a compensatory attempt at inhibition to overcome defective brain stem inhibitory pathways. Those schizophrenics who show a reducing response acutely might be expected to have a better prognosis.

6. Cerebral blood flow

a. Findings. Regional cerebral blood flow, which is considered to be a reflection of local neuronal metabolic activity, can be studied using the xenon 133 (Xe^{133}) inhalation technique. Local glucose metabolism by the brain can be measured more directly by positron emission tomographic (PET) scanning using 2-deoxyglucose labeled with 18 fluorine (18 F); all regions of the brain can be well visualized with this technique. Regional blood flow and metabolism vary with the age and sex of the individual, the medication status, the level of mental activity, and the type of task. Although chronic schizophrenics have normal total hemispheric flow, they have been found to evidence lower flow in frontal lobes and higher flow in the posterior sylvian and adjacent parasensory areas than do normal controls. While recent studies have not consistently demonstrated these anterior-posterior regional differences at rest, a significant percentage of chronic schizophrenic patients do show a reduction in frontal blood flow during activation tasks that are sensitive to frontal cortex integrity. PET scan results are consistent with regional blood flow studies. In addition, reduced frontal flow has been found to correlate with increased slow wave (delta) activity in frontal areas; similarly, the increased posterior fast beta activity and augmentation of some EPs observed in the postcentral, especially the left temporal-parietal, regions of schizophrenics may correlate with the increased flow to, and metabolic activity in, these same

areas. Recent flow studies have also shown lateralized abnormalities with high left hemisphere blood flow, which was most noticeable during activating tasks in unmedicated schizophrenic patients.
   b. Conclusions. The inferred hypofunction in frontal areas and hyperfunction in postcentral sensory areas has been thought to correlate with particular aspects of the clinical picture of schizophrenia. Specifically, apathy and diminished social awareness can be seen as the result of frontal brain dysfunction; the unusual sensory and perceptual experiences (e.g., illusions and hallucinations) in schizophrenia suggest dysfunction in the postcentral areas of sensory integration.

D. Neurologic and neuropathologic studies

   1. Neurologic findings. Minor nonlocalizing neurologic abnormalities have been detected in 60% to 70% of schizophrenic patients. These neurologic "soft signs" include defects in stereognosis, graphesthesia, coordination, balance and gait, and tremor. There is a high correlation between these signs and thought disorders, especially overinclusive thinking.

   2. Neuroradiologic studies
   a. An increase in lateral ventricular size, which is often expressed as the **ventricular-brain ratio (VBR)**, is the **most frequently observed abnormality** on CT scan; these findings confirm the ventricular enlargement noted in earlier pneumoencephalographic (PEG) studies. The increase in the VBR may be subtle and is similar to that observed in normal individuals at 70 years of age. Such ventricular enlargement is consistent with, although not diagnostic of, limbic pathology, diencephalic pathology, or both. While some recent negative studies have been reported and critiques of CT study methodology have been made, the majority of studies support this finding in at least some schizophrenic individuals.
   b. Dilation of cortical fissures and sulci, which suggests cortical atrophy, is the next most prevalent finding. Cortical atrophy appears to occur in a different subgroup of patients than those with ventricular enlargement; however, the abnormalities in both groups are present from a young age and early in the course of the illness, and they are not secondary to previous treatment. Furthermore, both ventricular enlargement and cortical atrophy correlate positively with neurologic soft signs, impaired performance on neuropsychologic tests, poor premorbid adjustment, and negative symptoms (e.g., apathy, anhedonia, and flattened affect). These patients have poorer responses to neuroleptic treatment and poorer long-term prognoses than schizophrenic patients without abnormalities demonstrable by means of CT.
   c. Atrophy of the cerebellar vermis has been observed in 5% to 40% of chronic schizophrenic patients and is rarely an isolated CT finding. In some studies, as many as 30% of affectively disordered patients (especially those with bipolar illness) have this abnormality; however, when histories of alcohol abuse are compared (alcohol is an established toxic agent for the vermis), only schizophrenic patients have significantly more vermian atrophy than medical control patients.
   d. In some schizophrenic patients without CT evidence of atrophy, there are **higher incidences of reversal of the normal frontal and occipital lobe asymmetries**. In the normal right-handed individual, the right frontal lobe and left occipital lobe should be larger on the CT scan. The finding of a symmetry reversal in some schizophrenics is the most controversial of the CT findings and presently has the least obvious clinical and theoretical implications.

   3. Postmortem studies. Gross neuropathologic studies correlate with the CT abnormalities previously described; some schizophrenics showed vermian atrophy, while others, especially those with neuropsychologic abnormalities during life, had large ventricles and lower brain weights postmortem. Recent microscopic studies have demonstrated increased fibrillary gliosis in the diencephalon and hypothalamus in up to 70% of chronic schizophrenic patients whose clinical pictures were dominated by negative symptoms. Gliosis is a usual response to neuronal loss or damage; the gliosis and focal neuronal dropout, which is maximal in subependymal and basal forebrain areas, are consistent with the CT findings of enlarged third and lateral ventricles in a certain percentage of schizophrenic patients.

   4. Conclusions. Despite some current controversy, evidence from these studies, especially the CT and histopathologic studies, appears to provide support for the concept of schizophrenia as a brain disease in a subgroup of patients. These findings correlate well with each other and are associated with negative symptoms, a poor response to drug treatment, and a poor prognosis. Evidence of neuronal loss and reactive gliosis is nonspecific but consistent with previous or low-grade inflammation from viral etiologies; this has not been established but provides a link to the viral and immunologic hypotheses described in sections VII B 6 and 7.

E. Psychological theories

1. **Overview.** A wide range of psychological functions have been studied, and schizophrenics have been found to perform differently from normals in a number of areas. Although often significant, these differences are not observed in all schizophrenics, evidence again for the heterogeneity of the disorder. A few of the more significant psychological theories are reviewed below. The schizophrenic's motivation and capacity to understand and engage the task are important variables in this sort of research.

2. **Phenomenology.** Some schizophrenics can describe the subjective experience of alterations in cognition and perception. In addition to noting changes in the intensity of perceptions, they frequently emphasize their distractibility, their feeling of being flooded by stimuli in acute states, and their thinking going in many directions at once. Symptoms such as withdrawal and catatonia can be seen as attempts to reduce the flood of stimuli; delusions could be a way of reorganizing these confusing stimuli, which cannot be differentiated with regard to relevancy.

3. **Attention.** There have been many studies in schizophrenic individuals demonstrating impaired reaction time, poor performance on tasks requiring sustained attention, and difficulty when a particular stimulus must be identified in the midst of other distracting stimuli. Some of these defects have been observed in schizophrenics in remission and in the children of schizophrenics. Schizophrenics may lack an adequate filtering mechanism to attend selectively; the signal-to-noise ratio is low, and there is too much "noise" in the system from irrelevant stimuli. Schizophrenics are unable to maintain a major response set toward a particular goal in the presence of distracting stimuli and alternative mental sets. They perform better on tasks with more external control and fewer opportunities for autonomous decisions. Another theory proposes a sensory input dysfunction, which causes states of stimulus overload and hyperarousal; these result in a lowered threshold for disorganization under increasing stress. There are some obvious parallels with these theories and the EP data.

4. **Cognition and information processing.** Various theories suggest that the primary defect exists in the system of constructs that an individual develops to deal with and predict events in his or her environment, resulting in impaired information processing. In addition to attentional deficits, problems with registration, integration, and retrieval of information have been proposed. These may occur because a high flow of information overwhelms the individual's limited capacity to assimilate and accommodate novel stimuli or because the constructs themselves have become loose (i.e., overinclusive) or idiosyncratic as a result of repeated invalidations of these constructs during development.

   Conceptual overinclusiveness diminishes with clinical improvement, while idiosyncratic and bizarre thinking persists, suggesting that the latter reflects a more primary defect. In addition, parents of schizophrenics are more deviant on projective tests than are parents of normal controls on measures of thought disorder and communication deviance. Whether biologic, psychological, or both in origin, there are identifiable deficits in perceiving and organizing the world found in the families of schizophrenics.

F. Psychoanalytic theories

1. **Overview.** Myriad psychoanalytic theories have been developed over the years since Sigmund Freud established that psychotic symptoms have meaning and can be understood in the same manner as can neurotic symptoms. Most psychoanalytic theories are derived from the observation and therapy of psychotic adults; early childhood experiences are inferred from adult memories and symptoms, which are viewed from a particular theoretical perspective. Some of the theories, however, are based on observations of children.

   a. **Strengths.** Whatever psychoanalytic theory is applied, there is an attempt to understand the individual and to make sense of his or her symptoms and behavior in the context of his or her personal history. The theory can direct treatment toward amelioration of symptoms and an improvement in the quality of life. Some psychoanalytic concepts generate testable hypotheses; some integrate well with data from other sources (e.g., psychological, developmental, and neurophysiologic) and provide a more comprehensive view of the patient.

   b. **Weaknesses.** Most psychoanalytic theories are descriptive rather than etiologic. Some of the concepts, particularly metapsychological formulations, are extremely complex, not testable, and in conflict with other data. Some of the theories are so focused on limited aspects of mental life and development as to preclude broader application. Lastly, there is more diagnostic uncertainty with regard to the patients in psychoanalytic literature from whom the theories derive; at times, all that can be said is that the patients are psychotic and may or may not be schizophrenic. In view of this multiplicity and complexity, several broad categories of theories and areas of emphasis in the study of schizophrenia are described below.

2. **Conflict theories** place schizophrenia on a continuum with neuroses and emphasize the role of unconscious conflict and defenses of unacceptable wishes and impulses. The schizophrenic differs from the neurotic in the extent of regression, the withdrawal of cathexis, and the kinds of defenses employed. The theories of Freud, Fenichel, and Arlow and Brenner fall into this category.

3. **Deficit theories.** These theories, although not clearly distinct from conflict theories, emphasize a weakness or deficiency in ego functioning, which distorts normal development in various ways and predisposes to psychosis in the face of conflict. The ego weakness may be innate or may be the result of deviant maturation secondary to conditions such as poor mothering, severe illness, and congenital anomalies. Theorists have emphasized different aspects of impaired ego development as central: a deficit in self-object differentiation (Federn), a deficit in primary autonomous functions and excessive unneutralized aggression (Hartmann and Jacobson), and the persistence of hostility and intense ambivalence in object relationships (Bychowski). Thus, schizophrenics would have a lowered resistance to all sorts of stress, uncertain boundaries between internal and external experience, poorly integrated and primitive defenses that compromise reality testing, and greater conflict over aggression. These theories allow for multiple etiologies in the derailing of ego development (e.g., genetic, congenital, and interactional). Some ego functions are more likely to be affected by organic factors, while others are more sensitive to interpersonal factors (Bellak).

4. **Interpersonal theories** describe the basis of schizophrenia in deeply disturbed interpersonal relationships from infancy onward, leaving the schizophrenic individual distrustful of and extremely sensitive to rejection by others. His or her sense of self is fragile and is threatened by previously dissociated elements of his or her personality. Social withdrawal and autistic thinking are maneuvers to maintain security, that is, to preserve self-esteem and reduce anxiety. However, these security measures also make social contact and intimacy more difficult and increase the likelihood of rebuff by others, which causes more frustration and threatens self-esteem. These theories, initially proposed by Sullivan and further developed by Fromm-Reichmann, Searles, and Arieti, allow for the correction of early disturbed relationships either in late childhood before the onset of overt psychosis if some intimacy and acceptance can be achieved or with intensive psychotherapy once the psychosis emerges.

5. **Object relations theories**
   a. **Klein** emphasized the importance of the first months of life in determining the quality of and the positive or negative feelings associated with internal representations of self and others. These disturbed self and object images are the basis for maintenance of Klein's "paranoid-schizoid position" and the persistence of the pathologic defenses of splitting and projection into adulthood.
   b. **Fairbairn** focused on "splits" in the ego, which interfere with its adaptive, integrative, and reality-testing functions. The immature object relations and splitting prevent transition from infantile oral dependence to mature dependence based on differentiation of self and others.
   c. **Winnicott** stressed the differentiation of self and others and the integration of separate ego states into a stable sense of self. A "good-enough" mother creates an environment where frustrations are titrated and the true self can develop. The preschizophrenic has a "not-so-good" mother and develops a false self, which, although initially protective, becomes entrenched and dominant. This false-self system breaks down in psychosis, and there is potential for strengthening the true self with intensive psychoanalytically oriented treatment.
   d. **Burnham and Gladstone** identify the faulty differentiation and integration in schizophrenics as resulting from disturbed early object relations. This leads to the **"need/fear dilemma,"** in which the schizophrenic is object-hungry and overly dependent on others to maintain his or her integrity; yet at the same time, he or she fears closeness, which signifies merger and loss of self.
   e. **Mahler** has studied normal and psychotic children through various phases of development and stresses the process of **separation-individuation**, wherein the child develops a sense of him- or herself as separate and autonomous and develops object constancy for the internal image of mother. The schizophrenic adult has accomplished neither of these tasks and remains overly dependent on a poorly differentiated mothering person.

6. **Summary.** The schizophrenic is an individual with ego functioning weakened to the extent that his or her development is distorted, his or her sense of self is unstable, his or her images of others are poorly differentiated and hostile, and his or her defenses are primitive. The result is an extreme vulnerability to external stress, especially in interpersonal relationships both

from too much closeness and too much distance, and significant difficulty in negotiating expected developmental crises. The schizophrenic's capacity to deal with his or her own drives is impaired, and aggressive impulses are a particular source of conflict and potential disorganization. The establishment of a supportive therapeutic relationship can permit the strengthening of ego functioning and analysis of internal conflicts.

G. Family theories

1. **Overview.** Interest in family pathology developed out of the interpersonal approach to schizophrenia. However, since observations are made and theories are subsequently constructed after schizophrenia has been diagnosed in a family member, the dysfunction observed in the family might be a consequence, rather than a cause, of the schizophrenia. Prospective studies of high-risk families should be helpful in this regard. Nevertheless, even families that appear normal on the surface manifest some or all of the following disturbances when examined closely.
   a. Family relationships are strongly ambivalent.
   b. Family roles are confused and variable.
   c. Family members have odd and private views of the world.
   d. Family members are unable to establish dependable and reliable identities.
   e. There is resistance to children growing up and moving away from the family.

2. **Lidz and associates** initially focused on factors that interfered with identity formation, particularly maternal overintrusiveness and lack of empathy. They determined that parents of male schizophrenics tend to have "skewed" relationships, wherein one parent, usually the mother, is seriously disturbed and the disturbance goes unacknowledged by the other parent. The mother's pathologic influence is not balanced by the passive ineffectual father. Parents of female schizophrenics were observed to have "schism" in their relationships; the parents compete with each other for loyalty, comfort, and support from the children in their ongoing but covert struggle. More recently, Lidz has suggested that the egocentric overinclusiveness seen in schizophrenics is an adaptation to a similar thought disorder in one or both of the parents.

3. **Bateson and associates** developed the concept of **"double bind" communications**, which are etiologic in schizophrenia and which have the following characteristics.
   a. The communications take place in an important and intense relationship from which the child cannot flee and in which a response is required.
   b. The two messages, which are expressed on different levels, such as verbal and nonverbal, conflict with or deny each other.
   c. The child is forbidden from commenting on the conflicting messages, which would clarify his or her response; thus no matter what the child says or does, he or she is wrong on one or another level. Psychosis develops as an attempt to deal with such situations. Double bind communications are apparent in everyday life but seem to have particular impact on vulnerable individuals in schizophrenic families.

4. **Jackson** elaborated a concept of **familial homeostasis**, in which the identified patient's illness is necessary for the maintenance of the family equilibrium. Change or improvement in one individual results in pathologic consequences for other family members as the family attempts to reestablish a new equilibrium.

5. **Wynne and Singer.** Wynne originally described **pseudomutuality** in family relationships of schizophrenics: Rigid roles are assigned to members at the expense of individuality, and superficial relatedness is maintained at the expense of genuine intimacy, which naturally requires the acknowledgment of individual differences. Later, in collaboration with Singer, Wynne identified a **transactional thought disorder**, which is predominantly amorphous or fragmented in any given family and which is present in parents and offspring; the thought disorder can be documented by psychological tests.

6. **Leff and Vaughan** as well as other investigators have studied relapse rates for patients in families that are rated for **expressed emotion (EE)**. EE is defined in terms of criticism and emotional overinvolvement. Patients returning to families with high EE had a relapse rate four times higher than that of patients returning to families with low EE. Maintenance neuroleptic treatment and reduction in total weekly face-to-face contact had an additive protective value for patients returning to families with high EE. The relapse rate was 92% for patients coming from families with high EE and who were not on neuroleptics and who did not reduce time spent with these relatives. These findings obviously have tremendous treatment implications.

7. **High-risk studies** are longitudinal prospective studies that follow particular variables in children at risk for schizophrenia, usually designated so on the basis of having a schizophrenic

parent or being referred to a child guidance center. The variables studied can be biochemical and neuropsychological or may include conditions such as pregnancy and birth complications, familial thought disorders, and familial communication deviance.

H. Social factors

1. **Findings.** There is a higher incidence of schizophrenia in lower socioeconomic groups and a higher density of schizophrenics in ghetto areas of large cities. However, this relationship is found only in cities with populations that are greater than 100,000, and it is not observed in smaller towns and rural areas. In India, the reverse is true: There is a greater incidence of schizophrenia in the higher-order castes. The hospital admission rates for chronic schizophrenics increases during periods when the economy is depressed.

2. **Conclusions.** Rather than being causally related, the higher incidence of schizophrenia in the lower classes appears to be secondary to a **drift downward**, which accompanies the illness because of pervasive deterioration in function. In addition, the psychotic phase of the disorder usually begins at a time when an individual would be receiving training or education towards an occupation. Difficult economic times cause stress in marginally compensated individuals as well as impede rehabilitation because of a constricted job market and increased competition.

I. Cultural factors

1. **Findings.** Most studies show approximately the same incidence of schizophrenia across cultures, with some exceptions (e.g., Irish Catholics have significantly higher rates for schizophrenia than do other groups). The extent of recovery varies considerably; schizophrenic individuals in developing countries have a better prognosis and a significantly greater likelihood of being symptom-free after a period of time than do patients in western countries.

2. **Conclusions.** Some cultural beliefs may become pathogenic for the individual when tested in a different context (e.g., increasing industrialization or immigration to another society). The cultures in developing countries are more likely to view schizophrenia as caused by an external agent or spirit, which can leave or be removed from the affected individual. Neither the individual nor the family is considered to blame for the condition; in fact, in some cases the illness is experienced as something wrong with the entire community. The absence of the attribution of personal responsibility and the communal effort to reintegrate the recovered individual rapidly into the social system, which itself is less complex, both probably contribute to the better prognosis of the illness in developing countries.

J. Conclusions regarding etiology

1. **Stress-diathesis model.** Given the wide-ranging and, at times, conflicting observations concerning the schizophrenic disorders, the most effective theoretical approach is a stress-diathesis model. Essentially it proposes a spectrum of vulnerabilities that might arise from multiple sources and that interact with myriad stress factors to result in pathology. A corollary of this approach is that appropriate environmental interventions, particularly during critical phases, could ameliorate or compensate for the vulnerabilities. For example, a genetically predisposed infant might have a neurophysiologic deficit of attention and arousal such that he or she cannot regulate and integrate the flow of sensory information. The capacity of the infant's caretakers to recognize this deficit and protect him or her from over- or understimulation might determine whether or not he or she develops stable and coherent internal representations of him- or herself and the world. Without such internal structures, the individual will have difficulty assimilating and adapting to further experiences, leaving him or her impaired socially and vulnerable to future life crises, even apparently mild ones. A variation of this example is a genetically normal child, who experiences stimulus overload during critical phases from traumatic and chaotic parenting. He or she might not develop the necessary internal structures to predict and deal effectively with the external environment. He or she too, is vulnerable to future stimulus overload, whether from internal or external sources. The severity, source, and developmental timing of the deficits and stresses not only relate to prognosis but also to the types of treatment that are most effective in a given individual.

2. **Summary of risk factors.** Listed below are some of the more established risk factors for schizophrenia: The list is not inclusive, and, alone, each factor is neither necessary nor sufficient for the development of schizophrenia.
   a. A schizophrenic family member—especially a schizophrenic parent or parents or a monozygotic twin who is schizophrenic
   b. A difficult birth with possible brain trauma
   c. A birth date in March or April in the United States

d. A deviant course of personality development, which includes being:
   (1) A shy, daydreaming, withdrawn, and friendless child
   (2) A child with idiosyncratic thought processes
   (3) A child particularly sensitive to separation
   (4) An anhedonic child
e. A parent who:
   (1) Is overpossessive and hostile
   (2) Is incapable of perceiving a child's needs
   (3) Has paranoid attitudes, disordered thinking, and deviant forms of communication
f. An inability to sustain attention and filter out irrelevant stimuli
g. Weakened ego functioning and the persistence of primitive defenses
h. Having taken a variety of drugs, especially LSD, amphetamines, and PCP
i. Celiac disease
j. Low levels of MAO activity in blood platelets
k. Abnormalities in dopaminergic, noradrenergic, and GABAnergic neurotransmitters and synapses
l. Elevated levels of urinary PEA
m. Rapid skin conductance recovery
n. Abnormal smooth pursuit eye movements
o. An augmenting or a nonsuppressing EP response
p. An EEG with more slow wave and less fast wave activity
q. Hypofunction of frontal lobes demonstrable on PET scanning or regional cerebral blood flow studies
r. A history of herpes simplex or another viral encephalitis
s. Minor neurologic abnormalities
t. Temporal limbic epilepsy
u. An abnormal CT scan demonstrating enlarged lateral ventricles or dilated cortical fissures

VIII. TREATMENT

A. Overview. The diagnostic heterogeneity and impairment of multiple psychological functions that are present in schizophrenia require a multifaceted approach to treatment. The specific combination of treatments should be individualized for any given patient and based on a thorough assessment of that patient's deficits and strengths.

B. Hospitalization

1. Indications. Hospitalization is not indicated simply by the appearance of symptoms but rather because of specific problems associated with the individual's decompensation. These include suicidal and homicidal ideation, command hallucinations, panic, significant confusion, inability of the patient to plan and care for him- or herself, and overtaxing of the family's capacity to care for the patient.

2. Goals
   a. Protection. The hospital should be a safe environment where physical needs are met, stresses are minimized, and impulses are controlled.
   b. Diagnosis. Twenty-four–hour care allows for extensive observation and evaluation of the patient's problems, strengths, history, supports, and responses to treatment. It is an opportunity to make descriptive, dynamic, and developmental diagnoses.
   c. Therapy. All aspects of the patient's treatment can be started in the hospital, including vocational rehabilitation and family visits, and can be adjusted, based upon the patient's tolerance and response.

3. Side effects. There are side effects, even with brief hospitalization. Despite experiencing tremendous distress before admission, patients often experience a loss of self-esteem and social stigmatization at being on a "mental ward." Their usual social supports may be disrupted or lost. The hospital rules and routines may promote excessive dependency, particularly with extended hospitalization.

C. Milieu treatment

1. Definition. A therapeutic milieu is usually one aspect of inpatient treatment. It is a structured and reactive environment, which is only present formally if it is actively cultivated and maintained by the staff; informally, patients always have their own subculture, which may or may not be therapeutic. An effective milieu for schizophrenics must have an adequate number of staff to meet the needs of very disorganized patients. The staff must be able to tolerate the chronicity of the disorder and to set realistic expectations, which take into account the residual.

2. Structure. One aspect of the staff's role is to shore up or temporarily substitute for severely impaired ego functions. Acutely schizophrenic patients may need help controlling their impulses, both sexual and aggressive, testing the reality of their perceptions and experiences, concerning both self and others, modulating affective responses, especially attempting to diminish anxiety, and reducing environmental stimulation. Thus, the milieu should be structured enough to provide both adequate controls on destructive and injurious behavior and a consistent routine and supportive setting for schizophrenics who are easily threatened and overwhelmed by stimulation in their environment. This includes allowing the patient privacy and time alone, avoiding intense or probing psychotherapeutic contacts, which can be overstimulating and disorganizing, and giving support, reassurance, and help with personal hygiene and self-care.

3. Flexibility. The milieu should also be flexible enough to respond to the changing needs of individuals with regard to length of stay, extent of restrictions, contact with family, involvement in groups, and interaction with other patients. For example, once the positive symptoms (e.g., hallucinations and delusions) associated with serious disorganization improve, the treatment of negative symptoms (e.g., apathy, blunted affect, and social withdrawal) involves active encouragement and stimulation, which should have been minimized before.

4. Ward community. The other patients as individuals and as a group are used as therapeutic agents in such a milieu. Open, direct communication and individual responsibility for behavior is encouraged. The feedback that patients give to each other can provide reality testing, support, and pressure with regard to maladaptive behavior. The more organized and improving patients can instill hope and act as role models for sicker patients. Generally, an attempt is made to minimize the hierarchical structure and to encourage decision making among the entire community in order to promote autonomy. The extent to which this occurs depends upon the staff's assessment of the collective ego functioning of the group and its capacity to handle such responsibilities.

5. Side effects. As with any therapeutic modality, there are potential side effects of a therapeutic milieu. The nurturing, tolerant environment may promote unnecessary regressions in some patients. Improved patients or the group as a whole may exert excessive pressure on disorganized patients, who may be overly compliant and unable to assert themselves, resulting in an unfair distribution of power unless the staff intervenes to maintain a balance. Excessive demands for interaction and participation may cause overstimulation and disorganization; this may prompt further withdrawal in schizophrenic patients. The structure and community of the ward is an artificial situation, and adaptation to it does not insure adaptation outside of the hospital. In fact, the transition to the total freedom and isolation of life on the outside can be abrupt, disorganizing, and depressing, unless actively worked through with the patients and eased by situations such as halfway houses.

D. Group therapy is used in both inpatient and outpatient programs. Schizophrenics generally do best in groups where concrete problems in daily living are addressed. Their social skills can be improved by facilitating interaction among members of the group and discussing interactions with others at work and at home. The group, better than anyone else, knows what it is like to have schizophrenia and can provide invaluable support and understanding for each other. Group therapy is most effective in conjunction with medication and other types of treatment intervention.

E. Individual psychotherapy

1. Establishing the relationship. There are many approaches to the psychotherapy of schizophrenia based on various theoretical conceptualizations of the disorder; however, all recognize the central importance of the therapeutic relationship. Establishing and maintaining a relationship with a schizophrenic individual who is suspicious, withdrawn, and prone to psychotic distortions of reality is a difficult task. This individual is sensitive to rejection, anxious with separation, uncomfortable with intimacy, and fearful of his or her imagined destructive potential. He or she has been repeatedly unsuccessful at having satisfying and secure relationships. It is important for the therapist to be active, interested, honest, warm, and empathic. The therapist and patient can share a view of the illness and its impact on the patient's life. This does not require agreement between patient and therapist about what is pathologic but only about the consequences to the patient of acting on his or her beliefs and perceptions. Still, some patients may not be able to tolerate the most cautious and distant individual relationship and prefer groups or brief, infrequent contacts based around medication adjustment.

2. Psychotherapeutic management uses the relationship in a supportive way; the therapist functions as an auxiliary ego for the patient with persisting deficits in multiple ego functions. The focus is to help the patient identify and deal with real life, including everyday problems such as renting an apartment, paying bills, and taking medication. Building an alliance around medication is essential to improve compliance. Working with families, employers, and boardinghouse managers may be crucial in helping the environment adjust in ways the patient cannot as well as in helping the patient negotiate potential conflicts with others and maintain him- or herself in the community. The therapist may also serve as a role model for the patient both in terms of interpersonal relationships and in dealing with life problems with less distortion of reality.

3. **Intensive psychotherapy.** While psychotherapeutic management is applicable to all patients, intensive insight-oriented psychotherapy requires the selection of appropriate patients. Some patients may tolerate intensive treatment from early in their illness, while other patients may tolerate it later, after there has been significant ego strengthening to the extent that they can withstand intense affects, control impulses, and discriminate among the transference aspects of the psychotherapeutic relationship. The patient can then gradually understand the multiple meanings of his or her psychotic symptoms and face fears and conflicts over sexual and aggressive impulses. The patient also learns to tolerate intrapsychic and interpersonal conflicts without resorting to regressive psychotic defenses and may achieve insight into the sources of the conflicts. The goal is to establish a stable sense of self and a capacity for intimacy and autonomous function; in short, to address and resolve the psychological causes of the individual's vulnerability rather than to help the individual and the world accept and accommodate them.

4. **Transference and countertransference issues** are present in all types of therapeutic relationships with schizophrenics but are more volatile in intensive psychotherapy. The patient's profound loneliness and despair may be quite discomforting for the therapist as may be the tremendous dependency and godlike idealization. Furthermore, the patient may have an uncanny ability to sense the therapist's unconscious conflicts and anxieties. The therapist must walk a line between pursuing unrealistic rescue fantasies and keeping the patient ill to preserve the gratification of a merged, idealized relationship.

5. **Side effects**
   a. **Dependency.** The therapist may unconsciously foster excessive dependency and fail to promote autonomous functioning when the patient is capable of it.
   b. **Acting out.** Psychodynamic exploration of inner conflicts represents a stress in itself, to which the patient may respond with regressive psychotic defenses. Destructive acting out, increased psychotic symptomatology, and even suicide can result if unconscious conflicts are explored without adequate ego strength to maintain some reality testing and contain affects.
   c. **Withdrawal.** The patient may withdraw further from interpersonal relatedness if the therapist is too confrontive or is unconsciously rejecting to the effect that the therapy relationship becomes an unanalyzed repetition of previous relationships.

6. **Summary. A psychotherapeutic relationship is the basis for all interventions in the treatment of schizophrenia**, including somatic and social intervention as well as psychological. As with the therapeutic milieu, structure and flexibility must be tailored to the individual patient's changing needs. Psychotherapy alone is neither effective nor possible for the majority of patients but is synergistic with other treatment approaches.

F. **Family evaluation and therapy**

1. **Evaluation.** For patients who are involved with their families, even at a distance, evaluation of the family system is crucial both from the viewpoint of diagnosing precipitating stresses and preventing future relapses.

2. **Interventions.** There are many types of interventions that can be made, depending upon the motivation of the family and the degree and kind of involvement with the patient.
   a. **Crisis orientation.** The family may be made to appreciate that the patient becomes psychotic in response to particular stresses, some of which may arise in the family. They can help the patient anticipate and avoid situations in which he or she is most vulnerable.
   b. **Alterations in the home environment.** Families that are overtly critical and overinvolved (i.e., families with high EE) substantially increase the frequency of relapse in patients. Both through education about the illness and identification with low EE families, they can reduce the level of critical and hostile interactions. For families who cannot or will not change, the amount of face-to-face contact can be reduced by involving the patient regularly in activities outside of the home; this also has a protective effect on relapse.
   c. **Adjustment of family homeostasis.** Although a schizophrenic family member can be very disruptive, some families establish an equilibrium that depends upon and actively, although covertly, maintains the patient's illness. Helping other family members work out

their personal and interpersonal difficulties must be done concurrently if they are to support the patient's progress.

    d. Language and communication. Some families have markedly disturbed patterns of communication and blurring of roles. Communication that is more focused and goal-directed can help all members establish separate identities and work through conflicts concerning separation and autonomy.

G. Occupational and rehabilitation therapy. Because of the onset in early adult life and chronicity of the disorder, a schizophrenic may lack basic knowledge and skills necessary to care for him- or herself and to function in the community. Simple tasks such as shopping become major stressors and sources of anxiety. Following a psychotic decompensation, the patient may not be able to return to his or her previous level of occupational or educational functioning and may require job retraining or new career goals. The structure and support of a sheltered workshop may permit constructive activity and a gradual return to work in more competitive and stressful situations.

H. Pharmacologic treatment and electroconvulsive therapy (ECT)

    1. Antipsychotic agents

        a. Overview. Neuroleptics are the mainstay of treatment for both acute psychosis and the maintenance phase of schizophrenia. There are several classes of antipsychotic agents, and all are clinically effective when given in adequate doses (Table 1-3).

        b. Efficacy

            (1) Acute psychosis. Neuroleptics have established efficacy for the following target symptoms: hallucinations, acute delusions, combativeness, anxiety, hostility, hyperactivity, negativism, insomnia, and poor general self-care. They are **not** directly effective for blunted affect, chronic paranoid ideas, grandiosity, asocial behavior, apathy, and anhedonia.

            (2) Maintenance. Neuroleptics also have a role in preventing relapse following remission of the acute psychosis. Fifty percent of patients relapse within 6 to 8 months of discontinuation of medication, and this increases to nearly seventy-five percent by 18 months. This is opposed to a relapse rate of only 25% of patients on medication within those 18 months.

        c. Choice of agent. The various neuroleptic agents differ in milligram potency and side effects but are equally efficacious when given in adequate doses. Although there is no evidence that certain subtypes of patients do better with certain medications, an individual patient may respond well to a particular drug; otherwise the physician should use a medi-

Table 1-3. Neuroleptic Medications

Generic Name	Trade Name(s)	Approximate Equivalent Oral Dosages (mg)	Usual Inpatient Oral Dosage Range (mg/day)
Phenothiazines			
Aliphatic	Thorazine	100	50–1500
Chlorpromazine			
Piperidine			
Thioridazine	Mellaril	100	50–800
Piperazine			
Fluphenazine	Prolixin, Permitil	2–4	2–60
Trifluoperazine	Stelazine	5	5–80
Perphenazine	Trilafon	10	16–64
Butyrophenones			
Haloperidol	Haldol	2–4	2–60
Thioxanthenes			
Thiothixene	Navane	5	5–80
Dihydroindolones			
Molindone	Moban, Lidone	10	20–225
Dibenzoxazepines			
Loxapine	Loxitane, Daxolin	10	20–225

cation with which he or she is familiar and attempt to minimize toxicity and side effects for any given patient (see Table 1-3).

d. Dosage

(1) **Acute psychosis.** At least 400 mg of chlorpromazine per day or its equivalent (e.g., 16 mg of haloperidol) are usually required for an antipsychotic effect. For certain extremely agitated patients, doses as high as 3000 mg/day of chlorpromazine or 150 mg/day of haloperidol may be necessary, but this is unusual. The usual dosage range is 400 mg to 1500 mg/day of chlorpromazine for a period of 3 to 10 days.

(2) **Stabilization phase.** Once there is relative resolution of the acute psychotic symptoms, the dosage of neuroleptics can be decreased gradually, still maintaining control of the symptoms. This may take 1 to 3 weeks.

(3) **Maintenance phase.** The goal is to maintain the patient relatively symptom-free on the lowest possible dose of antipsychotic medication. The dosage schedule usually can be consolidated in a single bedtime dose. The length of time on maintenance medication must be individualized but is generally in the range of 6 months to 2 years without a relapse before a medication-free trial.

(4) **Nonresponse.** If there is no response at an adequate dosage level, the physician should check compliance and absorption and obtain blood-level samples. If there is no response at therapeutic levels, a change to a different class of neuroleptics is indicated.

e. Route of administration

(1) **Oral medication**, either in tablet form or as elixir, is the usual method of administration.

(2) **Intramuscular administration** is available for most neuroleptics and is indicated when rapid treatment of an uncooperative patient is necessary or inadequate levels are obtained with oral administration.

(3) **Long-acting fluphenazine** is available for intramuscular injection as an enanthate or decanoate ester. Dosage is usually in the range of 12.5 mg to 50.0 mg intramuscularly every 1 to 3 weeks. Such infrequent and easily monitored administration can be quite helpful to poorly compliant outpatients.

f. Adverse effects

(1) **Extrapyramidal syndromes** result from blockade of DA receptors in the basal ganglia and occur more commonly with the high-potency neuroleptics.

   (a) **Acute dystonic reactions**, which are more common in younger male patients early in treatment, involve sudden tonic contractions of the muscles of the tongue, neck (**torticollis**), back (**opisthotonos**), mouth, and eyes (**oculogyric crises**). As well as being extremely frightening, such reactions can be dangerous if the patient's airway is compromised. They can be effectively treated acutely with benztropine 1 mg to 2 mg intramuscularly or diphenhydramine 25 mg to 50 mg intramuscularly or intravenously. Prophylaxis is accomplished with regular, orally administered anticholinergic medication.

   (b) **Drug-induced parkinsonism** is characterized by cogwheel rigidity, bradykinesia, tremor, loss of postural reflexes, masked facies, and drooling. It is more common in elderly patients, and although it usually occurs in the first few weeks of treatment, it may appear at varying times with varying doses. It can be effectively treated with any of the antiparkinsonian medications (Table 1-4) and may also respond to a decrease in neuroleptic dosage. Antiparkinsonian agents can generally be tapered and discontinued after 3 to 4 weeks of treatment in most patients. If the extrapyramidal syndrome remains unresponsive, a change to a different class of neuroleptics, usually one of lower potency, is required.

   (c) **Akathisia** is a syndrome of motor restlessness, which may involve the entire body but is often most obvious in the patient's inability to keep his or her legs and feet still. It can be mistaken for anxiety, agitation, or an increase in psychotic symptomatology. The akathisia may respond to antiparkinsonian agents, but if the patient responds poorly, a decrease in dosage or change to another neuroleptic is indicated.

Table 1-4. Antiparkinsonian Medications

Generic Name	Trade Name(s)	Usual Oral Dosage Range (mg/day)
Benztropine	Cogentin	1–8
Trihexyphenidyl	Artane, Tremin	2–10
Biperiden	Akineton	2–6
Amantadine	Symmetrel	100–300
Diphenhydramine	Benadryl	25–200

(d) Neuroleptic-induced catatonia occurs more commonly with the high-potency agents and is characterized by withdrawal, mutism, and motor abnormalities, including rigidity, immobility, and waxy flexibility. Although it can be mistaken for a worsening of the patient's psychotic symptoms, it is a complication of neuroleptic therapy. It may represent a variant of the neuroleptic malignant syndrome [see section VIII H 1 f (2)]. It should be treated by temporarily discontinuing neuroleptic therapy and, upon resolution, changing to a different class of neuroleptic. Amantadine, administered in an oral dose of 100 mg three times daily may also be helpful.

(e) Tardive dyskinesia is a late-onset movement disorder, which is thought to result from a disturbance in the DA-acetylcholine balance in the basal ganglia. Fasciculations of the tongue may be the earliest symptom, followed by lingual-facial hyperkinesias, which are persistent involuntary chewing, smacking, or grimacing movements. Choreoathetotic movements of the extremities and trunk, including the respiratory muscles, can be extremely disabling in severe cases. The symptoms often appear noticeably when there is a dosage reduction or discontinuation of neuroleptic medication, but they can usually be detected by close examination between neuroleptic doses. The syndrome can usually be reversed if it is detected early, and neuroleptics are discontinued. In severe cases, the movement disorder may be irreversible and can progress with continued neuroleptic treatment. Symptoms are worsened by anticholinergic medication, which should be discontinued if possible. Increased doses of neuroleptics may cause apparent temporary improvement by increasing the DA receptor blockade; however, this ultimately causes further progression of the movement disorder. Patients should be screened every 6 months for early signs and should be maintained on the lowest possible dose to minimize this serious complication of long-term neuroleptic use.

(2) Neuroleptic malignant syndrome is a potentially life-threatening complication of neuroleptic therapy and is characterized by muscular rigidity, fever, autonomic instability, and an altered level of consciousness. Onset of the full-blown syndrome is rapid over 1 to 2 days after a period of gradual progressive rigidity. Treatment involves immediate discontinuation of the neuroleptic medication and support of respiratory, renal, and cardiovascular functioning.

(3) Anticholinergic effects include blurred vision, dry mouth, urinary retention, and constipation.

(4) Cardiovascular effects most commonly include orthostatic hypotension resulting from adrenergic blockade. This occurs most frequently through the use of low-potency agents (e.g., chlorpromazine and thioridazine).

(5) Hypothalamic effects include changes in libido, appetite, and temperature regulation. Breast enlargement and galactorrhea can also occur.

(6) Jaundice of an allergic cholestatic type occurs most commonly with chlorpromazine and usually resolves following withdrawal of the medication.

(7) Agranulocytosis is a rare, unpredictable allergic reaction, which is potentially fatal but reversible if it is accurately diagnosed early so that the neuroleptic (usually chlorpromazine) can be discontinued and supportive measures introduced.

(8) Dermatologic effects include allergic rashes, which respond to discontinuation of the drug, and photo sensitivity, which can be treated with sunscreens.

(9) Ophthamologic effects include a pigmentary retinopathy associated with thioridazine in doses greater than 800 mg/day. Lens and corneal pigmentation has been reported with chlorpromazine, thioridazine, and thiothixene after long-term treatment, but this is rare. More common is blurred vision and worsening of narrow-angle glaucoma secondary to anticholinergic effects.

2. Barbiturates, such as 200 mg to 400 mg of amobarbital sodium, can be helpful for use as additional nonspecific sedation in extremely agitated patients.

3. Anxiolytic agents are generally not useful in the treatment of acute psychoses, although the efficacy of administration of high-doses of diazepam in conjunction with neuroleptics is currently under investigation.

4. Propranolol. There is some evidence that β-adrenergic blockers have a possible role in the treatment of schizophrenic disorders, but further studies are needed.

5. Lithium. When there is a significant affective component to the psychotic symptoms, lithium carbonate can be helpful in treating the illness. Although it can be used alone, it is usually used in conjunction with a neuroleptic. This combination appears to be particularly effective for the schizoaffective disorders and so-called good-prognosis schizophrenia; such patients often have family histories of affective disorders.

6. **Antidepressants** can be helpful when used in addition to neuroleptics in cases in which there is a mixture of depressive and schizophrenic symptoms. Antidepressants have not been found helpful in the treatment of negative symptoms in schizophrenia.

7. **ECT** has a secondary role in the treatment of the acute psychotic symptoms of schizophrenia. It is most likely to be effective in patients with catatonic and affective symptoms, and it is indicated in schizophrenia in the following situations:
   a. In the presence of immediate life-threatening circumstances, such as delirious catatonia or suicidal preoccupation
   b. When the patient requires massive doses of neuroleptics and can be treated with smaller doses following ECT
   c. When the patient is intolerant of or refractory to standard neuroleptic regimens

I. **Summary**

1. The **best treatment results** occur with a combination of psychosocial intervention and neuroleptic medication in the context of a trusting psychotherapeutic relationship; a small proportion of patients may not improve no matter what interventions are made.

2. Drug therapy should be individualized, with the patient maintained on the lowest possible dose and carefully observed for side effects.

3. Psychosocial interventions, both group and individual, are most effective when they are task-oriented and focus on specific target symptoms, behavior, and social interactions.

4. A reduction in the amount of critical, hostile comments made to a patient in a family with high EE or a reduction in the amount of face-to-face contact with family members decreases the likelihood of relapse.

BIBLIOGRAPHY

American Psychiatric Association: *Diagnostic and Statistical Manual of Mental Disorders*, 3rd ed. Washington, D.C., American Psychiatric Association, 1980

Grinspoon L (ed): Part II: The schizophrenic disorders. In *Psychiatry Update*, vol 1. Washington, D.C., American Psychiatric Press, 1982, pp 82–255

Kaplan HI, Sadock BJ: Schizophrenic disorders. In *Comprehensive Textbook of Psychiatry*, 4th ed., vol 1. Baltimore, Williams and Wilkins, 1985, pp 631–747

Schizophrenia 1980: An NIMH special report. *Schizophrenia Bulletin*. Washington, D.C., United States Government Printing Office, 1981, pp 2–158

STUDY QUESTIONS

Directions: Each question below contains five suggested answers. Choose the **one best** response to each question.

1.   All of the following are commonly observed features of schizophrenia EXCEPT

(A) auditory hallucinations
(B) decreased appetite
(C) blunted affect
(D) thought blocking
(E) delusions of influence

Questions 2–4

A 59-year-old woman with a history of chronic paranoid schizophrenia has become acutely agitated, and treatment with 40 mg of trifluoperazine is started. After 3 weeks, the woman is observed sitting motionless and unresponsive in a chair all day. When helped to walk, she has a shuffling gait.

2.   What is the most likely diagnosis?

(A) Exacerbation of the schizophrenic disorder with a catatonic stupor
(B) Hypothyroidism secondary to the trifluoperazine
(C) Akinesia secondary to the trifluoperazine
(D) Major depressive disorder with psychomotor retardation
(E) Apathy and dependency secondary to chronic hospitalization

3.   What is the most appropriate initial step in treating this woman?

(A) Increasing the dosage of trifluoperazine
(B) Encouraging the patient to participate in ward activities
(C) Adding an antiparkinsonian drug
(D) Decreasing the dosage of trifluoperazine and adding a thyroid hormone
(E) Adding a tricyclic antidepressant

4.   If the first treatment approach is unsuccessful, what is the next step?

(A) Changing to a different neuroleptic
(B) Changing to a different antidepressant
(C) Adding a stimulant such as dextroamphetamine
(D) Increasing the thyroid hormone
(E) Administering electroconvulsive therapy (ECT)

5.   A 22-year-old college student with many friends and good grades presents with an agitated, florid psychosis following news of the death of his mother. The most likely course for this patient's illness is

(A) chronic psychosis with a progressive downhill course
(B) chronic psychosis with remissions and relapses
(C) remission of the psychosis with a return to a good level of functioning
(D) remission of the psychosis with progressive residual symptoms
(E) none of the above

6.   Established complications of schizophrenia include all of the following EXCEPT

(A) multiple changes in jobs
(B) arrests for violent crimes
(C) failure in school
(D) multiple hospitalizations
(E) shortened life expectancy

7.   All of the following statements about the risk of genetic transmission of schizophrenia are true EXCEPT

(A) children with one schizophrenic parent who are raised by that parent have a risk of 12%
(B) children with one schizophrenic parent who are adopted at birth have a risk of 12%
(C) an identical twin reared with his or her twin has a risk of 50% if the other twin has schizophrenia
(D) an identical twin reared apart from his or her twin has a risk of 25% if the other twin has schizophrenia
(E) the more severe the illness, the higher the concordance rate

8.   Which of the following neurophysiologic findings in schizophrenic patients predicts a poor response to neuroleptic medication?

(A) Habituation of skin conductance
(B) Increased early delta waves in the electroencephalogram (EEG)
(C) Reducing responses of early evoked potentials (EPs)
(D) Abnormalities of smooth pursuit eye movements
(E) None of the above

9. Negative symptoms of schizophrenia are associated with all of the following findings EXCEPT

(A) increased ventricular-brain ratio (VBR)
(B) increased fibrillary gliosis in the diencephalon
(C) reduced blood flow in the frontal lobes
(D) reversal of normal cerebral asymmetry
(E) lower postmortem brain weight

Directions: Each question below contains four suggested answers of which **one or more** is correct. Choose the answer

A	if **1, 2, and 3** are correct
B	if **1 and 3** are correct
C	if **2 and 4** are correct
D	if **4** is correct
E	if **1, 2, 3, and 4** are correct

10. Observations that support the dopamine (DA) hypothesis of schizophrenia include

(1) a worsening of psychotic symptoms with dopamine-β-hydroxylase (DBH) inhibitors
(2) an improvement of symptoms in chronic schizophrenics with low doses of apomorphine
(3) an improvement of symptoms with neuroleptic treatment
(4) an improvement in negative symptoms with administration of L-dopa

11. True statements associating gluten metabolism with schizophrenia include

(1) there is an increased incidence of celiac disease in schizophrenic patients
(2) there is an increased incidence of psychosis in patients with celiac disease
(3) some schizophrenic patients improve on a gluten-free diet
(4) gluten-derived polypeptides have psychotogenic properties

Questions 12–16

A 19-year-old man has been described by his family as becoming increasingly withdrawn and spending much time alone in the basement over several months. He speaks little except to utter biblical references; when alone, he appears to mumble to and argue with himself. The family has become more concerned since they found that he cut the head off all the pictures of his older sister in the family album. During the psychiatric interview, he reveals to the psychiatrist that he has been hearing voices for several months and recently has been hearing the voice of God warning him of his sister's evil influence and ordering him to protect the family from her. The psychiatrist diagnoses paranoid schizophrenia. The family is concerned and supportive.

12. Appropriate initial treatment of this patient includes

(1) psychiatric hospitalization
(2) intensive individual psychotherapy
(3) thiothixene at 15 mg/day
(4) intensive family therapy

13. Despite appropriate initial treatment, the patient's level of agitation has increased. He was given thiothixene in a dose of 45 mg/day. He has indicated that the voices are less bothersome, but his pacing has increased, and he has some upper extremity stiffness. The next intervention should involve which of the following medications?

(1) Beginning lithium carbonate
(2) Increasing the thiothixene
(3) Beginning chlorpromazine
(4) Beginning benztropine

14. After 1 week, the patient no longer hears derogatory voices. His associations are more logical with some religiosity but no delusional ideas. He continues to pace the halls, and he sleeps poorly because he cannot find a comfortable position. The next step in treatment includes

(1) discontinuing the thiothixene
(2) increasing the frequency of the individual psychotherapy sessions
(3) beginning haloperidol
(4) beginning flurazepam

15. The patient stops pacing and begins sleeping regularly. He interacts appropriately with his family, and they are relieved at his improvement. The parents announce that they are going out of town in 2 weeks and that the patient cannot accompany them. The patient becomes extremely anxious and angry with his parents. Within a few days he appears more withdrawn and uncommunicative; his limbs are immobile and remain in whatever position they are placed for extended periods of time. What is the treatment approach?

(1) Beginning chlorpromazine
(2) Discontinuing haloperidol
(3) Beginning a tricyclic antidepressant
(4) Having a family meeting

16. The patient gradually improves over the next week. He is started on loxapine at 50 mg/day without any other medication. He does well over the next 2 months as the loxapine is decreased gradually to 30 mg/day. He then begins spending long periods of time in bed, eating poorly, and interacting less with his family. He expresses hopelessness about ever getting any better. The appropriate treatment response now includes

(1) increasing the loxapine
(2) discussing the feelings of hopelessness in individual psychotherapy
(3) beginning benztropine
(4) beginning imipramine

ANSWERS AND EXPLANATIONS

1. The answer is B. [*IV B 1 d, 2 c, 3 a (1), 4 a*] The range of symptoms observed in schizophrenia is extremely broad and includes disorders of thinking, feeling, perception, and behavior. Auditory hallucinations, thought blocking, and delusions of influence are common symptoms during the psychotic phase of the illness; a blunted affect may be present in the prodromal and residual phases as well as in the psychotic phase. Prominent vegetative symptoms such as decreased appetite should suggest an affective disorder, particularly if they occur in the presence of a significant mood disorder. While schizophrenics may frequently complain of feelings of depression, it is unusual for them to present with decreased appetite. They may have lost weight because of poor self-care or paranoid concerns about food, but this should not be mistaken for the appetite disturbance observed in depressive disorders.

2. The answer is C. (*VII H 1 f*) Elderly patients, particularly women, are relatively prone to drug-induced parkinsonism, which may present with cogwheel rigidity, bradykinesia, tremor, loss of postural reflexes, masked facies, and drooling. An individual may manifest one, several, or all of these symptoms, which usually occur in the first few weeks of treatment. The differential diagnosis is extremely important because an akinetic syndrome can easily be mistaken for a major depressive disorder or an exacerbation of the patient's psychosis in the form of a catatonic stupor. This may be particularly the case if other parkinsonian symptoms besides akinesia are not prominent. The diagnosis can usually be established by careful examination of the patient, which will demonstrate other parkinsonian symptoms such as cogwheel rigidity and the loss of postural reflexes. A test dose of an antiparkinsonian agent can produce dramatic results if the clinician remains in doubt. There is no hypothyroidism associated with trifluoperazine ingestion. While patients who are chronically institutionalized, particularly those with prominent negative symptoms, may appear apathetic, avolitional, and affectless, these symptoms should not be confused with those of neuroleptic-induced parkinsonism, as the latter is extremely responsive to specific treatment.

3. The answer is C. [*VIII H 1 f (1) (b)*] The appropriate treatment obviously depends upon the correct diagnosis. Neuroleptic-induced parkinsonian syndrome is usually extremely responsive to an antiparkinsonian agent such as benztropine or trihexyphenidyl. The peripheral and central anticholinergic effects of these agents may produce unwanted side effects themselves, such as blurred vision and urinary retention, which can be particularly troublesome in the elderly. Nevertheless, an antiparkinsonian drug would be the first step in treatment of this case. An additional initial approach might be to decrease the dosage of the neuroleptic in question, and sometimes resolution of the parkinsonian syndrome will follow. However, there is no indication to give the patient thyroid hormone unless there is a separate diagnosis of hypothyroidism. A major depressive disorder may follow the resolution of psychotic symptoms in a schizophrenic episode and, if significant, could be treated with an antidepressant along with a neuroleptic. There is no reason to believe that a major depressive episode is the most likely diagnosis in this case. Increasing the trifluoperazine might be indicated if there has been a clear worsening of the patient's psychosis; however, the clinician must be careful not to mistake neuroleptic catatonia, which is another complication of neuroleptic therapy, with a worsening of the patient's psychosis. Neuroleptic catatonia is treated by discontinuing the neuroleptic therapy. Encouraging the patient to participate in ward activities is a reasonable intervention; however, a patient with untreated akinesia would be unable to respond to such an approach.

4. The answer is A. [*VIII H 1 f (1)*] Some patients may be unable to tolerate high-potency neuroleptics such as trifluoperazine, even with the addition of an antiparkinsonian drug to the regimen. If the patient's psychosis cannot be managed on a lower dose, a change to a different class of neuroleptics is indicated. Such a patient is likely to do better on one of the lower-potency neuroleptics such as thioridazine or loxapine. Again, the proper treatment depends upon an accurate diagnosis. In the absence of a major depressive episode, neither an antidepressant, a stimulant, nor electroconvulsive therapy (ECT) is indicated. There is no evidence of hypothyroidism, the presence of which would indicate treatment with thyroid hormone.

5. The answer is C. (*V C 1 a*) While all of the other clinical courses have been observed in schizophrenia, this patient's symptoms and onset have a number of features that point to a good prognosis. Although the history is brief, the patient is noted to be a successful college student with friends, suggesting good premorbid adjustment. His psychotic symptoms have an acute onset following a major stress (i.e., the death of his mother). In addition, he is noted to be agitated with a florid psychosis, suggesting a predominance of positive symptoms such as hallucinations, delusions, and thought disorder. There is no mention of negative symptoms, which would be associated with a poor prognosis. Such patients are likely to respond well to neuroleptic treatment and often have a family history of affective illness. In the absence of a significant mood disturbance and with a course of less than 6 months, the patient's condition would be diagnosed as schizophreniform disorder. If this patient does not respond relatively quickly to neuroleptic treatment, consideration should be given to his having an atypical affective disorder. The notation of a careful family history would be extremely important in such a situation. If the family history is positive for an affective illness, treatment via an antidepressant or lithium is indicated according to the prominent clinical features.

6. The answer is B. (*V E*) While schizophrenic patients are frequently arrested for minor crimes related to their street living, such as disturbing the peace and trespassing, it has never been established that they are more likely to commit violent crimes than the general population; however, the violent crimes that are committed by schizophrenic patients may be quite bizarre and capture excessive media attention. Schizophrenic patients, if they are able to maintain employment, frequently require low-stress, isolated jobs. They lack the capacity to adapt and, if pressure is placed on them, will frequently change jobs. Difficulty in accomplishing educational goals is common due to either the general disruption produced by the psychotic episode or to the diminished ability to initiate and follow through on tasks if negative symptoms are present. Multiple brief hospitalizations are not uncommon, and prolonged hospitalization may result if the deterioration is severe. Lastly, in addition to having a significantly increased suicide rate, the life expectancy of schizophrenic patients is shortened because they may be quite isolated if living in boarding homes or on the street and may not be receiving adequate medical attention. Even those patients who are more closely involved with family and friends may be insensitive to their own health needs.

7. The answer is D. (*VII A*) Identical twins who are reared apart have the same concordance rate for schizophrenia as monozygotic twins who are reared together, which is in the range of 50%. The adoption studies support the notion of a genetic contribution to schizophrenia. Children with one schizophrenic parent have a risk of disease of about 12% whether they are raised by their biologic parents or not. Severely ill patients are more likely to have affected relatives than are mildly ill patients. In fact, the concordance rate for monozygotic twins who are severely ill is 77% as opposed to 27% for mildly ill monozygotic twins. The lack of a concordance rate of 100% for monozygotic twins establishes the importance of environmental factors; however, it is equally clear that significant genetic loading can have a powerful influence on the development of schizophrenia.

8. The answer is B. (*VII C 4*) Increased early delta waves, particularly when they are associated with less fast wave activity, predict a poor response to neuroleptic treatment. With regard to skin conductance, acute schizophrenics who do habituate have a positive response to neuroleptics; the nonhabituators have a poor response. Augmenting, not reducing, responses of early evoked potentials (EPs), particularly if they are persistent in the chronic state, correlates with a poorer prognosis. There is no established association between abnormalities of smooth pursuit eye movements and neuroleptic response.

9. The answer is D. (*VII D 2*) The negative symptoms of schizophrenia, which include apathy, anhedonia, and flattened affect, are associated with a poor prognosis. When predominantly present, they are also associated with an increased ventricular-brain ratio (VBR), increased fibrillary gliosis in the diencephalon, reduction of blood flow and glucose metabolism in the frontal lobes, and a lower postmortem brain weight. All of these findings are suggestive of a brain disease with neuronal loss and gliosis. Of all the neuroradiologic findings, the reversal of the normal frontal and occipital asymmetry is the most controversial, and there is no specific clinical correlation.

10. The answer is B (1, 3). (*VII B 1 a, 2 b*) The dopamine (DA) hypothesis of schizophrenia postulates a relative excess of dopamine in mesolimbic and mesocortical areas. Inhibition of dopamine-β-hydroxylase (DBH) causes an accumulation of DA and a worsening of psychotic symptoms; conversely, neuroleptics are potent dopaminergic antagonists, affecting certain psychotic symptoms. These findings do support the DA hypothesis. However, apomorphine, which is a DA receptor agonist, and L-dopa, which is a DA precursor, may produce some symptomatic improvement in certain situations. They produce a relative dopaminergic excess; therefore, they should cause a worsening of symptoms according to the theory. However, it is of interest that apomorphine and L-dopa may improve negative symptoms, which are generally not responsive to neuroleptic treatment.

11. The answer is A (1, 2, 3). (*VII B 5*) The complexity of individual and environmental factors that may produce schizophrenic symptoms is illustrated by observations about gluten. The incidence of schizophrenia was noted to drop with the decreased availability and consumption of wheat during World War II. Patients with celiac disease have an increased incidence of psychosis. Schizophrenic patients have an increased incidence of celiac disease, and a subgroup of schizophrenics have symptomatic improvement of their psychoses on a gluten-free diet. Although some gluten-derived polypeptides have been shown to have endorphin properties, they are not known to be directly psychotogenic.

12. The answer is B (1, 3). [*VIII B 1, H 1 b (1)*] This patient is having an acute decompensation with command hallucinations directed against his sister. This represents an emergent situation, all the more acute because of his symbolic attack on his sister via her pictures. The patient should be hospitalized to prevent harm to his sister, and it is likely that his agitation and hallucinations would respond to thiothixene. Although an empathic therapeutic relationship is important, intensive therapy, individual or family, is not indicated for most patients in this state. They require help with reality testing and impulse control and may become more disorganized with an intensive exploratory approach. This patient would likely experience intensive contact with his family, especially his sister, at this point as overwhelming and upsetting.

13. The answer is D (4). (*VIII H 1 f; Table 1-4*) There is evidence that the patient's psychotic symptoms (i.e., voices) are improving on thiothixene at a dose of 45 mg/day; therefore, neither an increase in this medication nor a change to chlorpromazine is indicated. If the patient's agitation is part of a manic psychosis, lithium carbonate would be indicated; however, there is no evidence of other affective symptoms. While the increased agitation can be confusing and may be due to a worsening of the psychosis, it may also be an akathisia secondary to neuroleptic treatment. The upper extremity stiffness supports this latter diagnosis of an extrapyramidal side effect; akathisia is more common with the high-potency neuroleptics like thiothixene and should be treated with an antiparkinsonian agent such as benztropine.

14. The answer is B (1, 3). [*VIII H 1 f (c)*] There is more evidence of continuing improvement of the psychosis but no resolution of the akathisia. Sometimes akathisia is poorly responsive to maximal anticholinergic treatment and requires a decrease in the neuroleptic dosage or a change to a different class of neuroleptics. Schizophrenics may be agitated, sleep poorly, and benefit from a hypnotic medication; however, the akathisia, not the psychosis, disturbs the sleep of this patient, and the akathisia should be treated directly. Likewise, intensifying the psychotherapy will not help the akathisia and may increase the patient's agitation.

15. The answer is C (2, 4). (*VIII F 2, H 1*) Again the primary differential is between a worsening of the psychosis, now with catatonic symptoms, and a side effect of the new medication, haloperidol. The patient is clearly disturbed at the prospect of his parents' departure and needs help to deal with this. The parents probably are quite concerned by the deterioration in the patient, and a family meeting would be helpful both to them and the patient. However, the high-potency neuroleptics may themselves cause a severe catatonic syndrome, which in some cases may progress to a neuroleptic malignant syndrome, a potentially life-threatening condition. The safest approach would be to discontinue all neuroleptics immediately, even though the psychosis may worsen. Once the catatonia has resolved, a different class of neuroleptics may be started if necessary. There is no evidence of a depressive syndrome to indicate the need of a tricyclic antidepressant.

16. The answer is C (2, 4). (*VI B 2, 3; VIII E, H 6*) At this point the patient appears to demonstrate depressive symptoms. The physician must rule out oversedation and akinesia from neuroleptic treatment; however, oversedation is unlikely because the patient is on a decreasing dose of loxapine. There is no evidence of other symptoms of drug-induced parkinsonism, while the hopelessness, withdrawal, hypersomnia, and anorexia do suggest a postpsychotic depression. A tricyclic antidepressant such as imipramine can be helpful in these cases in conjunction with neuroleptic treatment. Since the patient has had considerable resolution of his psychosis, talking about his feelings and attempting to integrate the psychotic experience may be very helpful at this point. The therapist should be alert to the possibility of suicide during this phase of the illness.

2
Affective Disorders
Jon A. Bell

I. **DEFINITION.** Affective disorders are clinical conditions of which the common and essential feature is a disturbance of mood. The term mood refers to persistent emotional states that affect how an individual acts, thinks, and perceives his or her environment. The *Diagnostic and Statistical Manual of Mental Disorders*, third edition, (*DSM III*) classification of affective disorders includes the **major affective disorders**, which are bipolar disorder and major depression, **other specific affective disorders**, which are dysthymic disorder and cyclothymic disorder, and **atypical affective disorders**, which are atypical bipolar disorder and atypical depression. Disturbance of mood is often accompanied by other signs and symptoms, including psychophysiologic, cognitive, psychomotor, and interpersonal difficulties.

II. **HISTORY.** Descriptions of depression in scientific and poetic literature date back to antiquity. Vigorous scientific investigation of mood disturbances has taken place primarily in the last century.

A. **Falret** described patients who became depressed and elated in a cyclic fashion—**la folie circulaire**—in 1854.

B. **Karl Ludwig Kahlbaum** made similar observations about mania and melancholia in 1882. He felt that these episodes were different stages of the same disease process, which he called "**cyclothymia.**"

C. **Emil Kraepelin** (1856–1926)

1. Kraepelin made painstaking observations of patients and described a number of affective disorders, including mania, melancholia, recurrent depression, and mild mood swings. In 1921 he concluded that all of these affective disorders are identical in certain ways. He called the underlying illness "**manic-depressive illness.**" This formulation of a single, underlying disorder with varied clinical manifestations was widely accepted for several decades.

2. Kraepelin's notion of a single affective disorder with varied clinical manifestations did not withstand scrutiny by clinicians in the 1930s and 1940s. By the mid-1950s it was suggested that some individuals suffered only from depression while others suffered from the cyclic disorder that Kraepelin had described—manic-depressive illness.

D. **Karl Abraham** (1877–1925) accepted Kraepelin's notion of a single affective illness. In his description of 6 patients, he presented a psychodynamic picture of affective illness, which emphasizes the role of loss in precipitating an affective episode and the element of regression in the clinical presentation.

E. **Sigmund Freud** (1856–1939)

1. **Freud emphasized the importance of loss in depression.** Instead of remaining angry with the lost individual, the anger is turned inward by the depressed person. Freud felt that this phenomenon accounted for the typical findings of guilt, lowered self-esteem, self-reproach, and suicidal ideation. He did not explain all depression in this manner, however. He clearly stated that **some depression is psychogenic in origin** (i.e., precipitated by loss) **and, in other cases, biologically determined**.

2. **Freud's conceptualization of two different types of depression gained favor. Depression was classified as either endogenous**, (i.e., biologically determined) **or exogenous** (i.e., precipitated by loss). It was felt that those patients who develop severe depression in the face of some acute precipitant suffer from a different disorder than those without recent loss in

their histories. Many advocated different treatments for the two groups. Psychotherapy with a focus on reactions to the acute precipitant was advocated for exogenous or reactive depression. Medication, electroconvulsive therapy (ECT), or both was prescribed for endogenous depression. This interpretation of depression was accepted well into the 1970s.

F. Investigation of the biologic features of these illnesses began in earnest in the 1950s.

   1. Research was triggered by a serendipitous observation made in hypertensive patients treated with the then new drug, **reserpine**. Many of these patients developed severe depression. It was soon realized that alterations in central nervous system biogenic amine functioning (which reserpine caused) altered affective states. Since that discovery, much of the research on affective disorders, especially depression, has focused on neurotransmitters and brain pathways.

   2. As research proceeded, controversy about the endogenous and exogenous classification of depression grew. Recognition of the clinical similarities between the two groups of depressed patients and laboratory studies, which did not distinguish between the groups, led to the current categorization. It is now felt that the presence or absence of a precipitant is less important diagnostically and therapeutically than the signs and symptoms of depression and their severity.

III. EPIDEMIOLOGY. Interpretation of the data on the epidemiology of affective disorders is complicated by variations in the type of classification used, in the parameters measured, and in the reliability of diagnostic categories. This is particularly true of dysthymic disorder and cyclothymic disorder, which are both relatively new categories.

   A. Major affective disorders have been studied extensively. Major depression is more prevalent than bipolar disorder.

   1. Studies in Great Britain, the United States, and the Scandinavian countries indicate that the risk of developing a major affective disorder ranges from 0.6% to nearly 25.0% over the course of a lifetime.
      a. Lifetime risk for bipolar disorder ranges from 0.6% to 2.0%.
      b. Lifetime risk for major depression ranges from 2% to nearly 25%. Most authorities agree that an accurate figure is in the range of 10% to 15%.

   2. The incidence of bipolar disorder is similar in men and women. Major depression is diagnosed about two times as often in women as in men. Some investigators have speculated that this difference reflects a bias on the part of clinicians in diagnosing depression more readily in women. In our society, women tend to be more emotionally expressive than men, and, therefore, they display sadness or unhappiness more easily than men. Recognition of depression in men is often more difficult. Investigators have pointed to the higher incidence of substance abuse among men and have identified it as a "**depressive equivalent**" or "**masked depression.**"

   3. Major affective disorders occur in all socioeconomic groups and do not appear to be more prevalent in one group than in another.

   4. Kraepelin first noted that **the risk for developing a major affective illness is greater for blood relatives of patients** with major affective disorders than it is for the population as a whole. Families of patients with bipolar disorder are much more likely to develop bipolar disorder than major depression. Families of patients with major depression are much more likely to develop major depression than bipolar disorder.

   B. Dysthymic disorder and cyclothymic disorder are relatively new diagnostic classifications. Data on the incidence and prevalence of these disorders are limited. However, some recent studies have been completed.

   1. Over a period of 1 year, investigators found dysthymic disorder to have a prevalence rate of between 4.5% and 10.5%. Few studies have been done on cyclothymic disorder. Some investigators have estimated that less than 1% of the population are affected, but further inquiry is needed.

   2. As is the case of major depression, dysthymic disorder is reported to be more common in women than in men in a ratio of two or three to one. There are no data regarding the ratio between men and women for cyclothymic disorder.

   3. No differences in the occurrence of either dysthymic disorder or cyclothymic disorder have been identified among socioeconomic groups.

   4. No conclusions can be drawn about familial patterns for either dysthymic disorder or cyclothymic disorder.

IV. DIAGNOSIS. The disturbance in mood seen in affective disorders usually involves either depression or elation, with symptoms characteristic of either a manic or depressive syndrome.

   A. The diagnostic categories of the major affective disorders include bipolar disorder and major depression, which are distinguished from one another on the basis of whether or not there has ever been a manic episode. Patients' conditions are diagnosed as bipolar disorder even if there has not been a depressive episode. Patients who have only suffered from depressive episodes are diagnosed as having a major depression. Major affective disorders are characterized by the presence of either a full manic or depressive syndrome.

   1. The essential feature of a manic episode is a distinct period when the predominant mood is elated, irritable, or expansive. The associated symptoms of a manic syndrome are also present.

   a. The **elevated or intensified mood** in a manic episode has various manifestations. Some patients are euphoric, extremely cheerful, or happy. An observer may find the individual's high spirits to be infectious, and only those who know the patient may recognize the excessive cheerfulness. Other patients are expansive: They involve themselves in a large number of activities and may have an insatiable craving for social interactions. They are not selective in their involvement and are propelled by seemingly boundless enthusiasm. Although it is common for the manic individual's mood to be elevated, some patients are predominantly irritable. They have little ability to tolerate frustration, and irritability may progress to hostility, belligerence, and assaultiveness.

   b. Hyperactivity is a common symptom of the manic syndrome. Affected individuals make elaborate plans and engage in numerous endeavors. They may have difficulty sitting down and relaxing. They are always doing something or anticipating what they will do next. Many activities are carried to excess. This agitation often makes it stressful for others to be around the manic patient. Under the pressure of an increased desire to be sociable, indiscriminate contacts with distant acquaintances occur. Late-night phone calls and visits are not uncommon. The inappropriate, intrusive, or threatening nature of these contacts is not appreciated by the manic. Expansiveness, grandiosity, impaired judgment, and boundless optimism frequently lead to wild spending sprees, reckless driving, unwise investments, and intense, exaggerated sexual activity. Behavior is often flamboyant or bizarre. The usual style of dressing may be replaced by more colorful or outlandish apparel. The individual may appear to be disorganized or out of control. Some manic individuals accost strangers and attempt to engage them in conversation or in unrealistic schemes.

   c. Speech is commonly rapid or pressured. Manic individuals speak loudly and are difficult to interrupt. Telling jokes, making puns or plays on words, and preoccupation with unimportant but amusing details are common. Dramatic or exaggerated forms of expression such as singing or gesturing may occur. The sounds of words may enchant the patient, leading to **clanging**, a phenomenon characterized by word selection based on sounds rather than meanings. The irritable individual is prone to hostile tirades when frustrated.

   d. The normal coherence of thought is compromised in the manic syndrome. Flight of ideas is a pattern of thought characterized by a rapid and continuous flow of speech with sudden changes in topic. These changes are usually based on comprehensible associations, distractions (e.g., noises), and plays on words. In its severe form, flight of ideas is difficult to follow, and the manic individual becomes incoherent and disorganized. Loosening of associations, a phenomenon characterized by rapid changes in topic that are not understandable, also occurs in disorganized manic patients.

   e. Typically, the manic individual is very distractible. This is evident in the shortened attention span of these individuals. Flight of ideas reflects distractibility. An inability to begin and complete a task because of distractions due to inadvertent and irrelevant stimuli is common. Signs, colors, lights, and sounds may be sufficient to disrupt concentration and attention.

   f. Just as the mood is elevated and exuberant, the manic individual's opinion of him- or herself is elevated. Some patients are uncritical of themselves; others have grandiose and delusional notions of their own worth and accomplishments. It is not uncommon for the manic to believe that he or she is an expert on a topic of which he or she is not: For example, manic individuals tell physicians how to practice medicine. Books are written. Jobs for which qualifications are lacking are actively pursued. In extreme forms, the manic patient is delusional. He or she believes that unique relationships with a deity or powerful political, religious, and entertainment figures exist.

   g. Manic patients have limited need for sleep. They go to bed late and are up early, often sleeping just 2 to 4 hours per day. Even with so little sleep they are full of energy. Sleeplessness for several days is not uncommon.

  h. **Rapid shifts in mood (lability) is commonly associated with the manic syndrome.** This phenomenon is characterized by an abrupt change from exuberance and elation to anger or depression. The anger or depression may last a few minutes or a few hours. When angry, the manic patient poses a significant danger to others. When depressed, he or she may act on sudden suicidal impulses. This mingling of manic and depressive syndromes is referred to as **bipolar disorder, mixed**, in which aspects of each syndrome become part of an ongoing clinical picture.

  i. **Psychotically disturbed manic patients experience delusions and hallucinations.** Usually, these phenomena are **mood-congruent** (i.e., consistent with the predominant mood). For example, an exuberant, euphoric patient believes that he or she has a special relationship with God (which is a delusion) and hears God's voice (which is an hallucination). Delusions of persecution may arise for the manic individual who imagines that others are jealous of his or her powers and relationships. Delusions and hallucinations that have no apparent connection with the predominant mood are **mood-incongruent**. The utility of the concepts of mood-congruence and mood-incongruence is open to question at this time.

2. **The essential feature of a depressive syndrome is either a dysphoric mood or a loss of pleasure or interest in usual activities.** This mood disturbance is prominent and persistent. It is accompanied by a number of typical symptoms and signs of a depressive syndrome. In making a diagnosis of major depression, weight is given to the severity and duration of symptoms. Two weeks of severe symptomatology is suggested as a guideline. A major depression may occur one time only or may be recurrent.

  a. **The depressed individual suffers from symptoms of a dysphoric mood.** He or she may complain of feeling "blue", sad, irritable, discouraged, hopeless, or depressed. Alternatively, the patient may express a loss of interest in and enthusiasm for everyday activities, saying such things as, "I just don't care about anything " or "Nothing makes any difference to me anymore." These symptoms are prominent and unaltering during the depression.

  b. **A change in appetite or weight is common in depression.** Typically, the patient loses his or her appetite. Interest in food is lost or food no longer tastes good. Food is consumed only when the depressed individual can force it down. In this situation weight is lost quickly, often 5 or 10 pounds in 1 week. Less commonly, individuals increase their food intake during a depressive episode. Frequent and large meals satisfy a craving for food, although there may be little gustatory pleasure. Weight may be gained quickly, up to 20 pounds in 2 or 3 weeks.

  c. **Disruption of normal sleep patterns is common in depressed individuals.** Some patients report difficulty in sleeping, which may take several forms. Difficulty in getting to sleep plagues many; they lie in bed for 1, 2, even 3 hours and cannot get to sleep (**initial insomnia**). Once sleep is achieved, it may be short-lived. Awakening in the middle of the night (**middle insomnia**) or in the early morning (**early morning awakening**) limits the hours of sleep. Overall, most depressed patients suffer from a lack of sleep. However, some sleep excessively, often 12 hours and more per day (**hypersomnia**).

  d. **The usual level of activity is altered for many depressed patients.** Most patients are less active than usual. The patient tells the examiner such things as, "I just can't get my work done " or "I spend my day sitting and can't get going." Observations of these patients reveal a lack of spontaneous movement and activity. They are motionless. They sit with hunched shoulders. They speak slowly and softly, sometimes so softly as to be inaudible. They are said to be **psychomotorically retarded**. Some individuals are strikingly more active than usual. They are restless and may not be able to sit still in a chair. Pacing, constant use of the hands, doing such things as pulling at clothing and hair, or incessantly smoking cigarettes may be prominent. Patients say that they "cannot sit still." They can be described as agitated.

  e. **Interest in sexual activity rarely persists in severe depression.** Typically, both the frequency and the enjoyment of sex are diminished. Men may become impotent. Women report an inability to feel aroused or excited.

  f. **Pleasure and interest in normal activities may be lost.** An individual who enjoys his or her work and hobbies no longer finds them satisfying. Little effort is made to participate or engage in activities. This loss of all pleasure is called **anhedonia**.

  g. **Fatigue is common in depression.** Individuals complain of low levels of energy, saying such things as, "I just get tired so easily " or "I don't have any energy."

  h. **Depressed individuals may be plagued by feelings and thoughts of worthlessness, self-reproach, and excessive guilt.** The patient may express an intense sense of responsibility for his or her thoughts and feelings or for events in his or her environment. He or she readily finds fault with him- or herself. Such ruminations may attain irrational proportions, and the patient may become psychotic (out of touch with reality). Delusions arise from the individual's preoccupations with self-worth, guilt, disease, death, and decay.

i. Cognitive impairment afflicts many depressed individuals. They find that they cannot think clearly. They are unable to concentrate. Tasks such as reading and calculating may become very difficult, if not impossible, to complete. A lack of attention during everyday activities such as cooking and watching television may leave the patient feeling frustrated and inept. Indecisiveness interferes with daily functioning when even minor decisions cannot be made. These cognitive disruptions are frequently apparent in the diagnostic interview.

j. Thoughts of death preoccupy many depressed patients. This phenomenon may take various forms. Some individuals wish for death or long to be reunited with a deceased loved one. Danger is more imminent for others. Plans for death are formulated. Some make wills and get their affairs in order. Others plan suicide. Reckless driving and excessive alcohol or drug use are examples of covert suicidal behavior that warrant attention.

B. Other specific affective disorders is a diagnostic category of long-standing conditions with minimal durations of 2 years. A sustained or intermittent disturbance of mood is associated with signs and symptoms of an affective syndrome. Unlike major affective disorders, only a partial affective syndrome is present. There are never any psychotic features.

1. The essential feature of a **cyclothymic disorder** is a chronic mood disturbance of at least 2 years' duration. **Numerous episodes of depression and hypomania occur in the course of the illness**. Depressive and manic syndromes are not of such severity or intensity to warrant a diagnosis of a full affective syndrome.

   a. Periods of normal mood may occur between episodes of depression and hypomania. Some individuals may have normal moods that last months at a time. Others may have limited or no periods of normal moods.

   b. When affected individuals are depressed, they suffer from a dysphoric mood or they have lost interest and pleasure in their usual activities. At other times they are hypomanic, a condition in which a muted form of a manic syndrome is present.

   (1) Signs and symptoms of the depressive periods include three or more of the following in addition to the mood disturbance (this information is according to the diagnostic criteria of the *DSM III*).

   (a) Insomnia or hypersomnia
   (b) Low energy or chronic fatigue
   (c) Feelings of inadequacy
   (d) Decreased effectiveness or productivity at school, work, or home
   (e) Decreased attention, concentration, or ability to think clearly
   (f) Social withdrawal
   (g) Loss of interest in or enjoyment of sex
   (h) Restriction of involvement in pleasurable activities or guilt over past activities
   (i) Feelings of being slowed down
   (j) Less talkativeness than usual
   (k) Pessimistic attitude towards the future or brooding about past events

   (2) Signs and symptoms of hypomanic periods include three or more of the following in addition to an elevated, expansive, or irritable mood (this information is according to the diagnostic criteria of the *DSM III*).

   (a) Decreased need for sleep
   (b) More energy than usual
   (c) Inflated self-esteem
   (d) Increased productivity, often associated with unusual and self-imposed working hours
   (e) Sharpened and unusually creative thinking
   (f) Uninhibited people-seeking (extreme gregariousness)
   (g) Hypersexuality without recognition of the possibility of painful consequences
   (h) Excessive involvement in pleasurable activities with a lack of concern for the high potential for painful consequences (e.g., heavy drug or alcohol use, spending sprees, and careless driving)
   (i) Physical restlessness
   (j) More talkativeness than usual
   (k) Optimism and an exaggerated sense of accomplishment
   (l) Inappropriate laughing, joking, or punning

   c. A review of these signs and symptoms reveals **paired symptoms**. An individual is socially withdrawn when depressed and extremely gregarious when hypomanic. Optimism and an exaggerated sense of accomplishment contrast with pessimism and brooding over past events. Paired symptoms indicate that the cyclothymic patient may present a history filled with apparent contradictions. "Sometimes I feel like I'm on top of the world, and other times I feel like I'm at the bottom of the heap " is a typical complaint.

2. A dysthymic disorder features a chronic disturbance of mood involving either a depressed mood or a loss of interest or pleasure in all, or almost all, usual activities. Associated symptoms of a depressive syndrome are not of sufficient severity or duration to warrant a diagnosis of major depression. This chronic condition must be present for at least 2 years in adults and 1 year or more in adolescents and children for diagnosis.

    a. Periods of normal mood may be present for a few days or weeks. The presence of a mood for a few months or more should lead to further evaluation; a diagnosis of dysthymic disorder is questionable in such a case.

    b. During depressive periods, signs and symptoms include three or more of those listed in section III B 1 b in addition to a chronic mood disturbance.

    c. To distinguish dysthymia from cyclothymia, the evaluator must determine if the patient returns to a normal mood (**euthymia**) or if the patient becomes hypomanic. The return to euthymia is such a change and relief for some individuals that it may seem to be a period of euphoria or exuberance. **The best clues to hypomania are abnormally high levels of activity, poor judgment, and impulsive behavior.**

    d. In many dysthymic individuals **depression is masked behind other complaints**. Chronic pain, insomnia, and chronic, unresolved somatic problems are common presenting symptoms to physicians. Hypochondriacal complaints represent the patient's experience of chronic depression.

    e. Alcohol abuse can produce a chronic depression or may represent an attempt to ameliorate dysthymia. The toxic effects of alcohol make it necessary for the patient to abstain before the depression can be fully evaluated.

C. Atypical affective disorders is a diagnostic category for individuals whose symptoms do not meet the criteria for major affective disorders or other specific affective disorders but who clearly have affective syndromes.

    1. Individuals who have manic features but whose symptoms do not meet the diagnostic criteria for bipolar disorder or cyclothymic disorder are classified as having **atypical bipolar disorder** (e.g., a patient who has full depressive syndromes and hypomanic episodes).

    2. Similarly, individuals with depressive syndromes whose symptoms do not meet the diagnostic criteria for a major depression or dysthymic disorder are classified as having **atypical depression**. A brief depression of mild or moderate intensity, which does not appear to be a reaction to a recognized stress, is one example of an atypical depression.

V. ETIOLOGIC FACTORS. Numerous studies have been made in an attempt to discover the causes of affective disorders. These studies have examined genetic, biologic, psychological, and sociologic variables. This remains an area of vigorous investigation.

A. Studies of major affective disorders suggest that these are a group of genetically influenced disorders. Shifts in an intrinsic activity cycle occur, and characteristic symptoms arise. Abnormalities at the synaptic and cellular levels appear to be part of the usual picture. Psychogenic and psychosocial factors appear to be significant in some cases, but their causation roles have not been determined.

    1. Genetic studies have shown the heritability of major affective disorders. There is a greater risk of developing a disorder for the monozygotic twin than for the dizygotic twin of an individual with a major affective disorder, suggesting the existence of a significant genetic factor. Families of both bipolar and unipolar (depressed) individuals have been studied.

    a. In families with histories of bipolar illness, some investigators have discovered an X-linked dominant pattern of inheritance. Others have discovered an inherited **abnormality of membrane lithium transport in red blood cells**, which suggests an autosomal dominant pattern of transmission with variable expression. Each of these two inheritance patterns has been further delineated. The X-linked dominant pattern features an early onset of bipolar disorder (around 25 years of age) with a positive family history. The autosomal dominant pattern has a later onset (around 40 years of age) with a negative family history. Not all patients fit into these two groups, and more studies are being conducted.

    b. Unlike bipolar disorder, **no markers have been discovered for major depression**. However, groups of depressed patients have been investigated by Winokur in his studies. One group includes women who have experienced a major depression before the age of 40 years. These women have experienced depression more often than the men in their families. There is an increased incidence of alcoholism and sociopathy in their male relatives. Winokur has called the depression experienced by this group **depressive spectrum disease**. The second group studied includes men who experienced their first major depression after the age of 40 years. Men and women in the families of this group experience depression at similar rates. There is little alcoholism or sociopathy among male relatives. The disorder suffered by this group is called **pure depressive disease**.

2. **In 1921 Kraepelin speculated that affective illness was due to biologic factors.** He considered psychological factors to be coincidental. He hypothesized that some inner control mechanism was accelerated or decelerated in mania and depression, respectively.
   a. The concept of **circadian rhythms** refers to various bodily functions that adhere to 24-hour cycles. Many circadian rhythms have been identified, including diurnal variations in mood, electroencephalogram (EEG) patterns, rest-activity cycles, and the regulation of neuroendocrine functions. Malfunctioning of an internal clock would explain several features of an affective illness. Difficulty in falling asleep, excessive sleep, early morning awakening, and variations in rest-activity cycles are some examples. The phenomenon of the mood switch in bipolar disorder may be indicative of a malfunctioning circadian rhythm.
   b. Studies of the effects of lithium and alcohol in animals have demonstrated that the intrinsic pacemaker is slowed by these drugs, which lengthens the circadian rhythm cycle. Exogenous estrogens accelerate the intrinsic pacemaker, thereby shortening the circadian rhythm cycle. Tricyclic antidepressants given to animals with abnormally prolonged circadian rhythm cycles accelerate the establishment of a normal cycle. Although these studies have not been conducted in humans, all of these drugs do effect affective changes in humans, leading to the hypothesis that disruption of human circadian rhythms produces affective illness.
   c. Recently investigators have identified a subgroup of depressed individuals who are afflicted only during months with fewer hours of sunlight. These patients have been successfully treated with increased exposure to light. Animal rhythms change in response to sunlight, and it is speculated that the same is true in humans.

3. **Levels of norepinephrine and serotonin have been implicated in the etiology of depression and mania.** These compounds transmit signals in the nervous system when they are released into the synaptic spaces.
   a. Deficiencies in the levels of norepinephrine and serotonin have been discovered in depressed patients. A biochemical profile of patients with these deficiencies has been developed in an attempt to identify subgroups of depression, although this has not significantly influenced clinical practice. Table 2-1 illustrates the two profiles.
   b. Levels of norepinephrine and its metabolites are elevated in mania. In addition, activity in dopaminergic neurons is increased.

Table 2-1. Biochemical Profile of Depressed Patients

Naturally Occurring Biochemicals	In the Presence of	
	Serotonin Deficiency	Norepinephrine Deficiency
5-Hydroxyindoleacetic acid [5-HIAA] (a serotonin metabolite)	Low levels	Normal or elevated levels
3-Methoxy-4-hydroxyphenylglycol [MHPG] (a norepinephrine metabolite)	Normal levels	Low levels
Growth hormone, in response to insulin	Normal levels	Low levels
Tricyclic antidepressant	Amitriptyline	Imipramine

4. **Some investigators have focused on psychological and sociocultural variables in their studies of affective illness.** These factors are difficult to measure with precision, thereby making much of this work highly speculative.
   a. Psychogenic theories are based on the notion of loss and speculations about the effect of loss on the individual. The hypotheses of Freud and Abraham have been described in section II D and E.
   b. Studies of families of bipolar patients were conducted by Fromm-Reichmann in 1954 and Gibson in 1959. Each found a similar family profile; however, the significance of these findings is unclear.

B. **Studies of causative factors of dysthymic disorder and cyclothymic disorder are few** in comparison to those for the major affective disorders. These diagnostic categories are relatively new, and data have not been accumulated.

1. **There is consensus that cyclothymic disorder is a muted form of bipolar disorder.** There are similarities in the clinical features. The family of a cyclothymic individual often has other cyclothymic members. Bipolar patients often have cyclothymic individuals in their families. These observations have led to the hypothesis that a lesser but similar disruption of circadian rhythms and cellular mechanisms is present in cyclothymic disorder.

2. **Dysthymic disorder has been studied more vigorously.** Some investigators point to its frequent association with other chronic conditions such as a personality disorder or chronic medical illness. The significance of this association is not clear. Most investigators have focused on psychological variables in their search for causation. Personality traits of dependency, a tendency to feel guilty or blameworthy, passivity, and a tendency to ruminate have been identified in dysthymic individuals. A difficult adaptation to adulthood is felt to be common in many of these patients. Further study is necessary to evaluate these findings. No biologic data have been accumulated.

C. **The etiology of atypical affective disorders** has not been studied. Serious study is hampered because the diagnostic category is ill-defined.

VI. COURSE AND PROGNOSIS. Data on the age of the affected individual at onset and the rapidity of onset, impairment and complications during acute episodes and long-term, and outcome with and without treatment provide a good picture of the course and prognosis of the affective disorders.

A. **The disease course of major affective disorders has been studied and chronicled since the early part of this century.**

1. A group of 208 patients was followed by Rennie from 1913 to 1916. Relapse (at 82%) was common among 17 manic individuals as it was (at 77%) among 121 depressed individuals. Initial manic episodes lasted an average of 3½ months. Initial depressive episodes lasted an average of 6½ months.

2. **Bipolar disorder usually becomes clinically evident before the age of 30 years.** Onset is typically sudden with a rapid escalation into the manic state. Manic episodes may last a few days or a few months and tend to be shorter in duration than depressive episodes. A depressive episode occurs at some point during the lifetime of most bipolar individuals, but the first episode of affective illness is frequently mania.
   a. **The frequency and sequence of episodes vary.** Some individuals have years of normal functioning between episodes. Others have episodes in clusters. In severe cases "cycling" occurs, which is a phenomenon characterized by alternations between mania and depression without periods of euthymia.
   b. **Manic individuals suffer significant impairment and complications.** Social and occupational functioning typically is severely affected. Impulsive and excessive behavior due to poor judgment and hyperactivity may lead to financial loss or ruin, legal difficulties, family disruption or disintegration, and death from accidents, suicide, or homicide. Substance abuse is common. The facts indicate that manics need protection from the consequences of their actions, which is often best provided in a hospital.

3. **Major depression may occur at any age, even early in childhood.** The pattern of onset is variable. Sudden onset may follow a severe stress. Signs and symptoms may develop over days to weeks and include such features as anxiety, phobic reactions, panic attacks, and mild depression.
   a. Recent studies have shown that **major depression is recurrent for about 50% of affected individuals**. Some investigators point to an increased risk for bipolar disorder in patients with recurrent major depression.
   b. Years of normal functioning may pass between depressive episodes for some individuals. Others have clusters of episodes. A chronic deteriorating course is unusual.
   c. **Impairment in functioning varies in major depression.** Relationships are disrupted. It may be difficult, if not impossible, to work. In severe cases the individual cannot take care of his or her own needs. Medical, financial, family, and occupational responsibilities are not fulfilled. The risk of suicide and, less frequently, homicide are the most serious complications.
   d. **Prognosis is good with proper diagnosis and treatment.**

B. **Dysthymic disorder and cyclothymic disorder are chronic conditions.** The clear-cut relapses and remissions observed in the major affective disorders are not observed in dysthymia and cyclothymia.

1. **Dysthymic disorder usually has its onset in early adulthood.** Acute, severe depressive episodes do not occur. There may be a family history of affective illness. Affected individuals have difficulty adjusting to the new tasks and responsibilities of adulthood. **Onset in middle-age is gradual and insidious.** An early history of good functioning in interpersonal, social, and occupational spheres stands in contrast to new difficulties. Failures at work, problems as a parent, and troubled relationships may be present. **Dysthymic disorder in the elderly occurs in conjunction with aging.** Mental deterioration may be hard to distinguish from depression in these individuals.

   a. **Chronically depressed individuals of all ages tend to experience more health problems than the population as a whole.** Some individuals delay seeking timely medical care; others seek health care frequently and become identified as chronic somatic complainers. The chronic patient may not be taken seriously and is more likely to have significant problems overlooked or misdiagnosed by physicians. Finally, some authorities have speculated that depression weakens the body and its normal defenses against illness.

   b. **Chronic impairment in several spheres of functioning is common in dysthymic individuals.** Relationships may be unsatisfying and lack intimacy. Interest in sex and the ability to perform sexually may be limited. Social activities provide little enjoyment or are avoided altogether. Divorce, unemployment, and professional failure occur.

   c. **Dysthymic individuals tend to be self-destructive.** The most obvious manifestations of this are suicide attempts. Another manifestation is a tendency to have accidents. Careful exploration may reveal ways in which an individual has guaranteed that he or she will fail at work or in a relationship.

   d. **The most significant variable for prognosis is recognition.** Many dysthymic individuals remain undiagnosed. Without diagnosis, chronic impairment, physical illness, and even death by suicide result.

2. **Cyclothymic disorder usually manifests itself in adolescence.** It can be recognized as a **change in personality.** An individual becomes moody. The duration and intensity of these periods of elation and depression vary.

   a. **Cyclothymic adults may be very successful during hypomanic periods.** They are optimistic, energetic, ambitious, creative, and gregarious. However, functioning is very different during depressive periods. Energy for work and interpersonal interactions is low. The contrast between these two periods may be marked, which leads to the perception that the affected individual is erratic and unreliable. Some cyclothymic patients do not even do well when they are hypomanic: Judgment is poor, and social interactions are inappropriate.

   b. **The prognosis is unclear at this time.**

VII. DIFFERENTIAL DIAGNOSIS. As defined in the *DSM III*, a diagnosis of an affective disorder cannot be made if the syndrome is due to a known organic factor or if it is superimposed upon schizophrenia, a schizophreniform disorder, or a paranoid disorder. Therefore, a search for organic causes or another psychiatric illness should be conducted in the diagnostic process.

A. **Major affective disorders may be difficult to distinguish from other psychiatric disorders.** Organic syndromes may be clinically difficult to distinguish as well.

   1. **Mania-like syndromes can be due to a number of causes.**

      a. Mania can result from the **ingestion of corticosteroids**, which are commonly administered for a number of medical illnesses. Collagen-vascular diseases such as rheumatoid arthritis and systemic lupus erythematosus and asthma are just two examples. **Tricyclic antidepressants** may produce a manic state in a susceptible individual. **Amphetamines and other stimulants** produce hyperactivity, pressured speech, and impulsive, excessive behavior, which are all features of mania.

      b. A neurologic disorder such as **multiple sclerosis** may produce a manic-like syndrome.

      c. A common diagnostic dilemma arises in the evaluation of the acutely psychotic patient. There may be signs and symptoms typical of manic psychosis or signs and symptoms that are not so typical. **An acute schizophrenic episode may appear to be mania and vice versa.** Because a psychotic individual appears to be schizophrenic acutely does not mean that he or she is not manic. The best allies of the clinician are time and history in making this differentiation. Some patients, however, have persistent features of schizophrenia and mania, a mixed clinical picture called **schizoaffective disorder.**

      d. Since **the intensity and duration of the syndrome differentiate mania from cyclothymia**, it is easy to see how this distinction can be difficult to make. Once again, history usually resolves the question.

e. An individual with a **narcissistic personality disorder** experiences highs and lows. Unlike those occurring in bipolar disorder, these peaks and valleys are short-lived and do not usually include the multitude of symptoms seen in manic and depressive episodes.

2. **Depressive syndromes can result from organic and functional disorders.**

a. A number of **antihypertensive medications** affect central nervous system amines. It should be kept in mind that the effect of reserpine on patients was an early clue to the role of amines in depression. A full depressive syndrome may develop with corticosteroids as well, particularly if they are withdrawn too quickly.

b. **Dementia** has many characteristics in common with depression, including lack of concentration, memory lapses, disorientation, and apathy. Both demented patients and depressed patients perform poorly on mental status examinations. Distinguishing between these disorders often requires treatment of the patient for depression. The depressed patient's mental status examination will show improvement, the demented patient's will not. The picture is further complicated by the fact that depression is a common secondary disorder in the demented.

c. **Cancer**, especially in its advanced stages, may produce a depressive syndrome. Pancreatic cancer presents as depression in 30% to 40% of all cases.

d. **Hypothyroidism** also mimics depression.

e. Very disturbed, psychotic depressive syndromes can include hallucinations, bizarre delusions, and very regressed behavior. This presentation would raise questions about **schizophrenia** as a diagnostic possibility. Time and history can be helpful in distinguishing one from the other.

f. The agitation, restlessness, insomnia, and dysphoria suffered in **anxiety disorders** can be similar to signs and symptoms of an agitated depression. For some patients, a period of anxiety precedes a major depression. Follow-up and treatment trials with medication may be necessary to make a diagnosis.

g. **Chronic use of depressants such as alcohol and barbiturates** makes it very difficult to assess depression. Many authorities feel that an affective illness cannot be evaluated adequately in this population.

h. Individuals with **somatization disorders** are often chronically depressed but do not describe themselves as such. Depressed patients who present with somatic complaints have similarities to this group. The severity of symptoms and the presence of other features of the depressive syndrome are helpful in making a diagnosis.

i. **There may be a fine line between major depression and dysthymia.** Signs and symptoms differ only in intensity and duration. Patient history is helpful, but follow-up may be necessary to differentiate the two.

B. **The differential diagnostic considerations for dysthymic disorder and cyclothymic disorder** are similar to those for the major affective disorders. Other chronic mental conditions such as personality disorders and substance abuse disorders warrant consideration in the diagnostic process.

C. **Bereavement** is the normal reaction to the death of a loved one. In response to loss, an individual sleeps poorly, eats poorly, loses weight, ruminates about the lost person, has trouble concentrating, is tearful, feels depressed, feels ill at ease, and has thoughts of dying. In short, **a full depressive syndrome is a normal reaction to the death of a loved one**. This syndrome usually lasts from 2 to 6 months, depending upon the cultural norms for grieving. Guilt about what was or was not done at the time of death may be prominent. A diagnosis of major depression is not made in this situation. If the syndrome is prolonged, if there is marked functional impairment, if marked psychomotor retardation develops, or if there is a morbid hopelessness and feelings of worthlessness and low self-esteem, a diagnosis of major depression should be entertained.

VIII. **TREATMENT.** In developing a treatment plan for a patient with an affective disorder, the clinician must consider the patient's lethality (i.e., suicide and homicide potential), resources (both internal, intrapsychic resources as well as external resources), past treatment successes and failures, and the specific diagnosis.

A. **The major affective disorders** are rewarding illnesses to treat because treatment is successful in most cases.

1. The **initial decision** in the care of patients with bipolar illness, manic or depressed, and major depression **is whether or not hospitalization is needed**. Whether the patient in question is manic or depressed, successful treatment depends upon the availability of adequate support to the patient. A loss of support systems or inadequate support may compel the clinician to hospitalize the patient.

    a. The **risk for suicide or homicide** is high for some patients with bipolar disorder. This may be due to an expressed and determined intent to kill oneself or another. Wild, impulsive behavior may create a dangerous situation as well. These patients need to be hospitalized.

    b. **Manic behavior** can be ruinous for the patient and others. Financial disaster, loss of career, and family disintegration are just three examples of tragic consequences. The hospital can provide a secure, protective environment, which minimizes the destruction that mania can bring to so many lives.

    c. **The agitated, driven behavior of acute mania can produce dangerous physiologic changes** (e.g., elevated blood pressure, elevated temperature, tachycardia, and dehydration). Unchecked, these changes could lead to significant and life-threatening medical complications. Hospitalization and sedation may be life-saving interventions.

    d. **Acutely depressed individuals may pose a significant risk for suicide or homicide**, and they should be hospitalized. It is estimated that 6% of women and 3% of men are hospitalized for depression during adulthood.

    e. **Severe depression may render a person unable to care for his or her basic needs**, in which case hospitalization may be necessary.

2. Most manic and depressed patients are treated as outpatients. This can be done even when patients are acutely disturbed if the following variables are evaluated.

    a. **Frequent contact is necessary** for the acutely ill individual. These illnesses can change suddenly and unpredictably. A turn for the worse can be quickly detected, and appropriate interventions can be made.

    b. Individuals treated as **outpatients should not be significant risks for lethal behavior**. Careful assessment for suicide and homicide potential is mandatory and should be an ongoing process.

    c. The patient's **support system** of family, friends, clergy, and co-workers should be evaluated for its adequacy relative to the patient's needs. Some individuals need more support than others. If a patient cannot bear to be alone, for example, the clinician must determine what his or her environment can provide.

    d. Once the setting for treatment has been determined, decisions about other specific interventions can be made.

3. Medication

    a. **Medication provides the clinician with a powerful tool for the treatment of mania.**

        (1) **The initial task in the treatment of acute mania is to quiet the agitation that commonly occurs.** This is usually accomplished with neuroleptic medications (e.g., phenothiazines and butyrophenones), although in rare cases barbiturates and ECT are used when neuroleptics fail to provide enough sedation.

        (2) **Lithium carbonate** revolutionized the treatment of mania. Its success is reported to be about 80% in most studies. It is beneficial in both the acute phase of mania and as a prophylactic agent.

            (a) Lithium should not be given until the patient's general medical health is evaluated because of its toxicity and metabolism. Of particular concern are renal, cardiac, and thyroid functioning. Once it has been established that the cardiac rhythm is stable, that renal clearance of lithium will be adequate, and that thyroid functioning is normal, lithium can be administered.

            (b) Lithium carbonate is given in high doses to patients with acute mania. Both the levels (0.8 mEq/L to 1.5 mEq/L) of lithium and the side effects (e.g., gastrointestinal upset, diarrhea, tremors, and muscular twitches) govern the dosage. In general, doses ranging from 1 g/day to 3 g/day are necessary.

            (c) It may be necessary to administer a neuroleptic agent along with lithium carbonate. This has been reported to be a dangerous combination in isolated cases; therefore, the combination should be administered cautiously, with attention to keeping the patient well hydrated.

            (d) As the acute phase resolves, the need for lithium diminishes. Therefore, with improvement, the dose is decreased. Once again, levels (0.6 mEq/L to 1.2 mEq/L) and side effects govern the dosage.

            (e) Once acute mania has resolved, the question of chronic treatment must be addressed. There is firm evidence to support the prophylactic efficacy of lithium. Decreasing the frequency and severity of episodes may favorably influence the long-term course of the illness. The risk of administering lithium on a chronic basis must be weighed against the potential disruption of another manic episode. Chronic administration of lithium has been associated with medical complications, which include diffuse goiter, decreased glucose tolerance, an elevated white blood cell count, nephrogenic diabetes insipidus, thyroid deficiency, parathyroid adenomas, and interstitial nephritis.

b. **Medications have also proven to be very useful in the treatment of severe depression.** They shorten the duration of the depressive episode in the majority of cases.

   (1) It should be emphasized that **diagnostic precision** aids in choosing the appropriate course of treatment. A bipolar depression is treated differently than a major depression in the patient without bipolar disorder. Lithium should be used in combination with the antidepressant in the bipolar patient.

   (2) **A history of success with a particular antidepressant should direct the clinician to use that medication for treatment of recurrent depression.** Similarly, a history of success with a particular antidepressant in a family member may point to the best choice in medication.

   (3) **Tricyclic antidepressants** are usually the first medications tried if the patient's health permits. Patients with cardiac disease should be evaluated before beginning the drugs.

      (a) Doses of tricyclic antidepressants vary widely among the different medications and within different patient populations. In general, elderly patients need about one-half of the dose needed by younger adults. The dose should be low at first (e.g., 25 mg of imipramine). These medications have powerful and unpleasant side effects (including dry mouth, blurred vision, dizziness, urinary retention, sedation, and orthostatic hypotension) caused by their potent anticholinergic effects. The dose should be raised slowly, always taking into account the patient's tolerance of side effects. The patient may become very uncomfortable with too rapid a rise in dose, which may affect his or her willingness to comply with treatment.

      (b) **Tricyclic antidepressants do not provide immediate relief**; rather, full therapeutic effectiveness usually is not realized for 2 to 6 weeks. Some symptoms respond more quickly. For example, insomnia may resolve with the sedating effects of amitriptyline in the first week of medication.

      (c) Most clinicians keep patients on antidepressant medication for 4 to 6 months after they have become symptom-free. At this point, the patient can be tapered off the medication over the course of 1 to 2 months.

   (4) **Some patients do not respond to tricyclic antidepressants.** In these cases the diagnosis should be reevaluated. The patient may have another disorder. A change in medication may be necessary if the physician is certain that the diagnosis is correct. Switching to a different tricyclic antidepressant is common practice. Failure of tricyclic antidepressants to work should lead to psychiatric consultation for the nonpsychiatric physician. The psychiatrist may prescribe a **monoamine oxidase inhibitor (MAOI)**, a second-line drug for depression. These medications are complicated to prescribe. They potentiate sympathomimetic agents, including tyramine and tryptophan, in the diet and interact with numerous other medications.

   (5) **Stimulants can alleviate depression.** However, they are not recommended because tolerance develops quickly and side effects at high doses are numerous.

4. **ECT** has been used for several decades. Recently, it has been viewed as inhumane; however, it remains an effective treatment for affective illness.

   a. **The precise therapeutic mechanism of ECT is not known.** Seizures are induced electrically in a medically cleared patient in a safe environment (often an operating room). The patient is paralyzed so that the seizure will do no harm. In most cases seizures are timed to last around 60 seconds for each treatment. A series of treatments, usually three per week, is given on alternating days. This is terminated when clinical improvement is evident. Memory loss, on a temporary basis, accompanies improvement.

   b. Properly administered, ECT is associated with very low morbidity and mortality. The success rate is greater than 90%.

   c. Patients selected for ECT fall into four groups:

      (1) Patients with a past history of good response to ECT

      (2) Severely depressed patients with psychomotor retardation, somatic delusions, delusional guilt, disinterest in the world around them, weight loss, and persistent suicidal intent

      (3) Patients who have not responded to medication or who cannot take antidepressants

      (4) Patients who are manic and who have not responded to other therapy

5. **Laboratory tests have recently proven to be useful in the diagnosis of depression.** It should be remembered that disrupted neuroendocrine functions may be etiologic in affective disorders. The **dexamethasone suppression test** measures the functioning of the hypothalamic-pituitary-adrenal cortical axis. A normal response to a dose of dexamethasone (which is 1 mg administered at 11 P.M.) is suppression of endogenous cortisol production, which is measured at 8 A.M., 4 P.M., and 11 P.M. on the next day. A significant number (around 50%) of depressed patients do not suppress cortisol production, and some depressed patients do respond normally to the dexamethasone suppression test. In addition, conditions such as

alcohol abuse and chronic medical illness can produce false-positive results. Nonetheless, the positive result can provide a reliable biologic marker to follow throughout treatment of depression. The response to dexamethasone should return to normal with successful treatment.

6. **Psychotherapy** is a useful and necessary adjunct to all of the previously described therapies. The form and intensity of psychotherapy varies from case to case. Some patients require supportive guidance from a therapist and nothing more; others have more pressing needs for indepth exploration of problems, relationships, and conflicts.

B. **Cyclothymia and dysthymia** are not as easily or successfully treated as the major affective disorders. Substance abuse is a common occurrence among dysthymic individuals. The physician must inquire about this and treat it when necessary.

1. Almost all cyclothymic and dysthymic individuals can be treated as outpatients. Suicidal behavior, however, may lead to **hospitalization**.

2. **Somatic therapies** are recommended by some authorities, but this type of treatment is controversial.
   a. Some investigators are optimistic about the response of cyclothymic individuals to **lithium carbonate**. Stable functioning is envisioned with chronic lithium treatment; however, more data are needed to draw any conclusions.
   b. **Antidepressants** are reported to be successful for some dysthymic patients. However, they do not work for all dysthymic individuals, and currently it is not possible to distinguish which patients might benefit and which will not.

3. **Psychotherapy** is a common treatment for these patients. Therapeutic techniques reflect theoretical considerations regarding the genesis of a chronic affective disturbance.
   a. **Psychoanalytically oriented theories** relate the development and maintenance of depression and maladaptive behavior to unresolved early childhood conflict. For example, an individual may have suffered the loss of a parent before the age of 18 years. Depression arises in adult life because the individual experiences a persistent vulnerability to loss, a tendency to feel as overwhelmed and helpless as she or he did when the parent died. Therapy would focus on the patient's vulnerability to loss and related behavior such as avoiding close relationships.
   b. **Cognitive theories** emphasize the role of how one thinks about oneself and the environment in the genesis of depression. Depression results from a series of "wrong" perceptions such as "I am a bad person," or "I can't change things." In this school of thought, therapy focuses on these incorrect perceptions and encourages the patient to think "correctly." Cognitive therapy is usually of short duration (a few weeks to months) and is reported to be efficacious.
   c. Some authorities argue that depression results from maladaptive personal interactions. Affected individuals have family backgrounds that are characterized by excessive dependency and sibling rivalry. **Therapy focuses on interpersonal relationships** and attempts to change associated maladaptive behavior.

BIBLIOGRAPHY

American Psychiatric Association: *Diagnostic and Statistical Manual of Mental Disorders*, 3rd ed. Washington, D.C., American Psychiatric Association, 1980

Cohen MB, Baker G, Cohen RA, et al: An intensive study of twelve cases of manic-depressive psychosis. *Psychiatry* 17, 2:103–137, 1954

Freud S: Mourning and melancholia. In the *Standard Edition of the Complete Psychological Works of Sigmund Freud*, vol 14. London, Hogarth, 1957, pp 243–258

Gibson RN, Cohen MB, Cohen RA: On the dynamics of the manic depressive personality. *Am J Psychiatry* 115, 2:1101–1107, 1959

Kaplan HI, Freedman AM, Sadock BJ: *Comprehensive Textbook of Psychiatry*, 3rd ed. Baltimore, Williams and Wilkins, 1980, pp 1035–1072, 1305–1358

Kolb LC: *Modern Clinical Psychiatry*, 9th ed. Philadelphia, WB Saunders, 1977, pp 438–479

Winokur G, Behar D, van Valkenburg C, et al: Is a familial definition of depression both feasible and valid? *J Nerv Ment Dis* 166, 11:764–768, 1978

STUDY QUESTIONS

Directions: Each question below contains five suggested answers. Choose the **one best** response to each question.

1. All of the following features are characteristic of mania EXCEPT

(A) hyperthermia
(B) alcohol abuse
(C) thyroid dysfunction
(D) dehydration
(E) suicide attempts

2. Although data on cyclothymic disorder are not sufficient to draw conclusions, many investigators feel that the disorder is

(A) a muted form of bipolar disorder
(B) more common than dysthymic disorder
(C) best treated with tricyclic antidepressants
(D) more common in women with alcoholic male relatives
(E) none of the above

Directions: Each question below contains four suggested answers of which **one or more** is correct. Choose the answer

A if **1, 2, and 3** are correct
B if **1 and 3** are correct
C if **2 and 4** are correct
D if **4** is correct
E if **1, 2, 3, and 4** are correct

3. Dysthymic disorder can be characterized by

(1) chronic fatigue
(2) social withdrawal
(3) insomnia
(4) hypersomnia

5. Side effects of tricyclic antidepressants include

(1) hypertension
(2) dry mouth
(3) diarrhea
(4) blurred vision

4. Drugs that are known to produce a manic-like syndrome include

(1) amphetamines
(2) tricyclic antidepressants
(3) corticosteroids
(4) reserpine

6. Long-term treatment with lithium carbonate can result in

(1) hypertension
(2) anemia
(3) leukopenia
(4) hyperparathyroidism

Directions: The group of questions below consists of lettered choices followed by several numbered items. For each numbered item select the **one** lettered choice with which it is **most** closely associated. Each lettered choice may be used once, more than once, or not at all.

Questions 7–10

For each contribution to the study of affective disorders, select the investigator with whom it is most commonly associated.

(A) Kraepelin
(B) Winokur
(C) Falret
(D) Freud
(E) Kahlbaum

7. The role of psychogenic factors, such as loss, in depression

8. The relationship between depression and alcoholism in families

9. Alterations in biologic rhythms

10. Manic-depressive illness

ANSWERS AND EXPLANATIONS

1. The answer is C. (*VI A 2; VIII A 1 c*) Thyroid dysfunction in the form of hyperthyroidism may produce a manic-like syndrome. It is important to remember, however, that a diagnosis of bipolar disorder, manic, can be made only if there is no organic cause (such as hyperthyroidism) of the disturbance. A thyroid deficiency may result from the treatment of bipolar disorder with lithium carbonate. Alcohol abuse and an ongoing risk for suicide are associated symptoms of mania. The agitated state of manic individuals can lead to dangerous physiologic conditions such as hyperthermia and dehydration.

2. The answer is A. (*IV B 1 b; V B 1*) The signs and symptoms of cyclothymic disorder differ from those of bipolar disorder in that they are less severe. The degree of disturbance is attenuated. There are probably similarities in the biology of the two disorders: Bipolar patients often have cyclothymic individuals in their families. There seems to be disruption of circadian rhythms and cellular mechanisms in cyclothymia but to a lesser degree than in bipolar illness. Treatment with lithium carbonate rather than tricyclic antidepressants is advocated for cyclothymia.

3. The answer is E (all). (*IV B 2*) Apathy and disinterest in normal activities are typical findings in chronic depression. Affected individuals suffer from low self-esteem, and they shy away from social interactions. These factors contribute to a lack of interest in sex. Sleep disruptions, whether in the form of insomnia or hypersomnia, are characteristic of depression, as are feelings of chronic fatigue.

4. The answer is A (1, 2, 3). (*VII A 1*) Reserpine produces a depression by depleting norepinephrine. Amphetamines are potent stimulants, which cause hyperactivity, pressured speech, and erratic, excessive behavior when used chronically. In susceptible individuals (i.e., individuals with bipolar illness), tricyclic antidepressants without lithium carbonate can bring on a manic episode. Corticosteroids produce depression or mania when given in sufficient doses.

5. The answer is C (2, 4). (*VIII A 3 b*) Tricyclic antidepressants may produce hypotension. The patient experiences dizziness or lightheadedness. If there are any bowel changes as a result of the medication, constipation is more likely to occur than diarrhea. The powerful anticholinergic effects of tricyclic antidepressants produce a dry mouth (through action on the salivary glands) and blurred vision (through action on muscles that control the eye's ability to focus).

6. The answer is D (4). [*VIII A 3 a (e)*] Lithium is a bivalent cation, as is calcium. Chronic administration of lithium can disrupt calcium metabolism and interfere with the normal actions of calcium. Parathyroid adenomas develop during chronic lithium use, leading to hyperparathyroidism. Blood pressure is not known to increase. Although anemia and leukopenia have not been associated with lithium use, leukocytosis has been.

7–10. The answers are: 7-D, 8-B, 9-A, 10-A. (*II C 1, E 1; V A 1 b, 2*) Freud noted that an individual reacts to a loss by becoming angry with the lost individual. However, to remain angry with someone who has died, for example, is not acceptable to most people. We begin to fault ourselves for feeling that way, and Freud speculated that the anger is turned on ourselves. He found support for this idea in typical symptoms of guilt, low self-esteem, and self-reproach.

Winokur has explored the genetics of depression. One pattern that he discovered was what he calls **depressive spectrum disease**. Women in this group suffer depression before the age of 40 years. Their male relatives have an increased incidence of alcoholism and sociopathy. In another group, men suffer depression after the age of 40 years. There is no increased incidence of alcoholism or sociopathy in male relatives. Winokur has called this **pure depressive disease**.

Kraepelin emphasized the role of biologic factors in affective illness. A malfunctioning inner control mechanism could either accelerate or decelerate, leading to mania or depression. However, little that is known of circadian rhythms today was known in 1921.

Based on his observations, Kraepelin felt that a single disorder with varied clinical manifestations must exist. He called this **manic-depressive illness**, a condition that corresponds to the current bipolar disorder. His ability to find associations between these conditions has promoted both research and improved treatment.

3
Organic Brain Syndromes
Jon A. Bell

I. INTRODUCTION. Disturbances of thoughts, perceptions, feelings, and behavior may be the result of organic or functional (nonorganic) factors or both. The disturbances in an organic brain syndrome are known or presumed to be due to some organic factor. In a functional disorder, other factors such as social and psychosocial stress are considered to be causative or the nature of a suspected organic disorder is unknown, as in schizophrenia.

An organic brain syndrome is the manifestation of brain tissue dysfunction. Brain tissue dysfunction may be transient or permanent. Psychological and behavioral abnormalities vary due to variability in the area of the brain that is affected, the mode of onset, the progression, the duration, and the nature of the pathophysiologic processes.

II. PATHOPHYSIOLOGY. In all cases of organic brain syndrome there is a failure of normal metabolic processes, **cerebral insufficiency**. The condition may be reversible or irreversible, depending upon whether or not cellular death has occurred. Derangement of cerebral functioning may result from a number of pathophysiologic or biochemical processes. These include the following.

A. Deficiency of fuels for oxidative metabolism can produce cerebral insufficiency. The brain uses glucose as the major substrate for metabolic processes, although it appears that some utilization of amino acids and protein may also take place. Oxygen is a second essential fuel. Any lack of fuel impairs brain function.

B. Mechanisms of release, conservation, and utilization of chemical energy may suffer impairment. Enzyme systems and metabolic pathways can be disrupted by toxic substances such as ammonia.

C. The process of synaptic transmission may be disrupted. Normally, information passes between neurons via synaptic connections. Pathophysiologic processes may deplete neurons of messengers such as dopamine and norepinephrine. Neurohumoral functions may also be disrupted.

D. Significant alterations in electrolyte content, hydration, pH, and osmolarity can impede brain function. As with other organs in the body, the brain functions best in a steady, stable environment. Whenever the body's internal environment is changed, optimal functioning is compromised. Changes are reflected at the cellular level as cell pH, electrolyte content, osmolarity, and hydration adjust to the internal environment.

E. Interference with macromolecular synthesis, which is necessary for cellular renewal and continued normal functioning, **can produce dysfunction**, due either to diminished substrate availability or disruption of cellular mechanisms.

F. Disruptions of brain anatomy or disequilibrium in functionally related systems produce an organic brain syndrome because brain function depends upon precise anatomical relationships. For example, a mass lesion compresses the brain and distorts anatomical relationships, leading to deficits in functioning pertinent to the affected locality.

III. CLASSIFICATION. Organic brain syndromes are divided into six groups in the *Diagnostic and Statistical Manual of Mental Disorders*, third edition, *(DSM III)*, including the following.

A. Disorders with generalized or global cognitive impairment

1. Delirium. The essential feature of delirium is a clouded state of consciousness, which reduces an individual's awareness of his or her environment. It occurs in all age groups, although the young and the elderly are most susceptible.

   a. Attention deficits. The patient has difficulty attending to both internal and external stimuli. He or she is easily distracted and has trouble conversing with others. The patient cannot shift, focus, or maintain attention without considerable effort and concentration. As the delirium advances, the patient can no longer overcome attention deficits. He or she becomes bewildered and confused.

   b. Sensory misperceptions. Early in a delirium, perceptions become blurred, hazy, and imprecise. Normal sensory cues such as sounds and sights become less reliable and accurate, sensations are not identified readily, and important perceptions cannot be acted upon (such as stopping at a red light or obeying a speed-limit sign). The patient may feel under a barrage of sensations, unable to screen out unimportant sensory information. As the delirium advances, the patient may experience hallucinations involving any sensory modality; visual hallucinations are common. He or she may become convinced of the reality of misperceptions, illusions, and hallucinations. Emotional and behavioral responses to these sensory disturbances arise. The patient may experience vivid dreams and nightmares as well.

   c. Fluctuations in the patient's behavior, emotional state, level of consciousness, perceptions, and thinking are typical findings in delirium. One moment the patient may be calm, relaxed, and able to think clearly; the next moment, he or she may be agitated, frightened, and confused. This state of agitation is not constant, however. The patient may become calm again or become lethargic and stuporous within a short period of time.

   d. Rapid onset is characteristic of delirium. A delirium may emerge more slowly if the underlying cause is a systemic illness or a metabolic imbalance. Usually the cause produces a more immediate, dramatic change, however. For example, drugs and alcohol have an impact within minutes to hours.

   e. A delirium rarely lasts more than a few days. Removal of the offending agent can end a delirious state as can treatment of the underlying cause, such as meningitis.

   f. Disordered thought processes are frequently observed in the delirious patient. Thoughts are not clear or coherent unless the affected individual exercises great care and effort. The patient is hesitant, vague, and uncertain. Thinking becomes concrete as delirium advances. Thoughts are fragmented and seemingly without direction or purpose. Switching from topic to topic without apparent transition (**loose associations**) also occurs. Reasoning is impaired. Without an ability to think clearly and without an ability to anticipate the consequences of his or her actions, the patient exercises poor judgment and acts in impulsive or dangerous ways. As delirium progresses, the patient may become irrational and may take hold of irrational beliefs (**delusions**). Actions based on these delusions jeopardize the safety of the patient and others, particularly if the delusions are paranoid in quality.

   g. Disorientation and memory deficits are common. Early in delirium the patient loses the ability to keep track of time and may lose track of the date. As delirium worsens, he or she becomes disoriented with respect to place and situation. It is very rare for an individual to forget his or her identity. Memories of immediate or recent events can be retained only with effort early in delirium. Confusion, bewilderment, and misinterpretation set in as delirium advances. Memory deficits lead to repetition in speech and behavior.

   h. Disturbances in psychomotor activity and in the sleep cycle are frequently observed. The patient may be agitated and hyperactive or appear to be quite restless. As delirium advances, he or she may become clumsy and awkward. He or she is unable to perform simple tasks and acts sluggishly, groping about in attempts to perform motor tasks. Impairment may be so severe that the patient cannot walk or sit. Speech may be pressured or limited early in delirium. Inarticulate, slurred speech is common. The patient may sleep excessively, fitfully, or not at all.

   i. Autonomic hyperactivity frequently is present in delirium. A number of causes of delirium produce changes in blood pressure, pulse, temperature, and respiratory rate. The presence of these changes should alert the physician to the possibility of an organic etiology for a behavioral disturbance. Alcohol withdrawal and meningitis are two examples in which vital signs would be abnormal.

   j. The patient's affective state varies in delirium. The predominant feeling may be fear or anxiety. Some patients are giddy or euphoric. Irritability and anger may be seen. Regardless of the patient's emotional state at any given moment, feelings may change rapidly. Such lability contributes to the unpredictability and impulsiveness of delirious patients. In a fearful frame of mind he or she may flee or fight. If the patient is depressed, suicide is possible.

2. Dementia. The essential feature of dementia is a loss of intellectual abilities of sufficient severity to interfere with social or occupational functioning or both. This disorder occurs predominantly in the elderly and usually affects both the personality and the cognitive functioning of the patient.

The course varies in dementia. When dementia is the result of trauma, losses appear suddenly and, in most cases, stabilize quickly. In dementia due to degenerative causes, the course is insidious and progressive. The demented patient is more susceptible to delirium. The ability to adapt to new situations is limited and leaves the patient vulnerable to stresses and changes in his or her environment.

a. **The most prominent loss is memory.** Early in the course of dementia the patient is forgetful of details. Such forgetfulness may be minor in scope and is frequently overlooked by others. However, the severity of memory loss increases, and more significant memory lapses occur, such as leaving the stove on. In the advanced stages, the patient may have no memory at all. Remote memories tend to be affected later, and recent memories are affected very early in this disorder.

b. **The demented patient loses the capacity to think abstractly.** He or she experiences difficulty with new tasks and may avoid doing anything new. The ability to generalize from past experience or to see the relationships between similar situations may be lost as well.

c. **Impaired judgment is common in dementia.** Behavior may be inappropriate for a given social situation. Coarse and obscene language may be used. The patient may not take care of him- or herself: He or she eats a poor, unbalanced diet, and no attention is given to cleanliness and grooming. The patient may live in squalor and filth. Impulsive actions occur: The elderly patient may become very active sexually in an exaggerated or inappropriate way, such as exposing himself to children; he or she may exercise bad judgment in business deals and squander savings impulsively.

d. **Personality changes tend to be either alterations or accentuations of the premorbid personality.** The patient who had been orderly and meticulous about cleanliness may become obsessively meticulous or quite slovenly. The active, socially involved individual may withdraw and become isolated and apathetic. The patient may become suspicious, guarded, or paranoid when his or her failing memory cannot provide information about the events of the day. A misplaced purse leads to the conclusion that someone has stolen it, an open window to the conclusion that someone has broken in. The patient becomes more dependent on others. He or she may become very anxious. Someone who has been congenial and friendly may become irritable and hostile.

e. **More subtle deficits in functioning eventually appear.** The demented patient may lose some ability to express him- or herself. Language is used in a vague, imprecise, or stereotypic fashion: A patient may use a few phrases again and again; the vocabulary may become limited, and the ability to name objects may be impaired (**dysnomia**). He or she may experience difficulty in performing routine, physical tasks such as shaving and dressing (**apraxia**). In the advanced stages of dementia, the patient may be mute and in need of assistance for most tasks, including eating.

f. **Depression is common in demented patients.** When dementia is mild, the patient is aware of his or her deficits, which creates both anxiety and depression. Severe depression and suicidal behavior are common. Other patients attempt to compensate for or conceal deficits by excessive orderliness, social withdrawal, or excessive attention to detail. Some patients elaborate and fill in details even when they do not remember (**confabulation**). This usually occurs unconsciously and is not intentional or planned by the demented individual. It does, however, obscure the fact that memory is impaired.

B. Disorders with relatively selective areas of cognitive impairment

1. **Amnestic syndrome.** The essential feature in this usually chronic and uncommon disorder is impairment of short- and long-term memory in an individual with a normal state of consciousness. This deficit is attributable to an organic factor, and impairment is moderate to severe. Damage to diencephalic and medial temporal lobe structures leads to this disorder. However, unlike dementia, **there is no loss of intellectual functioning**. Other features include the following.

   a. The affected individual is unable to learn new material (**anterograde amnesia**).
   b. The individual may be unable to recall the past (**retrograde amnesia**).
   c. Immediate memory may be intact.
   d. The individual may be disoriented.
   e. He or she may confabulate.
   f. The amnestic patient may become apathetic and lose initiative.
   g. He or she may have no insight into his or her deficits and exhibit little concern about them.
   h. Affect may become superficial.
   i. The disorder usually presents suddenly when caused by factors such as anoxia.
   j. Secondary complications arise because of a lack of memory. In severely impaired individuals, dangerous behavior may occur and supervision may be necessary at all times.

2. Organic hallucinosis. The essential feature is the presence of persistent or recurrent hallucinations due to organic factors in an individual with a normal state of consciousness. The
course depends on the etiology and may be brief or chronic. Other features are associated.
   a. Hallucinations may involve any sensory modality.
   b. Hallucinations may be as simple as the appearance of colors and as complex as the appearance of talking, moving, odd-looking creatures.
   c. The individual may recognize the hallucinations to be hallucinations or may believe that
   they are "real." If he or she cannot recognize an irrational basis for the hallucinations, the
   situation becomes delusional. However, there are no systematized delusions.
   d. The individual may find the hallucinations pleasant or upsetting.
   e. If the individual is distracted by hallucinations or predicates actions upon them, accidents
   may occur.

C. Disorders resembling other major disorders

1. Organic affective syndrome. The essential feature of this disorder is a disturbance in mood,
resembling either mania or depression, due to a specific organic factor. The patient has a normal state of consciousness. No loss of intellectual functioning is present. The same phenomena that are observed in an affective syndrome are present (see Chapter 2, "Affective
Disorders").
   a. The intensity of symptoms ranges from mild to severe.
   b. Impairment of functioning may be minimal but can be quite extensive.
   c. Mild cognitive impairment is frequently observed.
   d. The risks of an affective syndrome are present in this disorder: Impulsive, poorly considered behavior or self-destructive behavior may occur.
   e. Both toxic and metabolic factors can lead to an organic affective syndrome.

2. Organic delusional syndrome. The essential feature of this disorder is the presence of delusions due to a specific organic factor. The patient has a normal state of consciousness. Other
features include the following.
   a. Mild cognitive impairment is commonly seen.
   b. Speech may be rambling and voluminous.
   c. Delusional content is variable and related to the etiologic factors. Persecutory delusions
   are common.
   d. Although hallucinations may be present, they assume a secondary role in the illness; delusions are the predominant symptom.
   e. The patient can present with any number of symptoms. This condition is subjectively
   unpleasant in many cases: The patient may be perplexed and unkempt and dysphoric and
   anxious. The patient's level of activity may be increased (hyperactivity) or decreased
   (apathy). Ritualistic behavior, generated by delusional convictions, may be part of this syndrome.
   f. The degree of impairment is usually severe. The patient is not able to discern reality adequately and, therefore, cannot respond appropriately to real situations.
   g. The patient may harm him- or herself or others while responding to delusional ideation.

D. Organic personality syndrome. The personality may be affected in an organic personality syndrome, while impairment in other areas is relatively mild. **The essential feature is a marked
change in personality** due to a specific organic factor, usually structural damage to the brain.
The disorder may be transient or persistent; toxic factors generally produce short-lived disturbances, but structural factors (e.g., tumors) generally produce chronic disturbances. The differences in presentation reflect the differences in the nature and location of the pathologic process. The degree of impairment is variable; however, the presence of poor judgment may neces-
sitate supervised care. This disorder may prove to be the first sign of a developing dementia.
Observations may include the following.

1. The patient may be paranoid or suspicious.

2. Mild cognitive impairment may be observed.

3. Irritability is common.

4. Frontal lobe dysfunction is associated with:
   a. Emotional lability and unexpected outbursts of anger
   b. Impaired impulse control and poor judgment, such as sexually inappropriate behavior
   c. Apathy, indifference, and loss of interest in one's environment

5. Temporal lobe dysfunction is associated with:
   a. Verbosity in speech and writing
   b. Religiosity and overly aggressive behavior

E. **Substance-induced organic brain syndromes**

    1. **Intoxication.** The essential feature of this disorder is maladaptive behavior and a substance-specific syndrome due to either recent use or the lingering presence of the substance in the body. Other characteristics include the following.

        a. There is no evidence of one of the organic brain syndromes described previously in this chapter.

        b. The presenting symptoms depend upon the substance involved.

        c. The patient may suffer a number of functional disturbances in areas such as:
            (1) Perception
            (2) Sleep (wakefulness)
            (3) Emotional control
            (4) Attention
            (5) Thinking
            (6) Judgment
            (7) Psychomotor behavior

        d. Additional disturbances depend upon:
            (1) The individual's expectations
            (2) Environmental circumstances
            (3) The preintoxication personality
            (4) The individual's biologic state

        e. The course of an intoxication is usually brief. The duration depends upon the following factors:
            (1) The amount consumed
            (2) The rate of consumption
            (3) Tolerance of the substance by the individual
            (4) Body size (i.e., the volume of distribution)
            (5) The substance half-life
            (6) Gastric contents (if the substance is ingested)
            (7) The rate of absorption

        f. The degree of impairment is related to the demands of the affected individual's environment. If the intoxicated individual faces little or no responsibility, impairment is minimal; if the intoxicated individual faces significant responsibility, the impairment may be marked.

        g. Coma or seizures may occur in the severely intoxicated patient.

        h. Accidents are a common and, far too often, lethal complication of intoxication.

    2. **Withdrawal.** The essential feature of this disorder is the development of a substance-specific syndrome that follows the reduction or cessation of intake of a substance used to induce intoxication.

        a. There is no evidence for one of the organic brain syndromes described previously in this chapter.

        b. The array of symptoms is contingent upon the substance in use.

        c. The patient may experience a number of physiologic and psychological symptoms, including:
            (1) Malaise
            (2) Lability
            (3) Irritability
            (4) Anxiety
            (5) Restlessness
            (6) A change in sleep patterns
            (7) Impaired attention
            (8) A craving for the substance

        d. This condition may last from a few days to several weeks.

        e. The degree of impairment varies. Factors affecting the impairment include:
            (1) The physical health of the individual in withdrawal
            (2) Environmental elements, such as responsibility

        f. Criminal behavior may develop to acquire the substance.

F. **Atypical or mixed organic brain syndrome** is a residual category, which includes disorders that are due to a specific organic factor and do not meet the diagnostic criteria for another organic brain syndrome.

IV. ETIOLOGIES

A. **Epilepsy** is a symptom complex characterized by transient, episodic alterations in consciousness, which may be associated with convulsive movements or disturbances in feeling, behavior, or both. Features of epilepsy include the following.

1. **Seizures arise from disturbances of the electrophysiologic activity of brain cells**, which are produced by a variety of irritative stimuli. These physiologic changes are expressed in one or more of the following ways:
   a. Changes in electrical potential in an electroencephalogram (EEG). Although an EEG can localize the seizure focus in most cases, some disorders are missed due to a lack of abnormal electrical activity at the time of the recording or a seizure focus that is deep in the brain's interior.
   b. Variations in consciousness
   c. Disordered functioning of the autonomic nervous system
   d. Convulsive movements or psychic disturbances

2. **Various factors can precipitate seizure activity** in susceptible individuals, including:
   a. Hyperventilation
   b. Sleep deprivation
   c. Sensory stimuli, such as flashing lights, loud noises, and tactile sensations
   d. Trauma
   e. Fever
   f. Emotional stress
   g. Hormonal changes, such as those occurring during puberty and menstruation
   h. Drugs, such as alcohol, phenothiazines, tricyclic antidepressants, and antihistamines

3. **Seizures can be classified into three major groups.**
   a. **Grand mal–type seizures** have the following features.
      (1) The **aura** occurs seconds prior to the generalized seizure. The individual experiences motor (e.g., twitching) or sensory (e.g., smelling, seeing, and tingling) symptoms due to early seizure activity.
      (2) In the **tonic phase**, the individual suffers sudden and complete loss of consciousness. He or she may fall and be injured. All voluntary muscles contract for 10 to 20 seconds (the **tonic state**). The pupils are dilated. The corneal reflex is lost. Deep-tendon reflexes are decreased or absent. Inspiration ceases, and the face may take on a cyanotic look. Incontinence may occur. **Babinski's sign** is present.
      (3) In the **clonic phase**, muscles relax and contract intermittently, producing generalized jerking motions. Breathing is restored; saliva may froth up in the mouth. The tongue may be bitten due to the contracting jaw muscles.
      (4) A **postconvulsive coma** follows. The pupils are fixed. Deep-tendon reflexes are absent. The muscular tone is flaccid, and the face is congested. The individual is bewildered and confused upon awakening. He or she may perform semiautomatic acts or move about aimlessly. A clouded state of consciousness persists for a few minutes to a few hours, in most cases, but it may last for a few days after several seizures.
      (5) In rare cases, one seizure follows another without intervening regaining of consciousness (**status epilepticus**). Unchecked, this condition can lead to exhaustion, hyperthermia, rhabdomyolysis, dehydration, coma, and death.
      (6) **EEG tracings show a high-frequency, high-voltage pattern.**
   b. **Petit mal–type seizures** have the following features.
      (1) The individual experiences no aura because the onset is sudden.
      (2) The typical duration is 5 to 30 seconds.
      (3) The individual assumes a fixed posture. Eyes stare into space. He or she becomes inattentive to the task at hand. Muscle tone is lost, and things may be dropped. A rhythmic twitching of muscles may occur. There is an interruption of normal consciousness.
      (4) These seizures may also occur in rapid succession (**petit mal status**)
      (5) The age of onset is usually early in life, from 4 to 8 years. If the disorder persists beyond the age of 18 years (which occurs in two-thirds of those afflicted), a grand mal–type seizure disorder may develop.
      (6) EEG tracings reveal alternating fast and slow waves three times per second.
   c. **Psychomotor epilepsy is also known as temporal lobe epilepsy.** The features include:
      (1) Sudden onset
      (2) A brief duration of usually 30 seconds to 2 minutes
      (3) Various affective states, such as rage, terror, and alarm
      (4) A trance-like appearance
      (5) Seemingly planned outbursts, often aggressive in nature
      (6) Feelings of bewilderment, excitement, and confusion as well as loneliness, strangeness, and déjà vu
      (7) Involvement of the muscles of mastication, speech, and swallowing, producing twitching in the face and garbled speech
      (8) Hallucinations involving any sensory modality, such as flashing lights, repetitive sounds, and noxious odors

(9) Amnesia for the seizure and for the 30 seconds or so preceding the seizure
(10) More common occurrence in adults than in children
(11) Anterior frontal lobe EEG tracing with four to eight spikes per second
(12) Disordered thought formation with delusional ideation in some cases
(13) Resemblance to schizophrenic behavior with psychotic symptoms and erratic actions

4. In some cases, **deterioration in functioning has been observed in individuals with long-standing seizure disorders.** They seem mentally slow and intellectually compromised. Although there may be some organic damage, the psychological effects of low self-esteem and a constricted life-style should not be ignored.

5. In many cases, the diagnosis of a seizure disorder can be made by history and physical examination; in some cases, an EEG tracing provides confirmatory evidence. A few cases elude ready diagnosis. The diagnosis of seizure disorder should be considered when dealing with any acutely confused or delirious patient.

B. Neoplasms may be primary tumors of the brain parenchyma or the central nervous system or metastatic tumors from areas such as the thyroid or breast. The presence of a neoplasm is underdiagnosed. There is no consistent presentation.

  1. Signs and symptoms of a neoplasm may include:
    a. Signs of increased intracranial pressure, such as:
      (1) Headache
      (2) Impaired consciousness or level of energy
      (3) Papilledema
      (4) Vomiting
    b. Focal neurologic findings, such as weakness
    c. Psychiatric symptoms that fall into two groups:
      (1) Personality changes. An accentuation of preexisting traits may occur (e.g., the orderly individual becomes obsessed with cleanliness). The personality may be markedly changed, with a loss of inhibition leading to shameless, sexually inappropriate behavior.
      (2) Cerebral changes. Any and all functions may be affected. An individual may become absentminded or have frank memory deficits. The ability to reason or calculate may be impaired. Alterations in consciousness are seen; there is especially a tendency towards drowsiness. Interest in sex may be diminished. Perceptual difficulties including hallucinations may be present. The patient may be confused and confabulate to cover deficits. Simply paying attention to the task at hand may be difficult.

  2. Tumors in specific locations tend to present in specific ways.
    a. Occipital lobe tumors are associated with simple visual hallucinations.
    b. Parietal lobe tumors are associated with sensory deficits and agnosia. The individual may not recognize or perceive parts of the environment. For example, he or she may only perceive one-half of a clock face and be unaware of this deficit.
    c. Frontal lobe tumors tend to present as gradual, insidious changes in personality. The individual may become passive and apathetic and have a flattened affect. Another common presentation is irritability and anxiety in an individual who acts impulsively and in an uninhibited manner.
    d. Temporal lobe tumors usually present a clinical picture similar to that described for temporal lobe epilepsy. Paroxysmal motor, perceptual, and behavioral symptoms are the prominent features.

  3. Symptom intensity is related to the location and rate of growth of the neoplasm. A rapidly growing tumor can produce a delirious state. A slower growing tumor can produce insidious personality changes.

  4. Diagnosis of a neoplasm depends upon history, careful neurologic examination for focal abnormalities, and evidence of increased intracranial pressure. A sudden onset of seizures raises the possibility of a neoplasm. EEG tracings and radiographic techniques such as computed axial tomography (CAT) scans and brain scans are used to confirm the diagnosis.

C. Head trauma can cause both acute and chronic disorders, which affect cognition, personality, emotional expression, and physical health.

  1. Acute disorders commonly present a mixed clinical picture. Of particular concern is the possibility of progression. Close observation is warranted, with special attention given to signs of increased intracranial pressure. These disorders include the following.

    a. Concussion syndrome refers to a momentary interruption of normal cerebral processes following a severe impact to the head. Features are:
      (1) Rapid and complete recovery
      (2) Amnesia for the event and for the few seconds preceding the event
      (3) Variability in consciousness when the individual wakes up, which ranges from an alert, clear sensorium to a confused, clouded state of awareness
      (4) No neurologic or psychological sequelae, a determination that can be made only after observing for aftereffects

    b. Traumatic coma results from a more severe head injury, usually leading to damage to the brain parenchyma. Features are:
      (1) Contusion or laceration of the brain
      (2) A duration ranging from hours to days or, in some cases, weeks
      (3) A period of stupor, restlessness, and confusion following the coma
      (4) Amnesia or delirium possibly following the coma

    c. Traumatic delirium begins as an individual emerges from a coma. It is due either to tissue injury or increased intracranial pressure. Features include:
      (1) Bewildered, aggressive, or frightened behavior
      (2) Fluctuations in consciousness
      (3) Hallucinations, most often visual in nature
      (4) Variable duration, with a prolonged duration suggesting significant tissue damage
      (5) Gradual improvement for 12 to 18 months after the injury

    d. Amnestic-confabulatory syndrome is characterized by deficits in memory and perception. Features are:
      (1) Confabulation
      (2) Impairment of memory
      (3) Deranged, inaccurate perceptions

    e. Subdural hematomas occur in as many as 10% of individuals with head injuries. Venous blood accumulates between the dura and arachnoid membranes. Features may include:
      (1) Headache
      (2) Neurologic deficits reflecting the location of the hematoma
      (3) Variability in the level of consciousness
      (4) Irritability
      (5) Confusion
      (6) A predisposing condition such as alcoholism, senility, epilepsy, and paresis caused by syphilis that has spread to the central nervous system

2. Chronic disorders develop if recovery of damaged brain tissue is incomplete or if emotional and psychological difficulties linger after head trauma. These disorders are:
    a. Postconcussional syndrome. Symptoms may include:
      (1) Headache
      (2) Anxiety
      (3) Fatigue
      (4) Insomnia
      (5) Dizziness
      (6) Impaired memory
      (7) Impaired concentration
      (8) Narrowing of interests
      (9) Diminished tolerance of alcohol
     (10) Irritability
     (11) Lability
     (12) Decreased sexual potency or drive

    b. Post-traumatic personality disorder in adults. Symptoms may include changes in personality. An individual may become:
      (1) Irritable and quarrelsome
      (2) Aggressive
      (3) Impulsive
      (4) Irresponsible and unmotivated
      (5) Paranoid
      (6) Withdrawn

    c. Post-traumatic personality disorder in children. Family relationships, especially between parents and the affected child, may be troubled. Symptoms may include changes in personality. A child may become:
      (1) Impulsive
      (2) Destructive
      (3) Disobedient and disruptive

        (4) Overactive and restless
        (5) Cruel
    d. Post-traumatic defect syndrome. Symptoms may include:
        (1) Loss of initiative
        (2) Mental slowing
        (3) Impaired memory
        (4) Impaired concentration
        (5) Confabulation
        (6) Loss of motivation
        (7) Confusion
        (8) Impaired speech
        (9) Motor impairment
     (10) Seizures, especially following penetrating head injuries

D. Presenile and senile psychoses. With advancing age, presenile and senile psychoses develop in both men and women. **These conditions result from a progressive loss of neurons.** Changes observed in behavior, cognitive functioning, and personality differ from the normal changes brought on by aging both in degree and in kind. Features of these disorders are listed below.

  1. A variety of signs and symptoms may be present. These include:
    a. Loss of memory
    b. An impaired capacity to think abstractly
    c. Indifference to social norms
    d. Inappropriate sexual behavior
    e. Carelessness in or indifference about grooming and appearance
    f. Suspicion and distrust of others
    g. Irritability or hostility
    h. Anxiety
    i. Isolation and withdrawal
    j. Depression
    k. Preoccupation with bodily concerns
    l. Progressive loss of cognitive functions
    m. Paranoia or delusional thinking
    n. Impaired judgment
    o. Diminished sensory perception at night
    p. Confusion and agitation
    q. Physical symptoms, including:
        (1) Weight loss
        (2) Unsteady gait
        (3) Slowed speech
        (4) Hand tremors
        (5) Diminished sensory acuity
        (6) Atrophied skin
    r. Hypersomnia
    s. Hoarding of money or worthless objects
    t. Indiscriminate accumulation of animals
    u. Illusions or hallucinations

  2. Common clinical variations of presenile and senile psychoses include:
    a. Simple deterioration. A **slowly progressive course** is characterized by:
        (1) Progressive memory loss
        (2) Narrowing of interests
        (3) Loss of initiative
        (4) Sluggish thinking
        (5) Apathy
        (6) Irritability
        (7) Nocturnal restlessness
        (8) Eventual loss of contact with the environment
    b. Delirium and confusion. An **acute change** is evidenced by:
        (1) Changes in physical well-being, due to illness, drugs, or toxins
        (2) Perplexity and disorientation
        (3) Insomnia
        (4) Hallucinations
        (5) Restlessness

    (6) Fear and anxiety

    (7) Noisy behavior

  c. **Depression**, which may be the first recognizable feature of a dementing process. Patients may suffer the following:

    (1) Memory loss

    (2) Intellectual impoverishment

    (3) Agitation or withdrawal

    (4) Hypochondriacal preoccupations or delusions

    (5) Melancholia

  d. **Paranoia.** Features may include:

    (1) Irritability or hostility

    (2) Demanding, suspicious, mistrustful relationships with others

    (3) Paranoid delusions

    (4) Illusions or hallucinations, which are common

    (5) An undisturbed consciousness

    (6) An unimpaired orientation, which is usual

  e. **Presbyophrenia.** Features may include:

    (1) A defect in retention due to memory loss

    (2) Confabulation to cover memory loss

    (3) Talkativeness and apparent alertness

    (4) Being out of touch with reality

    (5) Restless, nonproductive activity

3. Various neuropathologic lesions have been identified, and different syndromes have been described.

  a. **Alzheimer's disease** was described by Alois Alzheimer (1864–1915). The onset of the disease is usually between the ages of 50 and 60 years. There is an insidious course of 5 to 10 years with no characteristic symptom complex. Alzheimer discovered the following:

    (1) Tangled, thread-like structures occupying much or all of the cell body of cortical ganglion cells

    (2) Involvement of up to one-quarter of the cells

    (3) Predominance in the frontal and temporal lobes but diffuse cortical involvement

    (4) Changes in the basal ganglia

    (5) Motor disturbances, including weakness, hypertonicity, facial paresis, or contractures in large muscle groups

    (6) Progression to a vegetative state

  b. **Pick's disease**, which usually afflicts individuals who are between 45 and 60 years old, was first described in 1892 by Arnold Pick in Prague. He discovered the following:

    (1) Atrophy and gliosis in associative areas of the brain

    (2) Little change in motor, sensory, and projective areas of the brain

    (3) Speech and thinking particularly impaired

    (4) Involvement of temporal and frontal lobes

    (5) Degenerative, not inflammatory, lesions

    (6) Severe atrophy, with a loss of 25% and more of the brain mass

    (7) Chromatolysis, which is loss of chromatic substance and displacement of the nucleus to the cell periphery

    (8) Changes in the basal ganglia, which are rare

    (9) Women afflicted twice as often as men

   (10) In many cases, the appearance of focal symptoms such as apraxia, aphasia, anomia, alexia, and agraphia before generalized dementia

   (11) Motor problems, which are rare

   (12) Hallucinations and illusions, which are rare

  c. **Creutzfeldt-Jakob disease** is a rare, presenile dementia caused by a slow virus.

  d. **"Senile plaques"** have also been observed in the brains of demented patients. The characteristics are:

    (1) Small areas of tissue degeneration throughout the cortex

    (2) The highest density in the frontal lobes

    (3) Axons with excesses of neurofibrils

    (4) Large dendrites

    (5) Dense, altered mitochondria

    (6) No absolute correlation with the severity of the clinical condition

4. Treatment. Given the progressive nature of these disorders and the grossly compromised capacity of affected individuals to adapt to new situations and to cope with stress, specific interventions are frequently required. Treatment should include:

  a. Provisions for the emotional well-being of the affected individual

    b. A home environment, if possible

    c. Structured care in a nursing home or hospital, if necessary

    d. Assistance to the family in the choice of environment and in understanding the illness

    e. Attention to nutrition and physical health

    f. Sensory stimulation at night, as needed

    g. Psychoactive medications such as neuroleptics or antidepressants, if indicated

    h. Correction of sensory deficits (e.g., eyeglasses and hearing aids)

E. Interruptions in intracranial blood flow compromise oxygenation and nutrition to the brain. Such interruptions may be sudden and catastrophic (e.g., a stroke or trauma) or may follow a more insidious course (e.g., progressive arteriosclerosis). However, these disorders are not always progressive. The onset of illness usually occurs between 50 and 65 years of age, with men afflicted more commonly than women. Dementia, depression, and delirium may present in similar ways. Therefore, careful attention to diagnosis is mandatory. Features of these disorders are listed below.

    1. Atheromatous plaques narrow or obliterate vessel lumina, which may cause:

        a. Hypoxia

        b. Disturbed metabolism

        c. Cell death

    2. Thrombosis causes 85% of this type of disorder versus the 15% caused by embolic phenomena.

    3. Prodromal symptoms include:

        a. Fatigue

        b. Headache

        c. Dizziness

        d. Impaired concentration

        e. Drowsiness

        f. Insidious physical or mental impairment

        g. Alterations in personality

    4. Individuals may develop overt **signs and symptoms of compromise**, which include:

        a. Confusion, which is the first obvious symptom in more than one-half of all cases

        b. Incoherence

        c. Restlessness

        d. Clouded consciousness

        e. Other deficits, such as muscular weakness or aphasia

    5. Early signs and symptoms of insidious disease include:

        a. Mental fatigue

        b. Loss of initiative

        c. Emotional instability

        d. Irritability

        e. Loss of finer sentiments, such as compassion, sympathy, and altruism

        f. Varying degrees of memory loss

        g. Mistrust of others

    6. Progression leads to more serious disturbances. Signs and symptoms may include:

        a. Nocturnal bewilderment

        b. Anxiety

        c. Violent behavior

        d. Lack of self-care

        e. Diminished judgment

        f. Loss of inhibitions

        g. Disturbances in thinking, including delusions

        h. Evidence of localized strokes

        i. Seizures

        j. Tremors

        k. Periods of delirium

    7. Treatment. The distinction between extracranial and arteriolar sources of disease indicates the course of treatment. Early recognition affords an opportunity for treatment with angioplasty or endarterectomy. Decreasing stress and physical exertion may slow the progression of the illness. Sedating medications tend to confuse affected individuals. Neuroleptics are effective in treating nocturnal restlessness.

F. **Significant psychiatric disturbances occur in approximately 3% of all patients taking medications.** These disturbances may be extensions of the desired effects of the medication or secondary effects. In addition, drugs are used in abusive patterns, which also leads to significant symptomatology.

1. **Several variables must be considered when evaluating the role that a drug plays in a behavioral disturbance.** These include:
   a. The drug and its actions
   b. The amount administered
   c. The duration of action
   d. The existence of medical illnesses
   e. The patient's age
   f. The cerebral functioning of the patient
   g. The patient's environment (e.g., does it lack stimulation?)
   h. Sociocultural factors, such as fears concerning medication
   i. Drug interactions
   j. The patient's personality

2. **Numerous drugs have been identified as etiologic agents in behavioral disturbances.** These disturbances may be mild or severe, transitory or prolonged.
   a. **Barbiturates** are useful as medications in addition to having high abuse potential. Organic mental disorders may arise acutely, with chronic use, or in withdrawal.
      (1) **Acute intoxication causes generalized central nervous system depression.** Signs and symptoms include:
          (a) Dizziness
          (b) Ataxia
          (c) Confusion
          (d) Slurred speech
          (e) A compromised level of consciousness, ranging from stupor to coma
      (2) **Severe intoxication** results from a dose of 200 mg to 1000 mg of pentobarbital. This may vary, depending upon tolerance or the presence of other sedatives such as alcohol. A fatal dose is 1000 mg to 1500 mg of pentobarbital.
      (3) **Chronic intoxication** leads to significant difficulties, although it may go undiscovered until a withdrawal crisis occurs. Symptoms of chronic intoxication include:
          (a) Fluctuations in the level of consciousness
          (b) Somnolence
          (c) Confusion
          (d) Slurred speech
          (e) Ataxia
          (f) Poor judgment
          (g) Hypomania, including irritability, euphoria, emotional lability, and querulousness
          (h) Carelessness about work
          (i) Social withdrawal
      (4) **Withdrawal** from barbiturates is hazardous and potentially life-threatening. Withdrawal may occur when the individual is cut off from his or her supply, as is the patient who is hospitalized for surgery. Features of withdrawal are:
          (a) Evidence of increasing central nervous system irritability about 8 hours after the last use of barbiturates
          (b) Muscular twitches
          (c) Tremor
          (d) Weakness
          (e) Dizziness
          (f) Nausea and vomiting
          (g) Sweating
          (h) Hyperactive deep-tendon reflexes
          (i) Headaches
          (j) Postural hypotension
          (k) Onset of grand mal seizures from 30 to 48 hours after the last use of barbiturates
          (l) Delirium with disorientation and elevated temperature lasting as long as 7 days
      (5) **Diagnosis of the magnitude of barbiturate addiction can be made with a pentobarbital tolerance test.**
          (a) A liquid dose of 200 mg of pentobarbital is given.
          (b) At 1 hour, the patient should be checked for signs of intoxication.
          (c) If the patient is intoxicated, the level of chronic use is low.
          (d) If the patient is not affected or continues to show signs of withdrawal, a high dose of pentobarbital is needed during the initial stages of withdrawal.

(6) Withdrawal should be undertaken in a hospital.
    (a) A **maintenance dose** is established, which may be as high as 300 mg of pentobarbital every 6 hours.
    (b) The dose is decreased 10%/day for 10 days.
(7) Individual psychotherapy, group therapy, or both should follow withdrawal to help the patient deal with stresses without reverting to drug abuse.
b. Hypnotics are given for sleep disturbances. Drugs such as chloral hydrate, glutethimide, flurazepam, methyprylon, methaqualone, and ethchlorvynol produce symptoms similar to those produced by barbiturates and are more potent and toxic than minor tranquilizers.
    (1) Between 1.0% and 3.5% of hospitalized patients suffer untoward reactions to these drugs.
    (2) Serious overdose may occur. Symptoms include convulsions, pulmonary edema, and coma.
    (3) Withdrawal syndromes may resemble delirium tremens with an elevated temperature, disorientation, agitation, hallucinations, clouded consciousness, and convulsions.
c. Minor tranquilizers are prescribed for relief of anxiety and for sedation; they are frequently abused as well. Included in this group are diazepam, oxazepam, meprobamate, chlordiazepoxide, lorazepam, and hydroxyzine hydrochloride. They are neither as toxic nor as potent as barbiturates and the synthetic hypnotics and offer a wider margin of safety. However, acute and chronic intoxication as well as withdrawal may occur.
    (1) Acute intoxication results from high doses. The individual may become delirious, hyperactive, and have attacks of rage.
    (2) Chronic intoxication leads to tolerance. Difficulties similar to those described for chronic barbiturate intoxication develop.
    (3) Withdrawal may lead to delirium with convulsions, hallucinations, and disorientation. Withdrawal symptoms may not be evident until 3 or 4 days after cessation of or decrease in the use of the drug and can last for 7 days. Upon evidence of withdrawal, a withdrawal schedule can be started, using pentobarbital.
d. Bromides were once commonly used as hypnotics but have been replaced by other drugs for the most part. However, over-the-counter preparations such as Miles Nervine and Bromo-Seltzer and Neurosine, a prescription drug, still contain bromides. Symptoms may arise from either acute or chronic bromide intoxication.
    (1) Acute intoxication is rare because very large doses tend to cause nausea and vomiting. Symptoms may include:
        (a) Confusion
        (b) Weakness
        (c) Ataxia
        (d) Depression
        (e) Delirium with hallucinations
    (2) Chronic intoxication results from the ingestion of large doses for an extended period of time or from impaired excretion of bromides due to renal disease. Levels of 150 mg/100 ml are found in the blood. Bromides act by displacing chloride ions. In so doing, the individual's hydration and electrolyte balance may be affected in the intoxicated state. **Chronic brominism may simply produce intoxication**. Signs and symptoms may include:
        (a) Forgetfulness
        (b) Diminished libido
        (c) Irritability
        (d) Slowed speech
        (e) Ataxia
        (f) Tremors
        (g) Sluggish, irregular pupillary reaction
        (h) Vertigo
        (i) Lethargy
    (3) Chronic brominism leads to delirium in about two-thirds of intoxicated patients. Signs and symptoms may include:
        (a) Disorientation
        (b) Restlessness
        (c) Anxiety
        (d) Insomnia
        (e) Hallucinations
        (f) Mood disturbances
        (g) Delusions
    (4) Some individuals may suffer a **transitory schizophreniform psychosis** with paranoid delusions and hallucinations but maintain a clear sensorium. A **bromide hallucinosis**,

that is, visual hallucinations without delusions or delirium, may also occur. **Many bromide abusers also abuse alcohol**. Brominism may be overlooked in the presence of this more common disorder.

   (5) Treatment for brominism must address both psychiatric symptoms and medical problems. Sodium chloride is given to eliminate bromide ions. Fluid intake must be maintained. Significant reduction of bromide levels takes several weeks.

 e. **Amphetamines** are chemically related to sympathomimetic amines and act primarily on the central nervous system. Included in this group are amphetamine sulfate, methamphetamine, dextroamphetamine sulfate, and methylphenidate. These drugs are widely abused because they produce euphoria and combat fatigue. Overdose, acute and chronic intoxication, and withdrawal all may occur.

   (1) Acute intoxication results from the alerting effects that amphetamines have on the central nervous system. Signs and symptoms include:
   (a) Mood elevation
   (b) Tireless, energetic feelings
   (c) Diminished appetite
   (d) Tachycardia
   (e) Elevated blood pressure
   (f) Dilated pupils
   (g) Dry mouth
   (h) Tremors
   (i) Sweating

   (2) An overdose of amphetamines may lead to a life-threatening medical crisis. Effects are short-lived, usually lasting 36 to 48 hours. Signs and symptoms include:
   (a) Restlessness
   (b) Irritability
   (c) Confusion
   (d) Disorientation
   (e) Auditory or visual hallucinations
   (f) Palpitations
   (g) Arrhythmias
   (h) Hyperactive, deep-tendon reflexes
   (i) Circulatory collapse
   (j) Convulsions
   (k) Coma

   (3) An **organic delusional syndrome** may develop after limited use of amphetamines, but this is rare. Most commonly, the syndrome develops after prolonged use and chronic intoxication. This condition often resembles paranoid schizophrenia. Signs and symptoms include:
   (a) Disorientation
   (b) Ideas of reference
   (c) Persecutory delusions
   (d) Hallucinations
   (e) Paranoid fears
   (f) Stereotypic actions, such as teeth gnashing and repetitive touching of the face

   (4) Chronic intoxication leads to marked tolerance. Cessation of use produces a **withdrawal syndrome** characterized by fatigue, depression, and apathy. In some instances, depression is severe and the risk of suicide is significant.

   (5) After chronic use, it may take up to 2 months for the effects of the drug to clear. An organic delusional syndrome may persist during this period, requiring treatment with haloperidol.

 f. **Anorectic agents** are used to suppress the appetite. These drugs resemble amphetamines but are less potent. Included in this group are phenmetrazine, diethylpropion, and chlorphentermine. Each can produce any of the conditions noted for amphetamines, including a paranoid psychosis.

 g. **Analeptic agents** are also chemically related to sympathomimetic amines and have an alerting effect on the central nervous system. Two commonly used drugs are aminophylline and caffeine.

   (1) Aminophylline is prescribed for many asthmatics and patients with other chronic pulmonary diseases. Both intoxication and overdose can produce delirium with nausea, vomiting, anxiety, agitation, and confusion.

   (2) Caffeine is the most commonly used stimulant, found in tea, coffee, and soft drinks. An overdose produces excitement, hyperactivity, flushing, insomnia, tremors, and tinnitus. An overdose may result from as few as 3 or 4 cups of coffee (300 mg of caffeine). Chronic intoxication produces a hypomanic condition with hyperactivity, insomnia, and rambling speech.

h. Hallucinogenic agents (psychedelics and psychotomimetics) are used and abused to obtain alterations of normal perceptual, emotional, and cognitive processes. Drugs in this group include: psilocybin, lysergic acid diethylamide (LSD), mescaline, marijuana, tetrahydrocannabinol (THC), and phencyclidine (PCP).

   (1) PCP produces a classic picture of delirium. Signs and symptoms include:
      (a) Depersonalization
      (b) Confusion
      (c) Disorientation
      (d) Isolation
      (e) Hostility
      (f) Negativism
      (g) Apathy
      (h) Catalepsy
      (i) Agitation
      (j) Violent outbursts

   (2) Other hallucinogenic agents do not compromise the level of consciousness but alter the form of consciousness. An organic delusional syndrome may develop with grandiose or paranoid delusions. An organic hallucinosis may develop with one or more sensory modality involved. Visual hallucinations are commonly vivid.

   (3) Treatment of unpleasant or untoward effects ("bad trips") begins with a calm, quiet, reassuring environment. Most patients improve as the drug effects subside within a few hours. Some patients may require tranquilizing with either benzodiazepines or butyrophenones.

   (4) Diagnosis of conditions caused by hallucinogenic agents depends upon both a good history and, when available, toxicologic screens. Screens are useful because many of these patients do not know what they have taken.

i. Major tranquilizers are used to treat symptoms of psychosis. Drugs in this group include phenothiazines (including thioridazine and chlorpromazine), butyrophenones (haloperidol), thioxanthenes (thiothixene), and others. They are most commonly prescribed for schizophrenic disorders for the reduction of anxiety and the inhibition of delusions, hallucinations, and psychomotor agitation.

   (1) These drugs tranquilize with minimal narcosis. However, large doses may lead to somnolence, stupor, and coma.

   (2) Acute delirious reactions have been observed when these drugs are taken with barbiturates or antiparkinsonian agents, probably due to the cumulative anticholinergic effects. Patients become confused, agitated, and disoriented.

   (3) In less than 1% of patients, seizures may develop. These drugs lower the seizure threshold.

j. Antidepressants produce many adverse effects. Drugs in this group include tricyclic antidepressants (including imipramine, amitriptyline, and doxepin) and monoamine oxidase inhibitors [MAOIs] (including phenelzine).

   (1) Common adverse effects of tricyclic antidepressants include:
      (a) Drowsiness
      (b) Fatigue
      (c) Tremors
      (d) Weakness
      (e) Confusion
      (f) Agitation
      (g) Anxiety

   (2) Overdoses of tricyclic antidepressants are usually severe, and only 1000 mg to 1250 mg of amitriptyline are sufficient for overdose. Initially, the patient becomes agitated, confused, disoriented, and experiences fluctuations in the level of consciousness. Seizures may occur. Stupor and coma eventually ensue. The patient is dangerously ill at this point with an elevated temperature and pulse rate, dilated pupils, and cardiac arrhythmias.

   (3) Combined use of MAOIs and tricyclic antidepressants can lead to a dangerous syndrome, which is characterized by agitated and delirious behavior, headaches, nausea and vomiting, hyperpyrexia, convulsions, and, possibly, death.

k. Lithium carbonate can produce toxic effects even at therapeutic levels (i.e., 0.6 mEq to 1.2 mEq/L). However, this is not common.

   (1) Levels of 2 mEq/L and more lead to a toxic confusional state. Affected patients are agitated, disoriented, and may have a multitude of physical signs and symptoms, including thirst, diarrhea, dizziness, slurred speech, weakness, and tremors. At very high levels (i.e., 4 mEq/L and more), coma and convulsions result.

   (2) Fluid replacement and administration of sodium chloride cause diuresis of excess lithium and reversal of the toxic condition.

l. Anticonvulsants all have potent effects on the central nervous system. In general, they slow down mental processes and tend to sedate the affected individual. They may produce either an acute or chronic organic mental disorder.

  (1) Hydantoin derivatives produce a variety of symptoms. An individual may be irritable or depressed with chronic use. He or she may experience drowsiness and tremors. Difficulty in walking (ataxia), talking (dysarthria), and seeing (diplopia) are common. Nystagmus may be noted. When very high levels of the drugs are present, full-blown delirium and delusions may occur.

  (2) Oxazolidinedione derivatives are used for petit mal seizures. At therapeutic levels, ataxia and vertigo (loss of the sense of balance or dizziness) have been observed. More symptoms appear at higher levels. An individual may become irritable and emotionally labile. He or she may be nauseated, may vomit, or both. Drowsiness and diplopia may be present. A common physical finding is nystagmus. With an overdose, the individual is sedated. Incoordination, dysarthria, as well as nystagmus occur.

  (3) Succinimide derivatives are also used for petit mal seizures. These drugs have numerous psychiatric effects. Side effects include irritability, drowsiness, dizziness, hyperactivity, euphoria, and headaches. Some patients report nightmares. Concentration may be impaired. An increase in aggressive behavior has been attributed to these drugs. Rarely, some patients develop an organic delusional syndrome with paranoid ideation. Some patients become depressed.

  (4) Clonazepam is a benzodiazepine derivative used for the treatment of petit mal, akinetic, and psychomotor seizure disorders. Patients develop tolerance to this drug and, as a result, may experience a withdrawal syndrome. A common effect is drowsiness. Some patients become atactic. At toxic levels, forgetfulness or confusion may be noted. Some patients develop psychotic symptoms, including hallucinations.

  (5) Phenacemide is a toxic medication that is rarely used. An individual may become depressed or very aggressive when taking this medication. Personality changes have been noted as well as psychotic disturbances.

m. Belladonna alkaloids and synthetic anticholinergic agents have wide therapeutic application and are sometimes used in abusive patterns. Compounds in the group include atropine, benztropine, scopolamine, propantheline, meclizine, diphenhydramine, and trihexyphenidyl. These drugs act by blocking acetylcholine activity in the peripheral nervous system. Scopolamine is readily available. It is a key ingredient in over-the-counter sleeping preparations. Abuse may be inadvertent or purposeful.

  (1) The effects of the drugs are numerous. They include sedation, decrement in bronchial and oropharyngeal secretions, decrement in gastrointestinal and urinary tract motility, mydriasis, and cycloplegia. Sweating is decreased, and heart rate is increased by these compounds. They are used in many medical specialties, including cardiology, ophthalmology, urology, gastroenterology, and psychiatry.

  (2) Effects on the central nervous system are varied. An individual may become restless and agitated. Emotional lability may be observed. Some individuals are confused and have memory deficits. Outright disorientation and unpredictable, wild behavior occur with toxicity. Convulsions and coma are seen in severe cases.

  (3) Gastric lavage and support of vital functions are indicated in an overdose.

n. L-Dopa. Idiopathic parkinsonism is commonly treated with L-dopa. This drug readily crosses the blood-brain barrier and is broken down to dopamine and norepinephrine, both pharmacologically active biogenic amines.

  (1) As many as 50% of patients taking L-dopa experience nausea, vomiting, and dyskinesias.

  (2) It is estimated that 20% to 30% of patients experience psychiatric symptoms. A variety of difficulties have been observed. Some patients suffer affective symptoms and become depressed or hypomanic. Others suffer cognitive and perceptual impairment. Individuals may be confused or disoriented. In more severe cases, delirious conditions develop. (Delirious conditions are more common in patients with underlying dementia.) Some individuals become psychotic with paranoid delusions, hallucinations, and psychomotor agitation.

  (3) Treatment is straightforward: The dose of L-dopa should be decreased.

o. Several agents used in the treatment of cardiovascular diseases can produce psychiatric disturbances.

  (1) Digitalis levels that are necessary to achieve therapeutic effects are close to the levels that produce toxicity. The toxic effects vary. Nausea and vomiting may occur. Affected individuals may become restless or apathetic. Some experience nightmares. In severe cases a delirium develops, with features of impaired concentration and cognition, irritability, distractability, delusions, and hallucinations. Effects of digitalis toxicity are greater in the elderly who have poor cardiac reserve and cerebral disease in some cases. The sensory deprivation experienced in the intensive care unit may exacerbate the toxicity of this drug.

    (2) Procainamide, an antiarrhythmic agent, has been noted to produce depression and weakness in moderate doses. Severe depression has been observed at higher doses. In rare cases, a psychosis with hallucinations may occur at high doses.

    (3) Propranolol, used to treat both hypertension and arrhythmias, may produce lethargy and drowsiness at moderate doses. Severe depression or a psychosis with visual hallucinations may occur at high doses.

    (4) Reserpine, an antihypertensive agent, acts in the central nervous system by depleting catecholamines (e.g., norepinephrine), which leads to depression, often of great severity.

    (5) Methyldopa, an antihypertensive drug, has been associated with depression and nightmares, even with usual doses.

    (6) Hydralazine, an antihypertensive agent, may produce headaches, gastrointestinal symptoms, and loss of appetite with moderate doses. At high doses more severe disturbances may occur, including anxiety, confusion, disorientation, depression, and an acute psychosis.

p. Diuretic agents such as hydrochlorothiazide and furosimide affect fluid and electrolyte metabolism. They may deplete sodium, potassium, and total body fluids with a brisk diuresis. Chloride ions may also suffer depletion, leading to a metabolic alkalosis. Symptoms may be mild, such as fatigue and weakness, or severe, including confusion, disorientation, cognitive impairment, and agitation.

q. Anesthetic agents act both locally and systemically with different effects.

    (1) General anesthetic agents are volatile inert gases, which are rapidly excreted. They **do not cause an organic brain syndrome** for this reason. The postoperative appearance of an organic brain disorder raises the question of anoxia occurring during surgery instead.

    (2) Local anesthesia may produce a toxic reaction when given intravenously. The central nervous system is stimulated by local anesthetic agents, leading to restlessness, tremors, or convulsions. Vital functions may be lost, and death may occur with severe toxicity.

r. Hormonal agents are given either to augment or to inhibit endogenous activity of the body. Changes in behavior and brain function are felt to be related to the metabolic alterations induced by these agents. Although there is some individual variation, the dose level correlates with the severity of toxicity.

    (1) Corticosteroids and adrenocorticotropic hormone (ACTH) produce increased glucocorticoid activity. At moderate doses the mood may be elevated; the patient may be euphoric. A degree of agitation, restlessness, or insomnia may be present. At high doses (> 40 mg/day of prednisone), a clinical picture consistent with mania or a psychosis with paranoid ideation may be observed. Confusion and disorientation may be seen. Curiously, some patients have an opposite reaction and become severely depressed. Dose reduction is indicated.

    (2) Withdrawal of corticosteroids may deprive the patient of sufficient glucocorticoid activity, which leads to depression, apathy, irritability, or psychosis.

    (3) Thyroid hormone (thyroxine) and synthetic preparations, when given in high doses, produce a syndrome that mimics hyperthyroidism. The affected individual experiences weakness, fatigue, tremors, palpitations, anxiety, agitation, insomnia, and heat intolerance. With severe toxicity, a dangerously rapid heart rate, elevated temperature, dehydration, diarrhea, vomiting, and a delirious state develop. The patient is severely agitated, confused, disoriented, and may exhibit psychotic features such as hallucinations and paranoid thinking.

    (4) Iodine 131 (^{131}I) and propylthiouracil may cause either a rapid or a slow, insidious onset of hypothyroidism. If hypothyroidism arises quickly, severe disturbances may be noted, including delusions, hallucinations, and a delirious state.

    (5) Insulin and orally administered hypoglycemic agents may produce either acute or chronic hypoglycemia. In mild-to-moderate acute hypoglycemia the patient may be irritable and difficult to interview; the history may be vague and imprecise. Evidence of impaired cognitive functioning or confusion may be found. The patient may be lethargic and complain of a headache. As blood glucose levels drop, the patient becomes more impaired. A delirious condition may develop with disorientation, agitation, and disturbances in perception and thinking. At low enough glucose levels, coma results. With chronic hypoglycemia the patient may develop an organic personality disorder with impaired judgment and impulse control, emotional withdrawal, and inappropriate outbursts of emotion. A dementia may develop over time.

s. Non-narcotic analgesics and antipyretics are commonly used. Toxic states may arise in-
advertently or intentionally with overdoses.

    (1) Salicylates (e.g., aspirin) produce agitation, confusion, tinnitus, hallucinations (usually
    visual), and a delirium at toxic levels.

    (2) At high doses **phenacetin** produces a depressed mood, lethargy, dizziness, feelings of
    detachment, and impaired concentration. A toxic delirious state may follow.

t. Anti-inflammatory agents also produce toxic states. **Phenylbutazone** has reportedly caused
headaches and psychotic reactions at low doses. At higher doses a delirious condition with
hallucinations, convulsions, and coma has been observed. **Indomethacin** produces headache in as many as 50% of patients. Severe reactions may include depersonalization, confusion, nightmares, depression, hallucinations, ataxia, and delirium.

u. Drugs used to treat infections may produce psychiatric disturbances.

    **(1) Among the antibacterials, sulfonamides, penicillin, and gram-negative agents (e.g.,
    chloramphenicol)** have produced psychiatric symptoms. Confusion, depression, and
    acute psychosis may occur with sulfonamides. Intravenous administration of penicillin
    has led to acute psychosis with agitation, anxiety, and hallucinations. Chloramphenicol
    has caused depression as well as a delirious condition.

    (2) Antituberculosis agents may produce symptoms due to either acute or chronic use.
    Acutely, **isoniazid** use may lead to anxiety and restlessness. With prolonged use, irri-
    tability, confusion, and paranoid thinking have been observed. A schizophrenic-like
    syndrome with hallucinations and delusions may arise in severe cases. **Cycloserine** use
    has been associated with confusion, agitation, and delirium. **Iproniazid**, a monoamine
    oxidase inhibitor (MAOI), may elevate the mood as well as produce additional manic
    symptoms. **Ethionamide** use may lead to somnolence and a depressed mood.

    (3) Amantadine, an antiviral agent, has produced agitation, aggressive behavior, halluci-
    nations, and delirium.

    (4) Chloroquine, quinacrine, and griseofulvin, which are antifungal and antiparasitic
    agents may produce a range of symptoms. Depressed mood, aggressive behavior, and
    changes in personality have been observed. More severe symptoms include hallucina-
    tions, delusions, paranoid ideation, and delirium.

v. Antineoplastic agents do not cross the blood-brain barrier. Thus, they rarely have any effect on the central nervous system. **Vinca** alkaloids have reportedly produced stupor, hallucinations, and coma, however.

w. Disulfiram, in normal doses, may reduce libido and sexual potency as well as levels of
energy. The patient experiences weakness, impairment of memory and concentration,
somnolence, disorientation, and confusion from acute toxic doses. Chronic ingestion leads
to carbon disulfide toxicity. The symptoms of this disorder include parkinsonism, depression, a peripheral neuropathy, and delirium. Of great concern with disulfiram is the acetal-
dehyde reaction that occurs when alcohol enters the body either by drinking or by absorption through the skin (e.g., when applying cologne or perfume) or mucosa (e.g., when using mouthwash). An acute and severe illness may result with palpitations, chest pain, and
possible circulatory collapse.

x. Alcohol is the most commonly abused drug.* This abuse produces varied clinical conditions ranging from intoxication to delirious states.

    (1) Alcohol intoxication (see Chapter 4, "Substance Abuse," section II A) is characterized
    by specific neurologic, psychiatric, and behavioral disturbances caused by recent in-
    gestion of alcohol. Blood alcohol levels are greater than 100 mg/dl and may be as high
    as 400 to 500 mg/dl. Intoxication may last from 2 or 3 hours to as many as 12 hours.
    Duration is related to the amount consumed and the rate of consumption. Chronic
    heavy drinkers metabolize alcohol at an approximate rate of 30 mg/dl/hr. Those who
    are not chronic heavy drinkers have a metabolic rate for alcohol of about 20 mg/dl/hr.

        (a) Neurologic signs of alcohol intoxication include slurred speech, motor incoor-
        dination, and an unsteady gait.

        (b) Psychiatric signs and symptoms include impaired concentration, memory, and at-
        tention as well as emotional lability, lack of inhibitions, loquaciousness, and ir-
        ritability.

        (c) Maladaptive behavior includes fighting, impaired judgment, impaired social and
        occupational functioning, and failure to meet responsibilities.

    (2) Idiosyncratic alcohol intoxication is a condition in which marked behavioral changes
    result from the consumption of a small amount of alcohol. Typically, the disturbance
    lasts a few hours.

        (a) Symptoms include aggressive or assaultive behavior that is atypical for the individ-
        ual concerned and are usually manifest early in life (i.e., in the late teens or early
        twenties).

---

*For more information on alcohol abuse, refer to Chapter 4, "Substance Abuse."

(b) Previous brain injury or current sedative use appear to be predisposing factors.

(c) Temporal lobe seizures may present in this way and should be looked for in any patient with this syndrome.

(3) **Alcohol withdrawal syndromes** vary in severity (for specific information, see Chapter 4, "Substance Abuse," section III A).

(4) **Alcohol withdrawal delirium (delirium tremens)** is a severe condition that arises within 1 week of cessation of, or significant reduction in, alcohol use. Delirium tremens is most common in individuals between 30 and 40 years of age, although all ages are susceptible. The presence of other illnesses such as infections or fractures predisposes an individual to this condition. Cognitive disturbances include impaired attention, memory, and concentration. Behavior is marked by impulsiveness and unpredictability, which is easily understood if it is recognized that cognitive and perceptual disturbances render these patients incapable of responding appropriately to the environment. As in all delirious states, these disturbances fluctuate. The patient may be quiet and calm one moment and wild and combative the next.

(5) **Alcohol hallucinosis** (see Chapter 4, "Substance Abuse," section III A 4) is a relatively uncommon condition in which there are persistent hallucinations when an individual, after a long binge, is abstinent from alcohol. This is not a withdrawal state. Typically, the affected individual has not been drinking alcohol for 1 to 2 weeks when hallucinations begin. They may last for weeks, months, or, rarely, years. No other signs of organic impairment are present. These patients do not have a thought disorder, as is found in schizophrenia.

(6) **Alcohol amnestic syndrome** refers to an impairment of memory secondary to prolonged alcohol use. It is rarely seen in individuals who are under 35 years of age. Other evidence of significant alcohol abuse, such as hepatic disease, is typically present in this disorder.

(a) **Wernicke's encephalopathy** develops over a period of a few days to a few weeks. The patient becomes confused and may have difficulty remaining alert. An atactic gait, nystagmus, and ophthalmoplegia (most often involving the sixth cranial nerve) are common findings. Evidence of a peripheral neuropathy includes decreased deep-tendon reflexes, weakness, and diminished sensation. **Thiamine deficiencies** cause pathologic changes in the mamillary body, the walls of the third ventricle, and other areas. A patient may recover from this condition spontaneously within a few days or progress to permanent deficits. These deficits often can be resolved rapidly with the administration of thiamine.

(b) **Korsakoff's psychosis** is the chronic condition that is also known as **alcohol amnestic syndrome**. Short-term memory losses are prominent. Long-term memory may also be affected. With little or no capacity to remember, behavior may be grossly disturbed. **Confabulation is common**. Interpersonal and occupational skills are lost. Depression and social withdrawal may occur. Korsakoff's psychosis does not respond to thiamine, and permanent, often severe, impairment exists.

(7) **Dementia** is frequently associated with alcoholism, even though alcohol has never been shown to be a causative agent for dementia. This "diagnosis" is usually made when a patient is alcoholic and no other cause can be found for the dementia.

y. **Cocaine**, an alkaloid derivative of the plant *Erythroxylon coca*, was first used in medicine as a local anesthetic in 1884. Use as a local anesthetic is its only current medical application. Abuse of this substance by the affluent has increased significantly in the last decade or so. The drug is inhaled (snorted), injected intravenously or subcutaneously, or smoked (which is termed free-basing). The latter two routes of administration are much more toxic than snorting. Both acute and chronic cocaine use may produce significant psychiatric disturbances.

(1) Acutely, **the drug produces a stimulated, euphoric feeling in the user**. This feeling lasts for a brief time, usually no more than 2 hours. Other effects are often present. These include:

(a) Severe, acute anxiety with paranoid ideation

(b) Irritability

(c) Elevated blood pressure and heart rate

(d) Dilated pupils, which are reactive to light

(e) Dry mouth

(f) Uncharacteristically aggressive behavior

(g) Hallucinations, usually tactile (e.g., formication—creeping sensations on the skin)

(h) Cardiac dysrhythmias

(i) Increased deep-tendon reflexes

(j) Respiratory arrest and death from high doses via the intravenous or free-basing route

(k) Craving for more cocaine

(2) Craving for cocaine leads to chronic abuse. Doses increase, and weekend use progresses to daily use. Chronic cocaine abusers are more likely to inject or smoke the drug because more cocaine can be delivered more quickly by these routes of administration. All of the acute effects listed above may occur. Additional effects include:

(a) Weight loss due to decreased food intake and poor self-care

(b) Impaired concentration

(c) Impaired erectile and ejaculatory function

(d) Hypersomnia, characterized by daytime sleepiness, frequent napping, difficult arousal from sleep, and the need for 10 or more hours of sleep each day

(e) Psychotic symptoms, including persecutory delusions, ideas of reference, and perceptual disturbances

(f) Hostility and aggressive behavior

(g) Nasal septal perforation from snorting

(h) Sepsis or bacterial endocarditis from intravenous use

(i) Seizures with an overdose

(3) Cocaine is not physically addictive, but a powerful psychological dependence develops in chronic users. Cocaine use governs the lives of cocaine abusers. Unfortunately, tragic financial, occupational, medical, interpersonal, and legal events often occur before the abuser is motivated to seek treatment.

G. Exposure to toxins. The environment has become a common source of exposure to toxins, with pollutants in the air and water. Industrial and occupational pollutants create hazards for workers as well as nonworkers in the area. Some of these toxins have become substances of abuse.

1. Gases may induce changes in brain function, generally when concentrations rise above tolerated levels.

a. Oxygen intoxication is the result of the inhalation of pure oxygen at levels of 2 atm or greater. Mood changes are noted. The individual becomes irritable and labile. He or she may complain of dizziness and paresthesias. Loss of consciousness may occur. Treatment is reduction of the oxygen being delivered to the individual.

b. The effects of **carbon dioxide** are related to its concentration. Levels between 2% and 10% of carbon dioxide tend to increase the respiratory rate and the depth of respiration. At higher levels headache, confusion, and delirium result.

c. Carbon monoxide forms carboxyhemoglobin in the blood, displacing oxygen and leading to hypoxia. Most individuals experience headache at levels of 20% or less of carboxyhemoglobin. At levels between 20% and 40%, severe headache, nausea, vomiting, dizziness, and dimness of vision result. At levels between 40% and 60%, tachypnea, tachycardia, syncope, and convulsions occur. Above 60% respiratory failure occurs followed by death. Changes in the globus pallidus and substantia nigra occur with acute, severe carbon monoxide intoxication, leading to parkinsonism and seizures. There is chronic intoxication in smokers and urban dwellers, who experience episodic depressions, withdrawal, apathy, impairment of perception and memory, and disorientation. Slowly, the globus pallidus and substantia nigra are affected. Seizures and movement disorders may develop.

2. Noxious vapors are encountered on the job, in the home, and in accidents and are abused for their effects. Exposure may have an excitatory effect. Affected individuals become hyperactive or agitated. Emotional lability may be evident. In others, apathy and disinterest may be prominent. Memory and concentration are impaired acutely. Some individuals become very aggressive. With chronic exposure, personality changes occur. Individuals may be apathetic or exhibit wide shifts in activities and interests. Significant cognitive difficulties and psychotic disturbances, such as paranoid thinking and hallucinations, have been noted in abusers. Many changes become irreversible with chronic exposure.

3. Exposure to heavy metals leads to widespread health problems, including psychiatric disturbances. Problems develop when the body's capacity to excrete a heavy metal is exceeded by the amount ingested. Intoxication can be either acute or chronic.

a. Lead may enter the body through the respiratory route, the gastrointestinal route, and through the skin. Toxicity is greater if vapors are inhaled than if some lead-containing compound is consumed (e.g., paint and moonshine liquor, which is often distilled in containers with lead solder). Symptomatology is mild with low levels in the blood (i.e., 100 μg to 150 μg/dl), and fatigue and anemia may occur. At higher levels (i.e., 150 μg to 200 μg/dl), constipation, loss of appetite, and lethargy may accompany abdominal pain. Encephalopathy has been observed when levels are above 200 μg/dl. Individuals experience dizziness and clumsiness and are irritable and restless. An excited delirious state develops, which can proceed to lethargy and coma. As many as 25% of severely intoxicated individuals die, and 40% of those affected who survive suffer severe sequelae.

b. Mercury poisons the body through the skin and through respiratory and gastrointestinal routes. In acute syndromes, the mercury usually has been swallowed. A gastrointestinal syndrome with diarrhea, dehydration, and bleeding occurs. Chronic intoxication usually results from inhalation of vapors. Early in the chronic illness, affected individuals may exhibit changes in personality (e.g., irritability, apathy, and lability) as well as tremors, gingivitis, and albuminuria. If the intoxication persists, insomnia, lethargy, depression, timidity, withdrawal from others, despondency and, in some cases, hallucinations occur. At the same time, physical signs and symptoms worsen. These include anemia, hypertension, colitis, renal disease, loosening of the teeth, and anorexia.

c. Thallium is found in rat poisons and in depilatory agents. Initially, intoxication causes pain in the legs, diarrhea, and vomiting. If a chronic condition (or severe acute condition) develops, depression, paranoid thinking, or choreiform movements may result. In severe cases a delirium develops with possible seizures and blindness. A clue to thallium intoxication can be alopecia.

d. Manganese exposure is rare, limited to specific contact with mines or battery casings. Vapors produce intoxication. Headaches, somnolence, and irritability may be seen initially. Later, emotional lability, nightmares, aggressive behavior, confusion, hallucinations, and compulsive and impulsive acts have been observed. Lesions in the basal ganglia and pyramis result, leading to gait impairment, tremors, rigidity of posture, monotonous speech, and micrographia. The recommended treatment is removing the source of exposure. Psychological symptoms resolve in 3 or 4 months in most cases.

e. Arsenic is found in insecticides, disinfectants, and rat poisons. Severe acute intoxication produces a life-threatening condition with fluid loss. Chronic, insidious intoxication produces lethargy, anorexia, and fatigue. Diarrhea and upper respiratory irritation may be present as well. Eventually an encephalopathic condition results, with loss of intellect, apathy, as well as personality changes.

f. Bismuth is found in salts used for constipation (this use is uncommon now). The salts may be absorbed, leading to a variety of psychological symptoms, including depression, anxiety, irritability, phobias, and paranoid delusions. Neurologic symptoms also occur, such as incontinence, dysarthria, ataxia, and pseudotremors.

4. Organophosphates are potent acetylcholinesterase inhibitors found in insecticides such as parathion and malathion. These compounds are introduced into the body via vapors and skin contact. Acetylcholine accumulates at synapses, blocking functioning. Mild acute intoxication produces headache, fatigue, numbness, gastrointestinal upset, dizziness, profuse sweating, excessive salivation, tightness in the chest, and abdominal pain. Severe acute intoxication leads to extreme weakness, difficulty in talking and walking, and muscle fasciculations. A flaccid paralysis may occur. Affected individuals may be delirious. Chronic intoxication may lead to diminished concentration, drowsiness, confusion, memory deficits, psychomotor slowing, slurring of speech, perseveration, depression, lethargy, anxiety, and irritability.

H. Nutritional deficiencies can disrupt brain functions. In addition to substrates such as oxygen, glucose, and amino acids, vitamins and minerals are essential for the proper functioning of enzyme and transport systems, maintenance of membrane integrity, and myelin formation. Vitamin deficiencies result from inadequate intake, impaired absorption, and increased metabolic requirements. These conditions are usually seen in impoverished people, food faddists, and alcoholics.

1. Thiamine is required for the formation of thiamine pyrophosphate, a coenzyme in the carbohydrate degradation cycle. Deficiencies occur in the malnourished or starving and in alcoholics.

a. Beriberi runs a subacute or chronic course. Affected individuals suffer from high-output cardiac failure with cardiac dilation, tachycardia, arrhythmias, edema, and dyspnea on exertion. A peripheral neuropathy results from demyelination of peripheral nerves and dorsal root ganglia. Psychiatric symptoms may include apathy, depression, irritability, impaired concentration, and nervousness. In severe cases memory and intellect may be permanently compromised.

b. Syndromes associated with chronic alcoholism are Wernicke's encephalopathy and Korsakoff's psychosis (see section IV F 2 w).

2. Nicotinic acid is necessary for the formation of coenzymes for tissue respiration. Skin rashes and atrophy of the mucous membranes result from a deficiency. In addition, headache, apathy, confusion, delusions, insomnia, and a clinical picture resembling dementia have been reported. These signs and symptoms respond promptly to administration of nicotinic acid.

3. **Pyridoxine (a form of vitamin B$_6$) deficiency** can lead to peripheral neuropathy. It should be noted that isoniazid, the antituberculosis drug, competes with pyridoxine and increases the chance of a neuropathy developing.

4. **Cyanocobalamin (vitamin B$_{12}$)** is absorbed from the gastrointestinal tract only when the required intrinsic factor has been produced by the gastric mucosa. Important functions of this vitamin include roles in hematopoiesis, nucleoprotein production, myelin production, and gastrointestinal epithelial cell maintenance. With vitamin B$_{12}$ deficiency, megaloblastic anemia and neurologic deficits develop over a period of weeks to months. Myelin is destroyed in the spinal cord, brain, and peripheral nerves. Parathesias are a common early sign. The gait may become unsteady. Deep-tendon reflexes are diminished. Apathy, depression, irritability, and moodiness are common. Less common are confusion, delusions, paranoid thinking, hallucinations, and a clinical picture resembling dementia. Although neurologic and hematologic symptoms are usually present, some patients present only with psychiatric symptoms. Most patients respond to vitamin B$_{12}$ administration, although the degree of disease progression is a factor to consider. Some patients have enduring deficits.

I. **Inborn errors of metabolism may produce psychiatric conditions.** The list of diseases in which either lipids, carbohydrates, or proteins are mishandled by the body is extensive. Mental changes including retardation are common elements of these diseases. These disorders are familial and usually appear early in life. Two disorders, Wilson's disease and acute intermittent porphyria, warrant further description.

1. **Wilson's disease (hepatolenticular degeneration)** is inherited as an autosomal recessive defect. Features of the disease are abnormal copper metabolism, degenerative changes in the brain, and cirrhosis of the liver. Copper is deposited in the liver, in the renal tubules, and in the brain (in the corpus callosum and putamen). Signs and symptoms appear in the second and third decades of life. Personality changes may be the first sign. Existing traits may become muted or exaggerated. Irritability and moodiness may be seen. Transient psychotic symptoms, including hallucinations, paranoid thinking, and even manic-like outbursts, have been described. A mild tremor and loss of coordination may be apparent in the handwriting of the affected individual. Speech may become indistinct or frankly dysarthric. Ataxia and chorea may develop. Facial immobility and dysphagia may occur. Cirrhotic changes in the liver and renal tubular damage result from copper deposition in these tissues. Treatment includes administration of D-penicillamine and a copper-restricted diet.

2. **Acute intermittent porphyria** is inherited as an autosomal dominant trait. The lesion is a defect in the regulation of the hepatic enzyme δ-aminolevulinic acid synthetase. An increase in this enzyme produces the episodic characteristic of this disease. Symptoms typically begin after puberty, usually between the ages of 20 to 40 years and occur more commonly in women than in men. Affected individuals may experience nervousness and emotional instability on a chronic basis. During acute episodes abdominal pain recurs. Confusion, disorientation, impaired concentration, or frank delirium may appear. Peripheral neuropathies, including cranial nerve palsies, are often seen. Some patients have convulsions and lapse into coma. These episodes can be stimulated by medications such as estrogens, sulfonamides, and barbiturates. Symptomatic treatment of the pain and psychiatric symptoms is recommended.

J. **Metabolic disorders are frequently reflected in rapid recent changes in behavior, thinking, and consciousness.** The earliest signs of metabolic irregularities are often compromised memory and orientation. Affected individuals may become agitated, anxious, hyperactive, or withdrawn. Failures in perception may occur as hallucinations, or illusions are experienced. Disturbances in thinking (e.g., delusions and paranoid ideation) may develop. Confusion and delirium develop in severe cases as do pronounced neurologic disturbances such as grand mal seizures. For the most part, EEG changes are nonspecific. The neurologic examination shows nonfocal involvement.

1. **Hepatic encephalopathy** results from severe, acute, or chronic liver disease. Ammonia and other toxins accumulate as a result of hepatic failure. Changes in personality, impairment of memory, intellectual deficits, and disturbances in consciousness ranging from apathy and drowsiness to coma can develop. A flapping tremor (**asterixis**) may appear. Individuals may hyperventilate, reflecting an acid-base disturbance common to hepatic failure. Triphasic wave patterns are seen on EEG. Limiting nitrogenous products in the body is the current treatment of this severe illness.

2. **Uremic encephalopathy** results from either acute or chronic renal failure. Urea and other metabolites, a metabolic acidosis, and alterations in normal electrolyte metabolism due to acidosis

produce the signs and symptoms of this disorder. Patients are restless. Memory, orientation, and the ability to maintain consciousness may be compromised. A peripheral neuropathy characterized by diffuse sensory and motor impairment and diminished deep-tendon reflexes may occur. Muscles twitch, and asterixis may appear. In severe cases seizures have been reported. Dialysis is indicated in most cases. Rapid dialysis can lead to a syndrome called **dialysis disequilibrium**, which is characterized by headache, confusion, changes in consciousness, and convulsions.

3. **Failure to maintain serum glucose at adequate levels can lead to an organic brain syndrome.** Glucose levels may be too high or too low.
   a. **Hypoglycemic encephalopathy** can result from causes as various as an islet cell adenoma of the pancreas, the administration of too much insulin, adrenocortical failure, hepatic necrosis, and a glycogen storage disease. Hypoglycemic episodes usually occur in the early morning or after exercise. The **rate of decline in serum glucose concentration seems to be crucial**. Premonitory symptoms include nausea, tachycardia, sweating, hunger, apprehension, and restlessness. As the encephalopathy progresses, disorientation, agitation, confusion, and hallucinations may occur. Diplopia, pallor, increased deep-tendon reflexes, clonus, and seizures may follow. Late in the course, stupor or coma is seen. Many of these symptoms can be confused with an anxiety attack. Treatment with intravenous dextrose is indicated.
   b. **Diabetic ketoacidosis** results from inadequately treated diabetes mellitus. The affected individual has too little insulin available to metabolize glucose properly. This is due either to insufficient doses of insulin or an ongoing condition that increases insulin demands, such as an infection or physical trauma. Early signs and symptoms of diabetic ketoacidosis include weakness, listlessness, fatigue, polyuria, polydipsia, headache, nausea, and vomiting. The patient's condition can worsen over a period of hours to days as ketonuria, ketonemia, dehydration, and acidosis persist. At any point a more rapid deterioration may occur as the patient becomes confused, stuporous, or comatose. Treatment with intravenous fluids and insulin is indicated. Care must be taken to maintain electrolyte balance as acid-base disturbances are corrected with treatment.
   c. **Hyperglycemic nonketotic coma** is a clinical syndrome seen in association with corticosteroid or diuretic therapy or peritoneal dialysis. It may be the first indication of diabetes mellitus in a patient or a complication arising from inadequately treated diabetes mellitus. It occurs in middle-aged individuals and in the elderly. The condition comes on slowly as the blood glucose level climbs as high as 1000 mg/dl. Unlike diabetic ketoacidosis, there is no significant formation of ketones. As the blood glucose level rises, the kidneys produce increased amounts of urine (polyuria) in an effort to correct the problem. Fluids move from tissues into the vascular space in an effort to lower serum osmolarity, causing intracellular dehydration. Serum sodium levels rise (**hypernatremia**). Patients become lethargic and easily fatigued. Memory difficulties and confusion develop. Coma and seizures may ensue.

4. **Failure to maintain serum sodium concentration in the normal range may lead to an organic brain syndrome.** Levels may be too high or too low. **A critical factor is the rate of change in the serum sodium concentration**. A rapid change has a more profound effect on the central nervous system.
   a. **Hyponatremia** is a condition in which there is a relative excess of total body water to total solute (sodium). It results from defects in the urinary dilution system brought about by conditions such as volume depletion, edematous states, adrenal insufficiency, a syndrome of inappropriate ADH (antidiuretic hormone) secretion as occurs with some malignancies (e.g., oat-cell carcinoma of the lung) and central nervous system infections, renal failure, psychogenic polydipsia, and exposure to medications including oral hypoglycemics, carbamazepine, and amitriptyline. Hyponatremia is usually of little consequence clinically. Symptoms rarely develop if serum sodium concentration is 125 mEq/L or greater. However, with a lower level of serum sodium concentration and rapid onset, marked central nervous system findings are present. Individuals become lethargic and inactive. Confusion develops, leading to erratic behavior and irrational thinking. As the condition progresses, stupor and coma develop. Central nervous system defects result from intracellular fluid accumulation (i.e., brain cells swell up and function inefficiently and erratically); once identified, this situation must be corrected slowly so that affected brain cells may adjust without another rapid change in cellular hydration.
   b. **Hypernatremia** is a condition in which there is a relative deficit in total body water to total solute (sodium). This condition is the result of losses of hypotonic fluids, which may occur with excessive sweating in the presence of inadequate fluid replacement, in burn victims who lose large volumes of hypotonic fluid through injured skin, and with diabetes insipidus. Brain cells become dehydrated when serum sodium concentrations rise, leading to impaired brain functioning. As with hyponatremia, confusion, lethargy, and alterations

in consciousness may develop. This condition should be corrected slowly with hypotonic fluids administered intravenously or orally to avoid further compromise of central nervous system functioning brought on by another rapid shift in cellular hydration.

5. Hypoxia has profound effects on brain functioning. Delivery of oxygen to the central nervous system depends upon the respiratory and circulatory systems, the supply of oxygen at the alveolar level, and the capacity of erythrocytes to transport and release oxygen. Numerous conditions can compromise the availability of oxygen to the brain. Cerebral vascular changes occur. Anemia reduces the oxygen-carrying capacity of blood because there are fewer erythrocytes available for transport. In pulmonary diseases such as emphysema, there is an impaired ability to exchange oxygen at the alveolar level, leading to reduced oxygen partial pressure (PO_2) in the blood and, therefore, to reduced delivery of oxygen to tissues. In congestive heart failure, circulation is impaired. Blood may be poorly oxygenated due to compromised pulmonary arterial circulation, and tissues may receive diminished amounts of blood. Toxins such as cyanide and toxin-caused diseases such as diphtheria interfere with cellular respiration, producing histotoxic hypoxia. Changes in levels and activity of 2,3-diphosphoglycerate (2,3-DPG), an intracellular enzyme in erythrocytes, affect oxygen transport and release as well. Carbon monoxide poisoning also produces hypoxia. Acute signs and symptoms of hypoxia include impaired judgment, confusion, loss of motor coordination, emotional lability, irrational thinking (e.g., paranoid ideation), and impulsive, erratic behavior. Some individuals are chronically hypoxic. These patients experience fatigue, drowsiness, inattentiveness, a delayed reaction time, diminished work capacity, and confusion. Severe hypoxia can lead to stupor, an obtundent state, and coma.

6. Elevated and depressed levels of potassium produce significant neuromuscular effects, especially cardiac arrhythmias, without any significant effect on brain functioning.

K. Endocrine disorders can lead to psychiatric symptoms. In general, changes may be evident in personality, mental functions, memory, and neurologic functions.

1. Tumors of the pituitary and hypothalamus can grossly alter neurologic and endocrine functioning. These tumors usually develop quiescently. Headaches are rare because intracranial pressure is not increased. Neurologic signs appear when the tumor is large enough to compress other brain structures. When the optic chiasm is compressed, bitemporal hemianopia develops. Memory and intellect are impaired by pressure to basal frontal and temporal lobe structures. Endocrine disturbances reflect the area of the hypothalamus or pituitary that is affected. Radiographic identification of these tumors is difficult because of their small size.

2. Tumors of the hypothalamus are associated with behavioral changes. A radical change in appetite leads to obesity or inanition. Sleep may be disturbed. The patient may become emotionally labile and be subject to rage reactions. Excessive water drinking arises in diabetes insipidus, a condition in which ADH is no longer secreted, leading to a failure to reabsorb water in the kidney. Conversely, the inappropriate and excessive secretion of ADH dilutes body fluids, leading to water intoxication and cerebral edema (see section IV J 4 a).

3. Elevated or depressed thyroid functions can lead to psychiatric symptoms.
   a. An individual with a hyperactive thyroid experiences weakness and fatigue. He or she may suffer insomnia. Weight loss occurs in the face of an increased appetite. Tremulousness and palpitations develop. The patient perspires excessively. Anxiety and restlessness are early signs of **hyperthyroidism**. As the condition progresses, impairment of memory, orientation, and judgment becomes apparent. In severe cases, a manic-like excitement is evident or a schizophreniform picture with delusions and hallucinations arises. Hyperthyroidism may be masked behind a state of apathy, confusion, and depression in the elderly. However, examination usually reveals eye signs (e.g., lid lag and exophthalmos) and other signs of the disorder. Treatment of the hyperthyroidism provides treatment of the associated psychiatric syndrome.
   b. Hypothyroidism (myxedema) may be caused by overtreatment with ^{131}I, diminished thyroid-stimulating hormone (TSH) or thyrotropin releasing hormone (TRH) levels, or thyroiditis. The patient is easily fatigued, often sleepy, and experiences weakness. Skin becomes dry and thick. Hair is brittle. Hot or cold temperatures are poorly tolerated. Speech is slowed and may be hoarse. The individual becomes irritable or appears depressed. As the disorder progresses, memory and intellect are impaired, so much so that a person appears demented. In severe cases, the patient becomes obtundent or comatose; if this occurs, the mortality rate is substantial (50%). Early recognition and treatment improves the outcome of hypothyroidism. Early treatment usually reverses all ill effects; left untreated, permanent cognitive deficits may develop.

4. Elevated or depressed parathyroid functions can lead to psychiatric symptoms.

    a. Hyperparathyroidism typically results from parathyroid neoplasms, which are usually benign adenomas. This disorder leads to elevated serum calcium concentration. (Hypercalcemia may also develop in disease processes affecting bones, such as Paget's disease, multiple myeloma, and metastatic carcinoma). The hypercalcemic patient experiences lassitude, anxiety, and irritability. He or she may become agitated, paranoid, confused, or depressed. Muscular weakness is common.

    b. Hypoparathyroidism occurs when parathyroid gland functioning is diminished or lost. This condition usually follows neck or thyroid surgery, when the parathyroid glands are excised. Hypoparathyroidism leads to hypocalcemia. Neuromuscular signs and symptoms include increased excitability, transient paresthesias, cramping, twitching, tetany, and seizures. Psychiatric signs and symptoms include confusion, agitation, drowsiness, hallucinations, and depression. Correction of serum calcium concentration eliminates the signs and symptoms.

5. Abnormalities of adrenal cortical functioning produce psychiatric symptoms.

    a. Adrenal insufficiency is a life-threatening condition when its onset is sudden. Vomiting, weakness, dehydration, hypotension, and impairment of consciousness may be present. Without prompt treatment, circulatory collapse and death will follow. Chronic adrenal insufficiency, **Addison's disease**, produces apathy, fatigability, irritability, and depression. Occasionally, a patient becomes confused or psychotic. Treatment with corticosteroids eliminates psychiatric symptoms.

    b. Cushing's disease is a state of adrenal cortical hyperactivity caused by either excessive ACTH secretion by the pituitary or an adrenal cortical adenoma that produces excessive amounts of corticosteroids. In modern medical practice, Cushing's syndrome is seen to develop in patients taking high doses of corticosteroids long-term for various conditions. Signs and symptoms vary. Some patients are restless, suffer from insomnia, have an elevated mood, and are hyperactive. Others feel anxious or depressed. Psychosis may develop with delusions and hallucinations. Suicide may occur. Treatment of a tumor or decreasing the dosage of prednisone is indicated and usually remedies the problem.

6. A pheochromocytoma is a catecholamine-secreting tumor of the adrenal medulla. The patient experiences severe anxiety as well as excessive perspiration, palpitations, tremulousness, lightheadedness, headaches, and pallor. These symptoms are very similar to those of panic attacks. Blood pressure is elevated in a sustained or a paroxysmal fashion. These tumors are often very small and difficult to locate. Once found, surgical excision is indicated in most cases.

L. Infections can produce changes in cognition, behavior, and emotional expression. Although these changes may occur with systemic infections, they are much more common with central nervous system infections.

1. A patient with a systemic infection such as pneumonia or typhoid often has an associated high fever. A delirium may be present. The affected individual is confused, agitated, and irritable. The level of consciousness fluctuates. Hallucinations may prove to be very troubling. Erratic, ill-considered behavior may occur. A safe environment with adequate provision for orienting the patient is necessary. As fever diminishes, signs of delirium typically remit.

2. A viral infection of the central nervous system produces encephalitis. Encephalitides may be acute or chronic.

    a. In acute viral encephalitis, inclusion bodies are formed in the brain. The patient may be excessively sleepy, lethargic, and confused. Other patients are irritable and hyperkinetic. Some experience anxiety, apprehension, and have outbursts of terror or rage. Fever, headache, and photophobia are common physical symptoms.

    b. Chronic viral encephalitides are much less common. Pronounced physical symptoms such as fever and headache may be diminished or absent. In adults, chronic encephalitis may present with extrapyramidal symptomatology or with a seizure. In children, alterations in behavior and character may be evident. A well-behaved child may become destructive and inconsiderate of others. There may be no neurologic or intellectual deficits. Viral titers and examination of the cerebrospinal fluid aid in diagnosis.

3. Tertiary syphilis has devastating effects on the central nervous system. As recently as 1920, 10% of all psychiatric hospitalizations were for general paresis, a form of tertiary syphilis. Currently, general paresis accounts for far less than 1% of admissions. The discovery of penicillin in 1943 provided definitive treatment, although cases are still occasionally seen. A second type of tertiary syphilis, syphilitic meningitis, warrants description also.

    a. General paresis occurs 5 to 30 years after an episode of primary syphilis, most frequently within 20 years.

(1) Diagnosis is made by examination of the cerebrospinal fluid and serum. Test results of spinal fluid are positive in more than 90% of untreated cases. Protein is elevated two to six times the normal levels. Globulins are disproportionately high. A cell count of more than 100 cells per ml indicates an active infection.

(2) Mortality rates are between 20% and 30%. Untreated individuals have an average life expectancy of 4 years. Active, adequate treatment with penicillin yields good results.

(3) Marked personality changes and neurologic signs may be noted. These include:
- **(a)** Irritability
- **(b)** Impaired concentration
- **(c)** Depression
- **(d)** Periods of confusion
- **(e)** Sleep disturbances
- **(f)** Headaches
- **(g)** Indifference or apathy
- **(h)** Impaired judgment
- **(i)** Grandiose delusions
- **(j)** Impaired memory
- **(k)** Erratic emotional reactions
- **(l)** Loss of muscle tone
- **(m)** Fatigue
- **(n)** Papilledema
- **(o)** Optic atrophy (in 65% of individuals)
- **(p)** Argyll Robertson pupils
- **(q)** Speech disturbances
- **(r)** Gait disturbances
- **(s)** Spasticity

b. Syphilitic meningitis primarily involves the meninges, unlike general paresis, which affects brain parenchyma. It usually arises 1 to 3 years after a primary syphilitic infection. In general, the personality is less affected when the brain parenchyma is not involved.

(1) Inflammation of the meninges around the base of the brain is **basilar meningitis**. The patient is usually clearly impaired, with neurologic signs. Headache, dizziness, sleepiness, confusion, and impaired memory are accompanied by pupillary abnormalities, ptosis, deafness, and a facial palsy.

(2) Vertical type results from inflammation involving the brain's convex surfaces (the cerebral hemispheres). Symptoms include severe nocturnal headaches, frequent dizziness, irritability, inability to sustain effort, slowed thinking, amnesia, aphasia, retarded speech, and seizures. Diagnosis by serology and examination of the cerebrospinal fluid should lead to successful treatment with penicillin.

4. Meningococcal meningitis may present as a delirium. The patient is confused, mumbles or rambles in his or her speech, and is restless and disoriented. Its course may be fulminant. Acutely, the patient may be noisy or violent. In subacute cases, drowsiness and confusion are prominent. Chronic cases present with impaired concentration, or, in children, impaired intellect. Meningeal irritation (i.e., a stiff neck) and fever are usually present. Gram stain of the cerebrospinal fluid reveals depressed glucose levels, purulence (i.e., the presence of leukocytes), and diplococci. Prompt diagnosis and treatment typically yield a full recovery.

5. Tubercular meningitis is a condition that develops when tuberculosis spreads from the lungs to the central nervous system. Its onset is insidious. Early symptoms include fatigue, irritability, peevishness, and disturbed sleep. If intracranial pressure increases, the patient experiences headaches, confusion, and clouded consciousness. As the disease progresses, meningeal irritation is evident. Examination of the cerebrospinal fluid reveals decreased glucose levels, elevated protein levels, an increased cell count, and the presence of tubercle bacillus upon stain or culture. Early treatment with isoniazid and streptomycin yields the best outcome.

6. Sydenham's chorea is a condition that develops following recurrent streptococcal infections (usually tonsillitis). Typically, a rheumatic condition accompanies the recurrent infections. In the brain, the cerebral cortex and basal ganglia are affected. Children are affected more often than adults, and females more often than males. The illness usually runs a 2- or 3-month course, although relapses may occur. Treatment with salicylates and bed rest is indicated. Signs and symptoms include:
- **a.** Emotional instability
- **b.** Impaired memory
- **c.** Impaired concentration
- **d.** Irritability
- **e.** Abnormal movement, including grimacing and jerky movements of the limbs

M. Demyelinating disease. The myelin sheaths that insure proper transmission of neuronal signals are destroyed, and the structural integrity of the nervous system is severely compromised in demyelinating disease. Neurologic and psychologic signs and symptoms result.

1. **Acute disseminated encephalomyelitis may involve both the brain and the spinal cord.** Its onset is abrupt, usually following either the exanthem of viral illnesses, such as measles, chickenpox, rubella, and smallpox, or vaccination against rabies or smallpox. In some cases there may be no preceding event.
   a. Initially, the patient experiences headaches, confusion, and a stiff neck. With spinal cord involvement, paralysis and sensory loss are prominent. Stupor, convulsions, and coma reflect brain involvement.
   b. Significant **neurologic findings** usually eliminate any question about an organic etiology when psychiatric symptoms, such as confused, erratic behavior, are present.
   c. Mortality rates range from 10% to 50%. Morbidity is high. Residual neurologic disturbances are common. Intellectual impairment may be present. Permanent changes in behavior, such as increased aggression or social withdrawal, may be observed.

2. **Multiple sclerosis (MS)** is a relatively common, chronic demyelinating disease. It features episodes of focal disturbances, which remit and recur. Women are afflicted more often than men. The peak incidence occurs in individuals between 30 to 35 years of age. It is about eight times more common in relatives of those with MS.
   a. The etiology of MS has been intensively investigated. **Most researchers believe that a viral agent is causative**.
   b. **Any part of the nervous system may be affected.** Therefore, signs and symptoms vary widely. The diagnosis is made when evidence for more than one lesion (i.e., more than one focal disturbance) is present and a remitting and relapsing course exists. Some patients present with psychiatric symptoms. Classically, patients have been described as euphoric or pathologically cheerful. Some patients, however, become irritable or depressed. The presence of fleeting neurologic signs and symptoms may raise the question of somatization. Diagnosis can be very difficult in patients who are somatically preoccupied.
   c. Signs and symptoms include:
      (1) Visual impairment (About 40% of patients experience visual impairment as an initial symptom. This is due to optic neuritis.)
      (2) Nystagmus
      (3) Dysarthria
      (4) Intention tremor
      (5) Ataxia
      (6) Impaired sense of position
      (7) Impaired vibratory sense
      (8) Bladder dysfunction
      (9) Weakness in limbs
      (10) Paraplegia
      (11) Spatial disorientation
      (12) Altered emotional responses
   d. MS typically runs a course of 20 years or more, although some patients suffer a more virulent form of the illness. Over the course of the disease, intellectual impairment may develop. Various psychiatric symptoms develop as well. Personality changes may be evident. Mood swings and depression have been observed frequently. An individual's behavior is altered. He or she may become isolated and withdrawn. Cases of paranoid personality changes are reported.

N. Autoimmune diseases are those conditions in which the body initiates an immune response against its own tissue (i.e., pathogenesis involves immunologic mechanisms). This process may involve the central nervous system and, therefore, lead to psychiatric signs and symptoms.

1. **Systemic lupus erythematosus (SLE)** is a disease of unknown cause. It is clear that a group of antibodies to substances found in cell nuclei are formed, so-called **antinuclear antibodies**. Antibody-antigen complexes form and are deposited in renal glomeruli and in blood vessels, leading to tissue damage. SLE occurs in women nine times as often as in men. Although it occurs in all age groups, it is more common in individuals between 20 and 50 years of age. Overall, between 2 and 3 of every 100,000 individuals are affected. The 5-year survival rate is about 80%.
   a. Some patients present initially with psychiatric complaints, especially affective symptoms. Emotional lability and psychotic symptoms, such as delusions and hallucinations also occur. Signs and symptoms include:
      (1) Arthritis and arthralgia
      (2) Fever

      (3) Malaise
      (4) Weight loss
      (5) Anorexia
      (6) Skin eruptions
      (7) Seizures
      (8) Cognitive deficits

  b. Of greatest concern in SLE are renal and central nervous system lesions. Patients with severe renal or central nervous system disease experience high morbidity and early mortality. Central nervous system lesions include necrotizing vasculitis of arterioles and capillaries, microinfarcts, and deposition of immunoglobulins and complement in the choroid plexus.

  c. A positive antinuclear antibody titer, evidence of renal disease, anemia, leukopenia, and thrombocytopenia, and biopsy aid in diagnosis, although other autoimmune diseases may be difficult to rule out.

  d. Some patients with SLE recover spontaneously. Some respond to steroids. Some are unresponsive to treatment. High doses of corticosteroids can also produce psychiatric symptoms, further complicating the evaluation of emotional and behavioral changes in these patients.

2. Vasculitides are autoimmune diseases that primarily involve blood vessels, often in the brain. Psychiatric symptoms may occur.

BIBLIOGRAPHY

American Psychiatric Association: *Diagnostic and Statistical Manual of Mental Disorders*, 3rd ed. Washington, D.C., American Psychiatric Association, 1980

Isselbacher KJ, Adams RD, Braunwald E, et al (eds): *Harrison's Principles of Internal Medicine*, 9th ed. New York, McGraw-Hill, 1980

Kaplan HI, Freedman AM, Sadock BJ: *Comprehensive Textbook of Psychiatry*, 3rd ed. Baltimore, Williams and Wilkins, 1980, pp 1035–1072, 1359–1482

Kolb LC: *Modern Clinical Psychiatry*, 9th ed. Philadelphia, WB Saunders, 1977, pp 239–373

STUDY QUESTIONS

Directions: Each question below contains five suggested answers. Choose the **one best** response to each question.

1. A 46-year-old woman has been found unconscious in the garage. The car was running, and all the doors to the garage were closed. Upon examination she is confused. The most likely cause of her confusion is

(A) lead poisoning
(B) hypoxia
(C) hypoglycemia
(D) gasoline inhalation
(E) none of the above

2. A 32-year-old man is noted to have an unsteady gait, a sixth cranial nerve palsy, and spider angiomas when examined in the emergency room. He is confused and agitated. He should be treated with

(A) haloperidol
(B) pentobarbital
(C) anticoagulants
(D) thiamine
(E) salicylates

3. All of the following statements about dementia are true EXCEPT

(A) demented patients are often depressed
(B) the ability to generalize from past experiences and to see the relationships between similar situations is lost
(C) inability to recall events of the distant past is an early feature of dementia
(D) demented patients may experience hallucinations
(E) Creutzfeldt-Jakob disease is a dementia caused by a slow virus

4. A 28-year-old woman presents with complaints of irritability and moodiness. She gives a history of brief episodes during which she hears voices and is excessively suspicious of others. Her speech is slightly slurred. Which of the following conditions is the most likely diagnosis?

(A) Hyperparathyroidism
(B) Lead intoxication
(C) Wilson's disease
(D) Folate deficiency
(E) Sydenham's chorea

5. A 29-year-old man presents with a history of three discrete episodes of elevated mood and hyperactivity; he has noted a tendency to get "lost" during these episodes. Once he experienced a loss of vision in the right visual field. Which of the following conditions is the most likely diagnosis?

(A) Multiple sclerosis (MS)
(B) Vitamin B_{12} deficiency
(C) Herpes encephalitis
(D) Systemic lupus erythematosus (SLE)
(E) General paresis

6. All of the following statements about alcohol abuse are true EXCEPT

(A) chronic, heavy drinkers metabolize alcohol at a rate of 30 mg/dl/hr
(B) rapid consumption of large amounts of alcohol may cause death due to respiratory arrest
(C) subdural hematomas are more common in alcoholics than in the population as a whole
(D) chronic, heavy alcohol use frequently causes dementia
(E) the duration of intoxication is typically 12 hours or less

7. A 23-year-old woman reports that she has been troubled by episodes during which she feels apprehensive and which usually occur in the morning. Her heart rate increases. She sweats excessively. Agitation and restlessness are prominent. Which of the following laboratory tests should be ordered?

(A) Measurement of serum glucose level
(B) A toxicologic screen
(C) Measurement of serum sodium level
(D) Thyroid function tests
(E) Measurement of serum ammonia level

Directions: Each question below contains four suggested answers of which **one or more** is correct. Choose the answer

A if **1, 2, and 3** are correct
B if **1 and 3** are correct
C if **2 and 4** are correct
D if **4** is correct
E if **1, 2, 3, and 4** are correct

8. A 67-year-old man is detained by the police after he has been caught exposing himself to school children. There is no past history of such behavior. Likely causes of this behavior include

(1) petit mal seizure disorder
(2) Alzheimer's disease
(3) digitalis toxicity
(4) intracranial neoplasm

9. A 16-year-old boy angrily accuses his father of spying on him and then assaults him. This is the first known episode of violent behavior on his part. At the hospital his condition fluctuates between apparent calm and extreme belligerence. Initial evaluation and treatment measures include

(1) a toxicologic screen
(2) a pentobarbital tolerance test
(3) seclusion and restraints
(4) naloxone administration

10. A 54-year-old woman has suffered a fractured hip. On the second day following surgical repair, she becomes agitated and uncooperative. On the third day, she appears to hallucinate and calls the nursing staff by the names of her children. She is febrile and tachycardiac. Causes for this behavior include

(1) alcohol withdrawal
(2) intravenous penicillin administration
(3) sepsis
(4) general anesthesia

11. Shortly after surgery for thyroid carcinoma, a 51-year-old woman becomes depressed. She complains of drowsiness and feels confused. Laboratory tests that should be ordered include measurement of

(1) serum cortisol level
(2) arterial blood gases
(3) hemoglobin level
(4) serum calcium level

Directions: The group of questions below consists of lettered choices followed by several numbered items. For each numbered item select the **one** lettered choice with which it is **most** closely associated. Each lettered choice may be used once, more than once, or not at all.

Questions 12–15

Match each sign or symptom below with the disease process with which it is most commonly associated.

(A) Frontal lobe neoplasm
(B) Occipital lobe neoplasm
(C) Temporal lobe neoplasm
(D) Parietal lobe neoplasm
(E) Pituitary neoplasm

12. Paroxysms

13. Apathy

14. Uninhibited behavior

15. Visual hallucinations

ANSWERS AND EXPLANATIONS

1. The answer is B. *(IV G 1 c)* Automobile exhaust contains carbon monoxide, and carbon monoxide poisoning produces hypoxia. Hypoxia leads to confusion, which may be transient or persistent, depending upon the degree and duration of oxygen insufficiency. Lead poisoning, hypoglycemia, and gasoline inhalation would not result from the circumstances in this case. Confusion can result from hypoglycemia, however.

2. The answer is D. *[IV F 2 w (6)]* The psychiatric findings of confusion and agitation are nonspecific. However, when considered in light of a gait disturbance and ophthalmoplegia in an individual with skin lesions that are found in chronic alcoholics, a presumptive diagnosis of Wernicke's encephalopathy can be made. Treatment with thiamine is indicated, which may reverse this patient's condition. Less fortunate patients develop Korsakoff's psychosis.

3. The answer is C. *(IV C 1–3)* Short-term memories, such as one's daily activities, register in the brain each day. Long-term memories, such as recollections from childhood, are already stored in the brain. In the initial stages of dementia, the ability to form enduring new memories is lost. Old memories persist until the later stages of the disease.

4. The answer is C. *(IV I 1)* Wilson's disease (hepatolenticular degeneration) usually presents symptomatically in the second or third decade of life. A personality change in the woman in this case is evident and is often the first sign of the disease. Transient episodes of psychosis may occur. The disease process involves the putamen and the corpus callosum, resulting in movement or muscular signs such as the dysarthria manifest here.

5. The answer is A. *(IV M 2)* This patient has experienced relapsing and remitting symptoms, a course that is characteristic for multiple sclerosis (MS). Different areas of the brain have been involved—the optic nerve, the parietal lobe, and unspecified areas related to mood. Optic nerve involvement is the most common finding in MS and would be uncommon in any of the other disease processes listed. The patient's age is also consistent with the diagnosis of MS, a disease with a peak incidence around the age of 30 years.

6. The answer is D. *(IV F 2 w)* There are many patients who present with dementia and who have a history of alcoholism. Often there is no alternative disease process that can be identified. The dementia is explained by attributing it to alcohol abuse, but no cause-and-effect relationship is established. Individuals who are severely affected with Korsakoff's psychosis are rare, and thiamine deficiency is implicated in the pathophysiology of that condition.

7. The answer is A. *(IV J 3 a)* The patient presents with an episodic disturbance that occurs at a characteristic time of day. Food intake during the day maintains the serum glucose at adequate levels but, without intake overnight, the level drops. Signs and symptoms of hypoglycemia are evident in the morning or after vigorous exercise. This syndrome could easily be mistaken for an anxiety disorder.

8. The answer is C (2, 4). *[IV A 3 b, B 1–4, D 1, 2, F 2 o (1)]* Alzheimer's disease and intracranial neoplasm may present in a variety of ways. Some patients have pronounced neurologic signs and symptoms, while others have marked changes in personality. One common change in personality is a loss of inhibitions, leading to coarse language or sexually inappropriate behavior. Petit mal seizures are brief in duration, usually lasting 5 to 30 seconds. The individual stares into space. The normal flow of thought is interrupted, and the individual experiences a disruption in consciousness. Muscular tone may decrease, or twitching may occur. No organized behavior, such as exposing oneself, would be evident. Digitalis toxicity presents a varied picture. Restlessness and apathy may be apparent. With severe toxicity, a delirious state develops. Cognitive impairment, irritability, and psychotic symptoms are observed. Although indiscreet behavior may occur, other, more pronounced, signs of disturbance will be present.

9. The answer is B (1, 3). *(III C 2; IV F 2 a, e, h)* The boy is paranoid and disturbed enough to predicate his actions on paranoid ideation. Evaluation of any episode of psychotic behavior must include consideration of organic factors. In this case drugs should be of particular concern and physical safety should be emphasized. Therefore, a toxicologic screen for drugs such as phencyclidine (PCP), cocaine, and amphetamines is indicated. Physical restraints and seclusion insure safety until diagnosis is made and specific treatment can be prescribed. A pentobarbital tolerance test is administered to assess the degree of addiction to barbiturates or other drugs in planning a withdrawal regimen. There is no evidence that this patient is an addict, and such a test could easily worsen his condition. Likewise, naloxone is administered in different circumstances: Specifically, if narcotics addiction is suspected in an unresponsive patient, naloxone can reverse the effect of the narcotic. This boy's agitation, however, is not typical of a narcotics overdose.

10. The answer is A (1, 2, 3). *[IV F 2 q (1), u (1), w (4), L 1]* The patient presents with a picture of delirium, and the fever and tachycardia may be clues to the etiology of the delirium. Certainly, a systemic infection is possible following major surgery, and sepsis often leads to delirious behavior, usually associated with a high fever. If this patient is alcoholic, she has been withdrawn suddenly. Intercurrent illnesses such as fractures and infections predispose an individual to severe alcohol withdrawal or delirium tremens. Penicillin is an antibacterial agent that has produced an acute psychosis characterized by agitation, anxiety, and hallucinations, all of which are present in this case. General anesthetic agents are volatile gases. They are excreted within hours, and an effect at 2 or 3 days is not possible.

11. The answer is D (4). *(IV K 4 b)* One complication of neck or thyroid surgery is inadvertent removal of the parathyroid glands. If this is done, the serum concentration of calcium falls, leading to the symptoms that this woman is experiencing. Although adrenal insufficiency, hypoxia, and anemia might produce similar symptoms, there is no reason to suspect any of these conditions from this history.

12–15. The answers are: 5-C, 6-A, 7-A, 8-B. *(IV A 3 c, B 2)* As does temporal lobe epilepsy, temporal lobe neoplasms cause outbursts of symptoms. Onset is sudden and unpredictable. Various affective states arise without warning, or a trance-like condition appears. Symptoms last for 2 minutes or less and then remit. The individual may not recall the paroxysm.

Frontal lobe neoplasms usually present as a gradual, insidious change in personality. A normally active and involved individual may slowly become passive. Interest in work, hobbies, and family diminishes until apathy and indifference are marked. Another personality change observed in frontal lobe disease is a loss of inhibitions. The socializing functions of the brain are carried out in the frontal lobes. People act in ways that are appropriate to social norms when these functions are intact. Neoplasms disrupt this.

The visual cortical areas of the brain are located in the occipital lobes. A neoplasm disrupts the structural integrity of these areas, which can result in misperceptions or simple visual hallucinations.

4
Substance Abuse
Steven L. Dubovsky

I. DEFINITIONS. Because they convey social disapproval and are subject to considerable cultural variation, terms such as drug abuse, addiction, and dependence require careful definition. Terms followed in this chapter by the designation *DSM III* are defined as they are in the current formal psychiatric nomenclature of the *Diagnostic and Statistical Manual of Mental Disorders,* third edition.*

A. Substance use disorders *(DSM III)* is a generic term referring to psychiatric disorders associated with regular use of substances that affect the central nervous system. The behavioral changes resulting from such disorders are generally viewed as socially undesirable.

B. Pathologic use of centrally acting substances is divided into the categories of **abuse** and **dependence** *(DSM III).*

    1. Misuse of substances must be present long enough for a pathologic pattern to be established for it to be considered **substance abuse;** sporadic excessive drug use is not technically abuse. Formal diagnosis requires that the following criteria exist for at least 1 month:
        a. Pattern of pathologic use, which may be manifested by:
            (1) Daytime intoxication
            (2) Repeated efforts to control drug use through temporary abstinence or attempted restricted use to certain times of the day
            (3) Inability to decrease or discontinue drug intake
            (4) Continued use of a substance despite the knowledge that it is worsening a physical disorder
            (5) Inability to function without daily drug intake
            (6) Complications of substance use such as blackouts, liver disease, and overdose
        b. Impairment of social or occupational functioning, as exemplified by:
            (1) Legal problems
            (2) Failure to meet important obligations
            (3) Missed work or inability to keep a job
            (4) Disruption of the family
            (5) Inappropriate fighting

    2. The term **dependence** denotes here **physiologic dependence,** which is characterized by the presence of **tolerance** and **withdrawal.** Dependence usually develops in individuals with a pathologic pattern of use and its social consequences, but it may occasionally occur in individuals who have not exhibited a pathologic pattern, as in the case of a patient who becomes dependent on a narcotic during the treatment of a medical illness.
        a. Tolerance has developed when the same dose of the substance produces a decreased effect or when increasing doses are necessary to produce the same effect.
        b. Withdrawal refers to the development of an **abstinence syndrome,** which is specific to the substance in use when it is withdrawn or the dosage is decreased.

C. Addiction is a term used by many researchers to refer to overwhelming involvement with seeking and using drugs or alcohol and a high tendency to relapse after withdrawal. It is therefore a quantitative description of the degree to which drug use pervades an individual's life rather than a condition that can be clearly defined. Insofar as **total preoccupation with a drug is a severe**

---

*American Psychiatric Association: *Diagnostic and Statistical Manual of Mental Disorders,* 3rd ed. Washington, D.C., American Psychiatric Association, 1980.

pattern of pathologic use, addiction may be said to be a form of substance abuse as defined in section I B. While some practitioners feel that all addicted individuals are physically dependent, many authorities state that it is possible to be drug-dependent and not be addicted in that one's life is not organized around finding and using the drug. Conversely, it may be possible to be addicted in the sense that drug-seeking behavior is paramount in an individual's life without that individual being physically dependent.

II. INTOXICATION SYNDROMES. Since the manifestations and treatment of the intoxication syndromes produced by different drugs vary drastically, it is crucial to be able to recognize the symptoms of intoxication produced by the commonly abused prescription and nonprescription drugs.

A. **Alcohol** is frequently combined with other substances. The odor on the patient's breath that is characteristically associated with alcohol intoxication is caused by impurities in the preparation used and is extremely unreliable in diagnosing intoxication. In addition, head injuries and metabolic encephalopathies are not infrequently mistaken for alcohol intoxication. Blood and urine screens are reliable means of diagnosis.

1. **Mild intoxication** is characterized by disorganization of cognitive and motor processes. The first functions to be disrupted are those that depend on training and previous experience. Central nervous system concentrations of alcohol parallel its concentrations in the blood. As intoxication becomes more noticeable, the following changes occur.
    a. **Overconfidence.** Only if performance is initially impaired by psychological inhibitions may an individual function more effectively after ingestion of small amounts of alcohol. Otherwise studies show that all aspects of physical and mental performance are decreased by alcohol. Nevertheless, the intoxicated individual tends to feel more efficient.
    b. **Mood swings,** emotional outbursts, and euphoria may occur.
    c. There may be **initial enhancement of spinal reflexes** as they are released from higher inhibiting circuits, followed by progressive general anesthesia of central nervous system functions.
    d. In addition to an **increased pain threshold** while other sensory modalities are unaffected, there may be distress in response to pain.
    e. Nausea, vomiting, restlessness, and hyperactivity may be present.

2. **Severe intoxication** is characterized by:
    a. Stupor or coma
    b. Hypothermia
    c. Slow, noisy respiration
    d. Tachycardia
    e. Dilated pupils (may be normal in some intoxicated individuals)
    f. Increased intracranial pressure
    g. Death (rare in the absence of ingestion of additional drugs, trauma, infection, or unconsciousness lasting longer than 12 hours)

3. **Treatment** depends on whether or not the patient is conscious.
    a. Nothing really needs to be done for the **conscious patient** beyond waiting for the alcohol to be metabolized. Stimulants and caffeine do not hasten sobriety. If the patient is very restless or agitated, restraint is safer than administration of tranquilizers or sedatives, which may potentiate the central nervous system depressant effects of alcohol. Antipsychotic drugs such as haloperidol in low doses may decrease hyperactivity without increasing sedation.
    b. The **stuporous or unconscious patient** should be kept warm. Care should be taken to prevent aspiration, especially if gastric lavage is performed. In addition to the normal management of overdoses of central nervous system depressants, it may be necessary to treat increased intracranial pressure with mannitol or by other measures. Alcohol can be removed by hemodialysis in extreme situations.

B. **Central nervous system depressants other than alcohol** include benzodiazepine tranquilizers (e.g., diazepam, oxazepam, chlordiazepoxide, lorazepam, prazepam, chlorazepate, and alprazolam), benzodiazepine hypnotics [sleeping pills] (e.g., flurazepam, temazepam, and triazolam), barbiturates (e.g., phenobarbital, amobarbital, pentobarbital, and secobarbital), chloral compounds (e.g., chloral hydrate), and drugs related to barbiturates (e.g., ethchlorvynol, glutethimide, meprobamate, methaqualone, methyprylon, and paraldehyde). Because they tend to produce abuse, tolerance, and dangerous abstinence syndromes, they are not as effective as benzodiazepines, and because they are lethal when taken in overdose, barbiturates and related compounds should not be used routinely as hypnotics or tranquilizers.

1. **Mild-to-moderate intoxication** with barbiturates and related compounds and benzodiazepines causes:
   a. Euphoria
   b. Hyperalgesia (increased pain perception)
   c. Increased seizure threshold
   d. Sedation or paradoxical excitement in susceptible individuals in certain circumstances, in children, and in the presence of organic brain disease
   e. Nystagmus, dysarthria, and ataxia
   f. Postural hypotension

2. Most cases of **severe poisoning** are due to purposeful overdoses in suicide attempts and accidental overdoses by addicts. A few patients, especially those with preexisting brain disease, may take too much medication because of drug automatism (i.e., confusion that is worsened by the drug), which results in the patient not remembering how much has been taken and continuing to take more pills, usually in an effort to get to sleep.
   a. **Severe intoxication** can cause:
      (1) Stupor and coma
      (2) Respiratory depression
      (3) Depressed reflexes
      (4) Hypotension
      (5) Decreased cardiac output
      (6) Hypoxemia
      (7) Bullous skin lesions and necrosis of sweat glands
      (8) Hypothermia
   b. **Death** from barbiturate intoxication is usually due to complications such as pneumonia and renal failure. Short-acting preparations such as amobarbital are more lethal at lower doses than long-acting compounds such as phenobarbital. Death from an overdose of benzodiazepines alone is extremely rare.

3. **Treatment** of central nervous system depressant intoxication involves emesis if the ingestion has occurred within ½ hour of admission and the gag reflex is intact; it involves gastric lavage if these conditions have not been fulfilled. A cathartic should then be given to decrease intestinal absorption of the drug. For severe poisoning, the following steps are taken:
   a. Protection of the airway
   b. Oxygen administration
   c. Ventilation when necessary
   d. Prevention of further loss of body heat
   e. Correction of hypovolemia and maintenance of blood pressure with dopamine
   f. Forced diuresis with **maximal** alkalinization of the urine
   g. Hemodialysis

C. **Central nervous system stimulants** include amphetamines, methylphenidate, cocaine, phenmetrazine, phenylpropanolamine, and many antiobesity drugs. Medical indications for their use include hyperactivity in children, severe nosebleeds, depression in elderly and medically ill patients, and possibly as short-term adjuncts in the management of obesity. Stimulants commonly cause tolerance and abuse.

1. **Mild-to-moderate intoxication** produces:
   a. Elevated mood
   b. Increased energy and alertness
   c. Decreased appetite
   d. Talkativeness
   e. Anxiety and irritability
   f. Insomnia
   g. Increased ability to perform repetitive tasks when the individual is tired or bored
   h. Hypertension in susceptible individuals
   i. Tachycardia
   j. Hyperthermia

2. **Severe intoxication** may produce a toxic psychosis. Although tolerance develops to many of the effects of stimulants, there is no tolerance to the tendency to develop psychotic symptoms, which may be indistinguishable from those of schizophrenia. Signs and symptoms include:
   a. Visual, auditory, and tactile hallucinations
   b. Delusions, especially of being infested with parasites
   c. Paranoia and loose associations in a clear sensorium
   d. Dilated pupils
   e. Elevated blood pressure and pulse (may be normal in some chronic abusers)

> **f.** Arrhythmias
> **g.** Seizures
> **h.** Exhaustion
> **i.** Coma (may occur in very severe cases)
> **j.** Intracranial hemorrhage (has been reported)

3. Treatment of psychotic symptoms is with haloperidol, which antagonizes the dopaminergic properties of stimulants. Hypertension and hyperthermia can be treated with phentolamine.

D. Hallucinogens and cannabis substances include lysergic acid diethylamide (LSD), psilocybin, mescaline, phencyclidine (PCP), 2,5-dimethoxy-4 methylamphetamine (STP), marijuana, hashish, and Δ^9-tetrahydrocannabinol (THC).

1. Results of **intoxication** depend on the substance.
   a. Most **hallucinogen** intoxication produces dilated pupils, increased heart rate and blood pressure, increased temperature, paranoia in a clear sensorium, illusions, hallucinations, depersonalization, anxiety, distortion of time sense, and inappropriate affect.
   b. **PCP** intoxication can also cause violent behavior, extreme hyperactivity, coma, mutism, analgesia, nystagmus, ataxia, and, rarely, intracranial hemorrhage.
   c. **Intoxication by marijuana and related substances** rarely produces hallucinations. More common are euphoria, anxiety, increased appetite, increased suggestibility, distortion of time and space, injected conjunctivae, and no change in pupils.

2. Treatment of intoxication and ''bad trips'' also depends on the substance.
   a. The psychological effects of the cannabis group of drugs and most hallucinogens are usually decreased by ''talking down'' (reassurance in a quiet setting). Oral administration of diazepam is sometimes a useful adjunct.
   b. Patients intoxicated with PCP may react violently to any environmental stimulation, including attempts at reassurance. They generally should be left alone in a quiet area. If they become violent, they may be sedated with intravenously administered haloperidol or diazepam. Seizures should be treated with intravenous administration of diazepam.

E. Narcotics include morphine, heroin, hydromorphone, oxymorphone, levorphanol, codeine, hydrocodone, oxycodone, methadone, meperidine, alphaprodine, and propoxyphene. Pentazocine has both narcotic antagonist and agonist properties. Many street preparations are adulterated with quinine, procaine, lidocaine, lactose, or mannitol or are contaminated with bacteria, viruses, or fungi.

1. Mild-to-moderate intoxication may produce:
   a. Analgesia without loss of consciousness
   b. Drowsiness and mental clouding
   c. Nausea and vomiting
   d. Apathy and lethargy
   e. Euphoria
   f. Itching
   g. Constricted pupils
   h. Constipation
   i. Flushed, warm skin due to cutaneous vasodilation

2. Severe intoxication is associated with:
   a. Miosis
   b. Respiratory depression
   c. Hypotension or shock
   d. Depressed reflexes
   e. Coma
   f. Pulmonary edema
   g. Seizures (may occur with propoxyphene or meperidine)

3. Treatment of severe intoxication is primarily supportive. Naloxone, a narcotic antagonist, can reverse coma and apnea; however, the effects of concomitantly self-administered drugs such as barbiturates are not altered, and detoxification from these drugs should also be undertaken if they are present. Naloxone may precipitate a severe abstinence syndrome in narcotic-dependent patients. It also frequently causes vomiting. Respiratory depression may recur up to 24 hours after apparent recovery from overdose with most narcotics and up to 72 hours after apparent recovery from methadone overdose.

F. Anticholinergic drugs include most over-the-counter cold and sleeping preparations, atropine, belladonna, henbane, scopolamine, antiparkinsonian drugs (trihexyphenidyl and benztropine), tricyclic antidepressants, some neuroleptics (especially thioridazine), jimsonweed, mandrake, and propantheline. Some anticholinergic substances grow wild, and some are included in various herbal medications.

1. **Intoxication** may produce:
   a. Confusion
   b. Delirium
   c. Hallucinations
   d. Amnesia
   e. Body image distortions
   f. Drowsiness or coma
   g. Tachycardia
   h. Decreased bowel sounds
   i. Fever
   j. Warm, dry skin
   k. Fixed, dilated pupils

2. **Treatment** is primarily directed toward protecting the patient and waiting for the drug to be metabolized. Intravenous administration of physostigmine can temporarily reverse coma or severe hyperpyrexia but should be used cautiously because of serious side effects, including vomiting.

III. ABSTINENCE SYNDROMES are substance-specific, physiologically determined syndromes that appear after abrupt withdrawal or decrease in dosage of the drug. Withdrawal from some compounds produces mild syndromes, withdrawal from others produces phenomena that are uncomfortable but not dangerous, and from a few substances life-threatening abstinence syndromes result. Blood levels are often zero in abstinence syndromes.

A. **Several alcohol abstinence syndromes** have been described.

1. **Alcohol withdrawal** *[DSM III]* (''**the shakes**'') usually appears within a few hours of stopping or decreasing alcohol consumption and lasts for 3 to 4 days and occasionally as long as 1 week.
   a. **Signs and symptoms** include:
      (1) Tachycardia
      (2) Tremulousness
      (3) Diaphoresis
      (4) Nausea
      (5) Orthostatic hypotension
      (6) Malaise or weakness
   b. **Treatment** involves tapering doses of a benzodiazepine such as chlorazepate beginning with a 60-mg divided dose on the first day, a 30-mg divided dose on the second day, a 15-mg divided dose on the third day, and none on the fourth day. Thiamine is usually administered parenterally at 100 mg/day for 3 days.

2. **Major motor seizures** (''**rum fits**'') occur during the first 48 hours of withdrawal in a small percentage of cases of alcohol withdrawal. Treatment is by means of intravenous administration of diazepam. Phenytoin is not administered unless the patient is an epileptic.

3. **Alcohol withdrawal delirium** *[DSM III]* (**delirium tremens**) begins on the second or third day, rarely later than 1 week, after withdrawal or decrease in intake of alcohol. It occurs in fewer than 5% of alcohol-dependent patients, usually after they have been drinking heavily for 5 to 15 years. If seizures occur too, they always precede the development of delirium. With appropriate treatment, mortality is extremely rare.
   a. **Manifestations** of delirium tremens include:
      (1) Delirium
      (2) Autonomic hyperactivity (increased pulse rate and blood pressure and sweating)
      (3) Agitation
      (4) Vivid hallucinations
      (5) Gross tremulousness
   b. **Treatment** involves hydration, parenteral administration of thiamine for 3 to 4 days, and a benzodiazepine (e.g., chlordiazepoxide) administered in a divided dose (i.e., 200 mg to 400 mg/day). In cases of severe agitation or psychosis, a neuroleptic such as haloperidol is given.

4. **Alcohol hallucinosis** *(DSM III)* is a rare condition that develops within 48 hours of cessation of drinking or at the end of a long binge with gradual decreases in blood levels.
   a. The **principal manifestation** is vivid auditory hallucinations without gross confusion.

Usually, the patient hears threatening or derogatory voices that discuss the patient in the third person or speak directly to him or her but never tell him or her what to do (i.e., command hallucinations are absent). Symptoms usually last a few hours or days but persist for weeks or months in about 10% of cases. Very occasionally, the syndrome may become chronic, in which case it may be indistinguishable from schizophrenia.

    b. Treatment. Neuroleptics may relieve agitation and hallucinations in patients who do not improve spontaneously.

B. Withdrawal from barbiturates, benzodiazepines, and related tranquilizers and sleeping pills produces syndromes that are similar in symptomatology but not in time of onset and duration to alcohol withdrawal. Abstinence syndromes are likely to occur after chronic use of 400 mg to 600 mg/day of pentobarbital, 3200 mg to 6400 mg/day of meprobamate, and 40 mg to 60 mg/day of diazepam or their equivalents. Withdrawal syndromes, which are usually less severe, have appeared in individuals taking lower doses for long periods of time.

    1. Symptoms usually begin within 12 to 24 hours, peak at 4 to 7 days, and last about 1 week after withdrawal from short-acting barbiturates. Withdrawal from longer-acting barbiturates and benzodiazepines begins later (i.e., 4 to 10 days after drug discontinuation) and reaches its peak more slowly (i.e., around the seventh day). Signs and symptoms include:

        a. Anxiety and agitation
        b. Orthostatic hypotension
        c. Weakness and tremulousness
        d. Hyperreflexia and clonic blink reflex
        e. Fever
        f. Diaphoresis
        g. Delirium (appears on the fourth to seventh day as the syndrome peaks)
        h. Seizures (may appear as late as the seventh day with withdrawal from short-acting barbiturates; later with long-acting preparations)
        i. Cardiovascular collapse

    2. Treatment. Withdrawal from central nervous system depressants can be life-threatening, and **treatment is mandatory** whenever the syndrome is suspected. Even if the patient seems only mildly anxious, he or she **must be hospitalized** to ensure adequate coverage if the condition worsens and to ensure compliance with the treatment protocol. A known compound (pentobarbital or phenobarbital) is substituted for the offending substance and is gradually withdrawn to suppress the abstinence syndrome. Treatment is not as effective if it is initiated after the appearance of delirium.

        a. Since all central nervous system depressants produce **cross-tolerance,** the amount of barbiturate or related compound to which the patient is tolerant can be calculated by administering 200 mg of pentobarbital or 60 mg to 100 mg of phenobarbital when the patient no longer appears to be intoxicated (usually within 12 to 16 hours after discontinuation of the offending substance).

            (1) If the patient becomes severely intoxicated or falls asleep with the test dose, he or she is not tolerant and does not need further treatment.

            (2) If the patient develops moderate symptoms after the test dose (e.g., dysarthria, nystagmus, and ataxia without sleepiness) he or she is moderately tolerant and requires 200 mg to 300 mg of pentobarbital or 60 mg to 90 mg of phenobarbital per day.

            (3) Absence of symptoms, or nystagmus without other signs of intoxication in response to the test dose, indicates significant tolerance. The patient should then be administered a total daily (divided) dose of 400 mg to 500 mg of pentobarbital or 150 mg to 180 mg of phenobarbital every 6 hours to suppress withdrawal.

            (4) Tolerance may also be tested by giving successive 60-mg to 100-mg doses of phenobarbital every 1 to 4 hours until the patient is intoxicated. The amount necessary to produce definite signs of intoxication, or a maximum of 500 mg/day, should then be administered in a divided dose every 6 hours to suppress the abstinence syndrome.

        b. Once the patient is stabilized, the dose of pentobarbital is decreased by 10% every 1 to 2 days. Phenobarbital, which is longer acting, may be withdrawn more quickly. Reappearance of abstinence phenomena indicates that the dose needs to be reduced more gradually.

        c. Since cross-tolerance exists between barbiturates and alcohol, phenobarbital or pentobarbital can also be used to suppress alcohol abstinence syndromes.

C. Stimulant withdrawal can produce increased sleep, nightmares due to rapid eye movement (REM) rebound, fatigue, lassitude, increased appetite, and depression, which may be severe. There is no observable physiologic disruption, however, and gradual withdrawal is not necessary. Imipramine is indicated for withdrawal depression (which is also called the "cocaine blues"); hospitalization may be necessary if the patient is suicidal.

D. Cessation of hallucinogens does not produce a significant abstinence syndrome. Flashbacks (brief reexperiences of the hallucinogenic state) may be precipitated by marijuana or antihistamine intake. Reassurance that symptoms will subside and administration of a benzodiazepine are usually sufficient therapy.

E. Narcotic withdrawal is not life-threatening; however, it may be extremely uncomfortable.

1. Symptoms usually appear 8 to 10 hours after cessation of morphine. The onset is slower when longer-acting drugs such as methadone have been used. Symptoms peak at 48 to 72 hours and disappear in 7 to 10 days. Disturbances include:

   a. Lacrimation and rhinorrhea
   b. Yawning and sweating
   c. Restlessness and sleepiness
   d. Gooseflesh
   e. Dilated pupils
   f. Irritability
   g. Violent yawning
   h. Insomnia
   i. Coryza

2. Treatment. Narcotic withdrawal is ameliorated by methadone substitution. When the patient demonstrates objective signs of withdrawal, a sufficient dose of methadone to suppress abstinence or a maximum dose of 20 mg to 50 mg/day is administered. The dose of methadone is then decreased by 10% to 20%/day. Clonidine, administered at 0.1 mg to 0.3 mg three times per day for 2 weeks may help to suppress withdrawal symptoms, although it may cause hypotension. Clonidine should be tapered rather than abruptly discontinued.

F. Anticholinergic drugs occasionally produce mania or seizures when they are withdrawn abruptly. Discontinuation of clinically significant doses taken for more than 1 month should therefore be gradual.

IV. ALCOHOLISM affects as much as 10% of the population. Alcohol abuse or dependence usually develops during the first 5 years of regular use of alcohol.

A. Three principal patterns of chronic alcohol abuse have been described:

1. Regular daily excessive drinking

2. Regular heavy drinking on weekends only

3. Long periods of sobriety interspersed with binges that last weeks or months

B. Genetic influences seem to play a role in the development of alcoholism, and a family history of alcoholism is a definite risk factor. In addition, individuals with a family history of teetotalism or who have an alcoholic spouse are at increased risk of being alcoholic.

C. Diagnostic clues to alcoholism include:

1. Inability to decrease or discontinue drinking

2. Binges lasting at least 2 days

3. Occasional consumption of a fifth of spirits or the equivalent in wine or beer

4. Blackouts (transient amnesia for events that occur while the patient is intoxicated)

5. Continued drinking despite a physical illness that is exacerbated or caused by drinking

6. Drinking a nonbeverage alcohol (e.g., shaving lotion)

7. Drinking in the morning

8. Abstinence syndromes

9. Apparent sobriety in the presence of an elevated alcohol level in the blood (which indicates tolerance to the sedative effects of alcohol)

D. Physical and psychiatric complications of alcoholism may develop.

1. Physical complications, which may be caused by associated nutritional deficiencies or by a direct toxic effect of alcohol, are not uncommon in patients who drink more than 3 oz to 6 oz of whiskey per day or the equivalent. More familiar syndromes include:
   a. Cerebral atrophy

   b. Wernicke's encephalopathy
   c. Korsakoff's psychosis
   d. Nicotinic acid deficiency encephalopathy
   e. Polyneuropathy
   f. Cardiomyopathy
   g. Hypertension
   h. Skeletal muscle damage of uncertain clinical significance
   i. Gastritis
   j. Peptic ulcer
   k. Constipation
   l. Pancreatitis
   m. Cirrhosis
   n. Impotence
   o. Various anemias
   p. Teratogenicity. (The fetal alcohol syndrome of mental retardation, microcephaly, slowed growth, and facial abnormalities may be a risk even if alcohol is consumed in only moderate amounts during pregnancy. Since safe quantities have not been established, abstention from all alcohol during pregnancy is most prudent. If the patient does drink, she should do so on a full stomach to minimize rapid rises in blood levels.)

2. Psychiatric complications
   a. Seventy-five percent of alcoholics have no other primary psychiatric diagnoses, although they may become depressed after withdrawing from alcohol when they realize that they have caused serious problems for themselves. Major depressive syndromes may also be caused by alcohol. **The major psychiatric complication of alcoholism is suicide:** more than 80% of individuals who kill themselves are depressed, alcoholic, or both.
   b. Alcoholism may be an attempt at self-treatment of another psychiatric disorder—usually depression, anxiety, or psychosis. This may be a possibility if psychiatric symptoms clearly preceded heavy drinking. However, the history is often undependable, and only a trial period of abstinence reliably distinguishes between primary alcoholism and alcohol abuse that is secondary to another condition. If psychological distress resolves after a period of abstinence, alcoholism is likely to have been a cause rather than a result of the psychiatric disorder.

E. Specific treatment approaches are geared toward the patient's preferences. In all therapeutic modalities about one-third of patients remain sober, one-third enjoy a period of sobriety followed by relapse, and one-third continue drinking. Useful interventions include the following.

   1. Confrontation of denial. The major obstacles to therapeutic success are the patient's denial of the severity of the problem and his or her wish to continue drinking. Repeated statements that the patient is not in control of the drinking and repeated confrontation with the complications of the alcoholism may be necessary before the patient will agree to treatment.

   2. Insistence on abstinence. Since it is not possible to identify in advance the very few patients who may be able to succeed with controlled drinking, total abstinence is the only realistic goal.

   3. Assessment of motivation. The patient who is willing to consider abstaining completely for at least 1 month is usually sufficiently motivated to give up alcohol completely. If the patient insists on some continued alcohol intake (usually with the assurance that he or she will be able to keep from drinking excessively), it is unlikely that the patient will be able to control his or her intake. Further therapeutic efforts may be unsuccessful until the patient is willing to attempt to give up alcohol completely for at least a brief period of time.

   4. Disulfiram (Antabuse). Most alcoholics' efforts at abstinence are supported by disulfiram, which causes severe nausea and vomiting when it interacts with alcohol. Even if the patient does not need the drug, his or her willingness to take it is a favorable prognostic sign. The only contraindications to the use of disulfiram are organic brain syndromes or other conditions that might interfere significantly with compliance. The usual dose is 500 mg at bedtime for 5 days followed by 250 mg at bedtime for at least 6 months. Vitamin C and antihistamines may abort the alcohol-disulfiram reaction.

   5. Involvement of family. The patient's family can be an important source of support, or they may openly or covertly encourage the patient to go on drinking. Occasionally, a statement by a spouse that he or she will not remain with the patient unless the patient stops drinking is the only force strong enough to convince the patient to agree to a trial of abstinence. Such threats should be mobilized only rarely and only when they are a true expression of the involved individual's feelings. Employers and other important individuals in the patient's life should also be involved in treatment whenever possible.

6. **Referral to specialized services.** Alcoholics Anonymous is the most effective treatment for patients who prefer a spiritual therapeutic approach. Other counseling programs also provide peer support and encouragement for the patient to stop drinking. Behavior therapy, which consists primarily of punishing drinking and rewarding sobriety, is useful to patients who consider their drinking a bad habit. Psychotherapy is appropriate for patients who feel that their drinking is motivated by unresolved emotional conflicts.

7. **Ongoing emotional support by the primary physician** is probably the most important factor in helping the patient to confront the problem and to maintain sobriety. The physician should accept periodic relapses in a nonjudgmental manner. If the patient refuses specific therapy for alcoholism, the physician should continue to be available to the drinking patient in case a psychosocial crisis precipitates a wish to become involved in treatment.

V. **NARCOTIC (OPIOID) ABUSE** is a major public health problem. The incidence of heroin use increased during the 1960s, and use of this substance is now a problem in smaller communities in the United States as well as in the large cities.

A. **Epidemiology** of narcotic, particularly heroin, use is important and deserves careful consideration. Two to three percent of adults aged 18 to 25 years have tried heroin at some time in their lives; additionally, abuse of narcotics usually occurs in the context of abuse of other drugs. Technically, narcotic abuse is a disorder lasting at least 1 month. It is characterized by a pathologic pattern of use (e.g., intoxication throughout the day, opioid use nearly every day, inability to decrease use, and episodes of overdose) and by impairment of social and occupational functioning. About 50% of the individuals who abuse narcotics become physically dependent on the drugs. Most addicts tend to abstain increasingly with time. They often finally discontinue drug dependence about 9 years after its onset.

1. **Patterns of narcotic abuse vary widely.** Some addicts, particularly those who are maintained on methadone, lead productive lives and enjoy good health. The need to obtain illicit drugs increases the incidence of prostitution and other crimes in order to support addiction; however, the behavior of the individual, once he or she is a narcotic abuser, is at least partially determined by his or her behavior and personality prior to drug use. The patient who develops an antisocial life-style as a result of drug abuse can be distinguished reliably from the antisocial patient who also abuses narcotics only after withdrawal and a period of abstinence, usually in a different environment. Because of physical complications of abuse and a life-style associated with violence, the death rate is much higher in addicts (10 per 1000) than it is in the general population. Patterns of narcotic use and dependence are as follows.
   a. A very **small percentage** of the addicted population **becomes dependent in the course of medical treatment.** If these individuals continue to receive narcotics from the physician, they are less likely to encounter the problems faced by other dependent individuals, who must obtain the drugs illicitly.
   b. More commonly, narcotic abuse develops when an adolescent or young adult who is engaged in experimental or recreational drug use progresses to more intensive use. Since 60% to 90% of adolescents experiment to some extent with drugs (and experimentation with drugs has been reported in children as young as 5 years of age), the number who actually develop a major drug abuse problem is not great. Problems are more likely to develop with use of central nervous system stimulants and depressants. Two determining factors appear to be the **context in which drug use takes place** and the **psychopathology of the abuser.**
   c. A significant number of individuals who have become dependent on narcotics now are receiving **methadone from organized treatment programs.**
   d. The incidence of narcotic addiction is much higher in physicians, nurses, and other health-care personnel than in any other group of individuals with comparable education and socioeconomic class. Most physician-addicts initially use a narcotic to relieve depression, fatigue, or a physical ailment rather than for pleasure. However, with the exception that they are more likely to make drugs available to themselves through prescriptions and through use of narcotics ordered for patients in hospitals, the pattern and consequences of the addiction are no different than they are for other addicts, even though the personality characteristics of health-care personnel (and probably of medical patients) who develop narcotic abuse are probably different from those of the urban heroin addict.

2. **Heroin abuse tends to be transmitted in an epidemic fashion** among individuals who know each other. These epidemics begin slowly, peak rapidly, and then decline quickly. They tend to abate completely after 5 to 6 years.

a. Populations at risk have varying susceptibilities to heroin addiction. Young black males are at highest risk, and women seem to be at lowest risk.

b. Abuse is initiated in a susceptible individual by someone personally known to him or her who is already addicted. The risk of such initiators exposing their acquaintances to heroin abuse continues for about 1 year. Drug "pushers" actually cause few new cases of dependence, although they obviously are a major source of the drug.

c. Heroin abuse tends to spread until all susceptible individuals within a given group have been exposed. New addicts then tend to expose their friends in other circles, who produce a third generation of abusers.

3. When **cultural norms support heroin use** and relatively pure preparations are available, a large percentage of users become dependent.

a. For example, more than 40% of the United States Army enlisted men stationed in Vietnam reported trying narcotics at least once, and about one-half of these became physically dependent at some time during their stay in Vietnam.

b. Very few individuals who became dependent on narcotics in Vietnam continued drug abuse when they returned to the United States, suggesting that removal of peer group support for drug abuse, removal of the easy availability of drugs, and, possibly, removal of major environmental stresses leading to intense anxiety ended the reasons for continued abuse.

c. Most individuals in this country who become dependent on narcotics tend to remain in a peer group that encourages abuse and tend to be psychologically predisposed to develop abuse. The majority of these individuals develop a chronic behavioral disorder that may remit when access to the drug is denied but has a high tendency to relapse when the individuals return to an environment in which drugs are available and friends and colleagues condone abuse.

4. Up to 50% of drug abusers suffer from another psychiatric illness, especially depression, anxiety states, and borderline and antisocial personality disorders. Individuals from disorganized social backgrounds are also more susceptible to abuse. A combination of a susceptible psychosocial constellation, availability of narcotics, an environment that encourages abuse, and friends or colleagues who already are users may be necessary for the development of addiction.

B. Medical complications of narcotic abuse may result from contaminants of illicit preparations and the patient's life-style.

1. Female drug abusers have a high incidence of **venereal disease** because of the need to engage in prostitution to obtain the narcotic.

2. Fatal overdose due to fluctuations in the purity of available compounds is not uncommon.

3. Intravenous injection of some impurities may cause **anaphylactic reactions.**

4. Hypersensitivity reactions to impurities may also cause the **formation of granulomata** and neurologic, musculoskeletal, and cutaneous lesions.

5. Infections commonly caused by contaminated products and shared needles include hepatitis, endocarditis, septicemia, tetanus, and formation of pulmonary, cerebral, and subcutaneous abscesses.

6. Suicide and death at the hands of associates are more common in narcotic abusers than in the general population.

C. Treatment of narcotic abuse requires a multidisciplinary approach.

1. If the patient has strong psychosocial supports available and is highly motivated to discontinue drug use, he or she can be **withdrawn immediately using methadone** (see section III E 2).

2. If supports are weak or motivation to undergo withdrawal is uncertain, a period of **methadone maintenance** is instituted to strengthen supports, motivation, and the relationship with the treatment team. The usual dose of methadone is this setting is 40 mg to 80 mg/day.

a. Although methadone can be prescribed for acute or chronic pain by any appropriately licensed physician, methadone maintenance for the treatment of addiction can only be carried out by a federally approved program. Methadone maintenance is only permissible if the patient has clearcut signs of addiction, such as intoxication, needle tracks, and medical or psychosocial consequences of abuse.

b. Periodic unscheduled urine and blood screens are performed to test compliance with the program. Persistent noncompliance (i.e., continued self-administration of narcotics) results in dismissal.

   c. Very gradual withdrawal from methadone is attempted when the patient seems ready. Most addicts note some abstinence symptoms when the dosage is reduced below 20 mg/day, and reduction in dosage by as little as 1 mg/week below this level may be necessary for the treatment of long-term methadone users.

  3. *l*-Alpha-acetylmethadol (LAAM), also known as methadyl acetate, a long-acting preparation, suppresses narcotic withdrawal for 72 hours. When it is used instead of methadone for maintenance, less frequent administration of the drug is necessary. Compliance does not seem to be influenced significantly if the patient visits the drug maintenance center less frequently.

  4. Therapeutic communities play an important role in the treatment of narcotic addiction. Confrontation by fellow addicts has more credibility to an addict than therapies that are administered by professionals.

  5. If outpatient therapy is not successful, **residential treatment** is necessary to remove the patient from easy access to the drug and from associates who encourage continued abuse. Group confrontation and support are utilized extensively in these settings. Compliance with treatment is higher when it is mandated by the courts than when it is voluntary and the patient is free to withdraw at any time.

  6. Narcotic-abusing physicians increasingly are being identified by state licensing bodies and medical societies. Treatment programs have been extremely successful when the problem is identified early and when continued licensure for medical practice is made contingent on ongoing treatment and surveillance.

D. Since **very few addicts are created in a medical setting,** it is extremely important that health-care providers not permit fears of addiction from interfering with the administration of appropriate doses of narcotics to patients in pain. The following guidelines apply.

  1. Adequate doses of narcotics should be administered to patients with bona fide pain syndromes. Addicts generally require higher doses than other patients.

  2. Narcotics should be administered regularly rather than on an as-needed basis. This approach prevents the patients from becoming preoccupied with pain and its relief and provides a constant blood level that results in lower individual doses being necessary.

  3. An addict should not be withdrawn when he or she is physically ill.

  4. Prescriptions should not be written for outpatients with suspicious complaints or those with a high abuse potential, as indicated by:
    a. Losing prescriptions or running out of medication early
    b. Requests for a specific drug
    c. History of abuse of alcohol or other drugs
    d. Physician shopping
    e. Claims that a physician who originally wrote a prescription is unavailable
    f. Threats when narcotics are not prescribed
    g. Dishonesty with the physician for any reason

VI. ABUSE OF TRANQUILIZERS AND SLEEPING PILLS, unlike problems with other centrally acting drugs, may be created or encouraged in everyday medical practice.

A. Barbiturates and related compounds are particularly prone to abuse. Benzodiazepines are more effective and less habituating than barbiturates. While they may relieve anxiety or insomnia temporarily, tolerance quickly develops to the antianxiety or sedative effects of the latter drugs. The diagnosis may only first be suspected when an abstinence syndrome that responds to phenobarbital or pentobarbital appears in a patient who is admitted to the hospital and is denied access to the abused substance.

  1. Because they suppress REM sleep, barbiturates and related sedatives such as secobarbital, glutethimide, and ethchlorvynol subject the patient who uses them to a rebound of REM sleep, usually in the form of nightmares, when the drug is discontinued. Although it seems to the patient that he or she cannot sleep without the drug, within a few weeks, continued drug use serves only to prevent withdrawal and suppress REM rebound, and escalating doses often are needed to accomplish this result.

  2. When barbiturates and related compounds are used as tranquilizers, drug withdrawal tends to be mistaken for a return of anxiety, occasioning an increase in dosage to suppress the symptoms. Fear of withdrawal symptoms then leads to continued drug use and inability to function without the drug as well as other manifestations of abuse.

3. Sedative abuse often complicates abuse of other substances.

B. Abuse of sedatives and tranquilizers can be minimized if barbiturates are not prescribed routinely for insomnia and anxiety and benzodiazepines are not prescribed for patients with a high abuse potential. **Identification and management of abuse** are facilitated by the following.

1. A detailed history of amounts and kinds of all prescription and nonprescription drugs that have ever been taken should be obtained. Often the patient continues to take drugs that were prescribed by a physician that he or she is no longer seeing.

2. Prescriptions for a patient who has terminated treatment must be discontinued.

3. Drug screens in patients who abuse any drug should be performed to identify mixed abuse. Drugs will not be present in the blood of a patient who is experiencing an abstinence syndrome.

4. Regular appointments should be scheduled for the patient who has been taking barbiturates for years and who is reluctant to discontinue them. When the patient is assured of an ongoing relationship with a physician whom he or she trusts, he or she may be willing to taper drug intake gradually.

5. All patients who agree to be detoxified should be hospitalized. This permits adequate treatment of what may be a life-threatening withdrawal and ensures compliance with the withdrawal protocol.

STUDY QUESTIONS

Directions: Each question below contains five suggested answers. Choose the **one best** response to each question.

1. None of the following drugs should be administered to patients who are intoxicated with alcohol EXCEPT

(A) diazepam
(B) phenobarbital
(C) disulfiram
(D) glutethimide
(E) haloperidol

2. An overdose of narcotics causes all of the following abnormalities EXCEPT

(A) dilated pupils
(B) hypotension
(C) depressed reflexes
(D) coma
(E) respiratory depression

3. Amphetamine psychosis is characterized by all of the following EXCEPT

(A) mania
(B) loose associations
(C) clear sensorium
(D) tactile hallucinations
(E) paranoia

4. Treatment of alcohol abstinence syndromes may utilize all of the following regimens EXCEPT

(A) thiamine supplementation
(B) benzodiazepine administration
(C) caffeine ingestion
(D) intravenous hydration
(E) neuroleptic administration

5. Which of the following abnormalities is a manifestation of barbiturate intoxication but not of barbiturate withdrawal?

(A) Confusion
(B) Nystagmus
(C) Postural hypotension
(D) Disorientation
(E) Agitation

6. What is the **most** effective treatment of narcotic abuse?

(A) Administration of narcotic antagonists
(B) Antidepressant therapy
(C) Administration of long-acting agonists
(D) Removal of the addict from his or her environment
(E) Ongoing psychological support

7. A 40-year-old businessman from another city arrives in the emergency room complaining of severe, chronic migraine headaches, which are relieved only by meperidine. His primary physician is unavailable by telephone. The emergency room physician should ask about all of the following conditions EXCEPT

(A) hallucinations and delusions
(B) legal problems
(C) losing prescriptions
(D) loss of consciousness
(E) use of alcohol

8. A middle-aged woman has been treated for a number of years by various physicians for insomnia. On the night of admission to the hospital for elective surgery, she becomes anxious and agitated. There is no evidence of bleeding, infection, or neurologic disease, but the patient develops postural hypotension and fever. Administration of which of the following substances might be appropriate at this point?

(A) Diazepam
(B) Haloperidol
(C) Disulfiram
(D) Phenobarbital
(E) Thiamine

Questions 9 and 10

9. A patient hospitalized for gastritis is found during his last outpatient appointment to have a slightly enlarged liver. Appropriate initial blood tests would include all of the following EXCEPT

(A) hemoglobin
(B) blood alcohol level
(C) blood cultures
(D) drug screen
(E) bilirubin

10. Although the blood alcohol level of the patient in question is 100 mg/100 ml, there is no evidence of intoxication. It is a reasonable assumption that the patient

(A) is tolerant to narcotics
(B) is dependent on alcohol
(C) has pancreatitis
(D) is impotent
(E) has cerebral atrophy

Directions: Each question below contains four suggested answers of which **one or more** is correct. Choose the answer

A   if **1, 2, and 3** are correct
B   if **1 and 3** are correct
C   if **2 and 4** are correct
D   if **4** is correct
E   if **1, 2, 3, and 4** are correct

11. Stimulant withdrawal may be associated with

(1) increased appetite
(2) paranoia
(3) suicide
(4) insomnia

12. The relationship between alcoholism and depression is characterized by which of the following statements?

(1) Nonbeverage forms of alcohol are most frequently associated with depression
(2) Depression may occur when the patient is sober
(3) Alcohol intoxication provides an easy means of suicide
(4) Suicide is most common in alcoholics

13. True statements about hallucinogens include which of the following?

(1) Hallucinogens are not associated with abstinence syndromes
(2) Intoxication causes depersonalization and anxiety
(3) Most "bad trips" can be ameliorated by reassurance
(4) Tolerance develops to hallucinogenic effects

14. The differences between phencyclidine (PCP) and other hallucinogens are characterized by which of the following statements?

(1) PCP is more likely to produce neurologic abnormalities
(2) PCP is more likely to produce hallucinations
(3) An individual intoxicated with PCP is less likely to respond to "talking down"
(4) PCP intoxication is less likely to be associated with violence

15. Anticholinergic poisoning is characterized by

(1) warm, dry skin
(2) mydriasis
(3) psychosis
(4) tachycardia

Directions: The group of questions below consists of lettered choices followed by several numbered items. For each numbered item select the **one** lettered choice with which it is **most** closely associated. Each lettered choice may be used once, more than once, or not at all.

Questions 16–20

Match the drug-induced condition with the appropriate treatment.

(A) Haloperidol administration
(B) Forced diuresis
(C) Physostigmine administration
(D) Supportive care
(E) Naloxone administration

16. Narcotics-induced coma

17. Anticholinergic-induced psychosis

18. Amphetamine-induced psychosis

19. Barbiturate intoxication

20. Alcohol intoxication

ANSWERS AND EXPLANATIONS

1. The answer is E. *(II A 3, B; IV E 4)* Central nervous system depressants such as diazepam, phenobarbital, and glutethimide augment the central nervous system depression caused by alcohol. In addition, glutethimide produces dangerous abstinence syndromes and may be lethal when taken in overdose. Disulfiram produces severe nausea and vomiting when combined with alcohol, and patients taking this medication must be cautioned against even eating foods cooked in wine. Although restraint is the safest approach to the agitated patient who is intoxicated with alcohol, a nonsedating neuroleptic such as haloperidol may be administered if the patient continues to struggle when he or she is restrained.

2. The answer is A. *(II E 2)* Like alcohol, barbiturates, and benzodiazepines, narcotics produce central nervous system, respiratory, and cardiovascular depression when they are taken in large amounts. In contrast to many other substances, narcotics cause constricted rather than dilated pupils unless cerebral hypoxia has supervened. Improvement with intravenous administration of naloxone helps to confirm the diagnosis of narcotic intoxication.

3. The answer is A. *(II C 2)* Amphetamine psychosis is associated with disturbances such as paranoia and loose associations, which may make it indistinguishable from schizophrenia; the only means of differentiating between the two conditions is to observe the patient in a drug-free state. Tactile hallucinations and delusions of infestation with parasites also may occur. Mania is more likely to be produced by a number of commonly prescribed drugs, including antidepressants, administered to patients with past histories or family histories of mania.

4. The answer is C. *(III A)* Benzodiazepines suppress alcohol withdrawal ("the shakes"), seizures, and delirium tremens. Thiamine is usually given because glucose administered for an alcohol abstinence syndrome in the presence of thiamine deficiency can precipitate Wernicke's encephalopathy. Hydration and sedation are the mainstays of treatment of severe abstinence syndromes, and neuroleptics may ameliorate the few cases of alcohol hallucinosis that do not improve spontaneously. Caffeine is not useful in the treatment of abstinence from or intoxication with alcohol.

5. The answer is B. *(II B; III B)* Both intoxication with and withdrawal from barbiturates may cause confusion, delirium, anxiety, agitation, disorientation, and postural hypotension. If the patient is thought to be withdrawing and a barbiturate is administered, these signs should improve, and nystagmus, which is a sign of intoxication but not withdrawal, may appear.

6. The answer is D. *(V A, C)* Narcotic antagonists precipitate severe abstinence syndromes in patients who take narcotics. Satisfactory long-acting antagonists analogous to disulfiram have not been developed. Although narcotic abusers may become depressed or may attempt to treat depression with narcotics (this is especially true of physician addicts), antidepressants are not helpful unless the patient stops abusing the narcotic. Psychological support may also be helpful, but it is usually an insufficient reason for the patient to abstain from use. Removal of the patient from the environment that supports abuse is the most reliable means of encouraging abstinence.

7. The answer is A. *(V D 4)* Suspicion of narcotic abuse is increased by demands for a specific opioid, losing prescriptions, requests for prescription refills when the physician who allegedly wrote the prescription is unavailable, legal, occupational, or psychosocial consequences of abuse, and threatening behavior when a requested prescription is not written. A history of loss of consciousness might indicate central nervous system disease, intoxication with any substance, or abstinence from central nervous system depressants. Abuse of multiple drugs is common in narcotic abusers. Psychosis is not a common cause or result of narcotic abuse.

8. The answer is D. *(III A, B; VI)* The history of treatment of insomnia by multiple physicians suggests that the patient probably has been receiving more than one hypnotic (sleeping pill). Since she has been treated for years, she probably has received at least some barbiturates or related compounds, which were in widespread use before benzodiazepines were introduced. It is also not unlikely that she has continued whatever medications have been prescribed over the years in a continued attempt to sleep. If she is dependent on barbiturates, she will experience an abstinence syndrome when they are withdrawn, as would occur upon admission to the hospital and with the prescription of insufficient doses. In view of the rapid onset of symptoms, barbiturate withdrawal is a more likely diagnosis than abstinence from benzodiazepines. In either case, phenobarbital would be likely to suppress withdrawal symptoms if it is administered before the patient becomes delirious. Most neuroleptics, especially haloperidol, lower the seizure threshold and increase the possibility that this manifestation of withdrawal will occur. Diazepam also suppresses a barbiturate abstinence syndrome, but its long duration of action makes it difficult to regulate clinically. Thiamine is appropriate for alcohol withdrawal, which could conceivably be a factor here too. However, the first step is to suppress the abstinence syndrome, which can be accomplished with phenobarbital or pentobarbital administration regardless of whether the cause of the syndrome is alcohol, barbiturates, or benzodiazepines. Disulfiram is not indicated unless alcoholism is diagnosed and discussed.

9. The answer is C. *(IV D 1; VI)* The patient has two indicators of possible alcohol abuse—gastritis and an enlarged liver. In addition to investigating these possibilities with hemoglobin and bilirubin tests, a blood alcohol level test is indicated to provide further evidence of alcohol abuse (i.e., no evidence of impairment with an elevated blood alcohol level). Since many patients abuse multiple drugs, a blood screen is also appropriate. Such investigations are much more common means of uncovering alcoholism in a medical setting than is information volunteered by the patient. Blood cultures would be more appropriate to the workup of an unexplained fever, especially in an abuser of intravenously administered drugs.

10. The answer is B. *(IV C 9)* Absence of intoxication in the presence of a high blood alcohol level indicates that the patient is tolerant to the central nervous system depressant effects of alcohol, thereby meeting a major criterion for alcohol dependency. (It may also be assumed that an abstinence syndrome is likely to occur if alcohol intake is discontinued abruptly). Pancreatitis, impotence, and cerebral atrophy are complications of alcoholism that should be investigated; however, there is as yet no evidence that the patient suffers from them. Since narcotics and alcohol are not cross-tolerant, tolerance to alcohol does not provide any information about tolerance to narcotics.

11. The answer is B (1, 3). *(III C)* Increased appetite, fatigue, depression, and suicidal ideation may occur with stimulant withdrawal. Although nightmares may occur, the patient usually sleeps more because he or she has been deprived of the stimulant. Paranoia is a symptom of stimulant intoxication, not withdrawal.

12. The answer is C (2, 4). *(IV D 2)* Any form of alcohol may produce depression as a direct effect of abuse. Alcoholics may drink in an attempt to treat an underlying depression; when they are sober, the depression may become more evident or they may simply appreciate their problems more clearly. Although intoxication with alcohol alone is not commonly fatal, the overall suicide rate is increased in alcoholics.

13. The answer is A (1, 2, 3). *(II D; III D)* Hallucinogens are not known to produce physical dependence (i.e., tolerance and withdrawal do not occur). The depersonalization, anxiety, hallucinations, and severe dysphoria produced by most hallucinogens can be ameliorated by reassurance in a quiet setting and by administration of benzodiazepines if necessary.

14. The answer is B (1, 3). *(II D)* Unlike other hallucinogens, phencyclidine (PCP) may produce neurologic disturbances such as seizures, coma, analgesia, nystagmus, and ataxia. It is, however, no more likely to produce hallucinations than other drugs in this class. Patients who are intoxicated with PCP are more likely to become violent than those intoxicated with other hallucinogens, and attempts to reassure them may make them even more violent. A more effective treatment of intoxication is to leave the patient alone in a quiet place and sedate or restrain him or her if agitation does not abate.

15. The answer is E (all). *(II F)* Because so many psychotropic and over-the-counter drugs have anticholinergic properties, it is extremely important to be able to differentiate anticholinergic toxicity from other types of organic brain syndromes and poisoning. Any psychiatric symptoms, especially delirium and psychosis, that are accompanied by tachycardia, warm, dry skin, and dilated pupils should raise the suspicion of anticholinergic poisoning and prompt a careful history of use of prescription and nonprescription drugs. Intravenous administration of physostigmine temporarily reverses coma and fever but is not a useful treatment for the other manifestations of toxicity.

16–20. The answers are: 16-E, 17-C, 18-A, 19-B, 20-D. *(II)* Narcotic-induced coma is reversed by naloxone, a narcotic antagonist. Anticholinergic-induced coma and fever may temporarily be improved by physostigmine. Nonsedating neuroleptics (e.g., haloperidol) may relieve amphetamine-induced psychosis and agitation. If the urine is alkalized maximally, excretion of barbiturates can be hastened by forced diuresis. Alcohol intoxication is treated with supportive care until the alcohol is metabolized.

5
Anxiety
Steven L. Dubovsky

I. DEFINITION. Anxiety is an abnormal fear that is out of proportion to any external stimulus. Ten to fifteen percent of general medical outpatients and ten percent of inpatients experience significant anxiety. Of the healthy population, 75% are anxious at some time in their lives; symptoms become severe in 2% to 5%. Until recently, anxiety was viewed primarily as a psychological response to internal or external stress; however, biological factors now also are felt to play a role in some types of anxiety.

A. Endogenous and exogenous categories of anxiety

1. Endogenous anxiety occurs spontaneously without any identifiable precipitating stress. Physical and psychological symptoms of anxiety persist for at least 1 month, and no specific medical or psychiatric disorder explains the symptoms. Eight stages of endogenous anxiety include:
   a. Spontaneous and sudden anxiety attacks
   b. Gradual progression to full-blown panic attacks
   c. Hypochondriacal fears of occult disease
   d. Development of **anticipatory anxiety** that unpredictable anxiety will result
   e. Phobic avoidance of situations in which panic attacks occur
   f. Generalized phobic avoidance
   g. Abuse of drugs or alcohol to control anxiety
   h. Depression as a result of increasingly disabling anxiety

2. Exogenous anxiety is precipitated by environmental stress.
   a. Spontaneous anxiety or panic never occurs if anxiety is truly exogenous.
   b. The anxiety can always be explained by specific external stress or psychological conflict.
   c. Symptoms are more irregular than those of endogenous anxiety and demonstrate a relatively consistent relationship to psychosocial stressors.

B. Diagnostic categories of anxiety [information is taken from the *Diagnostic and Statistical Manual of Mental Disorders*, third edition, (*DSM III*)].*

1. Panic disorder. At least three spontaneous panic attacks, characterized by sudden apprehension or fear (see II A, B, and C), which are not precipitated by physical exertion, a life-threatening situation, or a phobic stimulus, occur within a 3-week period.

2. Generalized anxiety disorder. Persistent, generalized anxiety is present for at least 1 month in a patient over 18 years of age.

3. Obsessive-compulsive disorder. Previously called obsessive-compulsive neurosis, this disorder is characterized by persistent, intrusive, recurrent ideas, thoughts, feelings, images, or impulses (**obsessions**), which are experienced as senseless or repugnant, and repetitive sterotyped actions (**compulsions**), which the patient recognizes as senseless and tries to resist. These actions, which are performed with a subjective sense of necessity to prevent some future event, often are a significant source of distress or interfere with the patient's ability to function.

4. Post-traumatic stress disorder. Long after the initial psychologically traumatic event (e.g.,

---

*American Psychiatric Association: *Diagnostic and Statistical Manual of Mental Disorders*, 3rd ed. Washington, D.C., American Psychiatric Association, 1980.

war, rape, or accident), the patient continues to experience considerable distress due to the trauma.

    a. Symptoms. Some patients with marginal premorbid adjustment may develop psychotic symptoms in association with post-traumatic stress disorder. Differentiation from schizophrenia, mania, and depression may be difficult. In addition to continuing or recurrent preoccupation with the event, the patient experiences:

        (1) Decreased responsiveness to the present environment, with diminished interest in usual activities, feelings of detachment or estrangement from others, and constricted emotional responsiveness

        (2) Signs of distress that were not present before the traumatic event, including hyperalertness, easily startled reactions, insomnia, nightmares, guilt about having survived or about what actions were necessary in order to survive, difficulty in concentrating, avoidance of activities that recall the event, and increased symptoms when the patient is exposed to situations that symbolize or resemble the original trauma

    b. Treatment of this condition can be more difficult than that of a more acute adjustment disorder. Adjunctive techniques (e.g., biofeedback) and medication [especially monoamine oxidase inhibitors (MAOIs)] may be useful.

  5. Phobias. The patient has persistent, irrational fears of benign situations, accompanied by a compelling need to avoid them. The patient realizes that this behavior is unreasonable and is disturbed by it. Phobias may develop spontaneously (endogenous) or develop after a specific traumatic event (exogenous). Common examples include:

    a. Simple phobias. The patient fears and avoids animals, heights, closed spaces, or any object or situation that does not primarily involve being alone, being in public places, or being in certain social situations.

    b. Agoraphobia. The patient's life is increasingly constricted by fear and avoidance of being alone or being in crowds or public places and in tunnels, on bridges, and in public transportation, from which escape might be difficult or help not available in case of sudden incapacitation.

    c. Social phobia. The patient suffers from a persistent, irrational fear that he or she will humiliate him- or herself in a social or public situation, leading to what he or she realizes is an irrational avoidance of such situations.

  6. Primary psychiatric disorders may be associated with anxiety, which may be prominent or even the presenting complaint.

    a. Depression. About 70% of depressed patients also feel anxious, and 20% to 30% of apparent cases of anxiety are caused by an underlying depression.

    b. Psychosis. As control of mental processes is lost, a patient experiencing psychotic disorganization due to mania, schizophrenia, or borderline (brief reactive) psychosis often displays considerable anxiety, which initially may obscure the underlying severe disturbance of thinking, affect, or behavior.

    c. Organic brain syndrome. Anxiety is the most common emotion experienced by patients with acute organic brain syndromes (delirium), who are frightened by a sudden disruption of cognitive abilities, and by demented patients, whose brain syndromes are made worse by an intercurrent illness or by a sudden change in the environment (e.g., a change in the roommate of a hospitalized, demented patient).

    d. Adjustment disorder with anxious mood. The patient experiences symptoms in excess of those that would normally be expected or suffers impairment of social or occupational functioning within 3 months of exposure to an obvious stress. In contrast to post-traumatic stress disorder, anxiety and other symptoms appear soon after the onset of the traumatic event and are expected to resolve when the stress abates or when the patient achieves a new level of functioning.

    e. Factitious disorder. Rarely, a patient will consciously simulate a mental disorder, including anxiety, apparently for the sole purpose of becoming a patient. The patient often relates an improbable history and has been hospitalized numerous times, often under different names. In contrast, **malingering** refers to the conscious simulation of a condition for some obvious gain. It is more common in a patient with a history of lying, drug abuse, and antisocial behavior.

II. SIGNS AND SYMPTOMS. A subjective state of anxiety may be obvious, or it may be concealed by physical or other psychological complaints.

  A. Psychological symptoms

    1. Apprehension, worry, fear, and anticipation of misfortune

    2. Sense of doom or panic

   3. Hypervigilance

   4. Irritability

   5. Fatigue and lack of energy

   6. Insomnia

   7. Predisposition to accidents

   8. Derealization (the world seems strange or unreal) and depersonalization (the patient feels unreal or changed)

   9. Difficulty in concentrating

B. Somatic complaints

   1. Headache

   2. Dizziness and lightheadedness

   3. Palpitations and chest pain

   4. Upset stomach and diarrhea

   5. Frequent urination

   6. Lump in the throat

   7. Motor tension or restlessness

   8. Shortness of breath

   9. Paresthesias

   10. Dry mouth

C. Physical signs

   1. Diaphoresis

   2. Cool, clammy skin

   3. Tachycardia and arrhythmias

   4. Flushing and pallor

   5. Hyperreflexia

   6. Trembling, easily startled reactions, and fidgeting

III. ILLNESSES CAUSING ANXIETY. Before investigating psychological causes of anxiety, it is important to exclude the possibility of physical disorders in which anxiety may be a presenting complaint even before other signs of disease become evident.

A. Cardiovascular disorders

   1. Arteriosclerotic heart disease

   2. Paroxysmal tachycardia

   3. Mitral valve prolapse

   4. Hyperdynamic β-adrenergic circulatory state

B. Pulmonary disorders

   1. Pulmonary embolism

   2. Hypoxemia

   3. Asthma

   4. Chronic obstructive lung disease

C. Disorders of the endocrine system and metabolism

   1. Hypoglycemia

   2. Hyperthyroidism

3. Hypocalcemia

4. Cushing's syndrome

5. Porphyria

D. Tumors

1. Insulinoma

2. Carcinoid tumor

3. Pheochromocytoma

E. Neurologic disorders

1. Multiple sclerosis

2. Temporal lobe epilepsy

3. Organic brain syndrome of any etiology

4. Meniere's disease

F. Infections

1. Tuberculosis

2. Brucellosis

G. Drug-related disorders

1. Abstinence syndromes (e.g., abstinence from alcohol, tranquilizers, and sleeping pills)

2. Intoxication with sympathomimetics

3. Akathisia

4. Caffeinism

5. Chinese restaurant syndrome, resulting from ingestion of monosodium glutamate

IV. ANXIETY THAT MIMICS DISEASE STATES. Anxiety may also mimic disease states; for example, in **hyperventilation syndrome,** the patient who complains of shortness of breath, weakness, paresthesias, headache, and carpopedal spasm is often unaware of the psychological stresses that lead to hyperventilation and may either adamantly deny feelings of anxiety or feel that any anxiety that is experienced is secondary to not being able to breathe.

Symptoms abate when the patient is calmed and the respiratory rate decreases. Treatment consists of instructing the patient to breathe into a paper bag, which is held over the nose and mouth. Carbon dioxide accumulates and reverses the respiratory alkalosis caused by hyperventilation.

V. PSYCHOLOGICAL FACTORS. Patients who are encountered in nonpsychiatric practice often display anxiety that reflects specific combinations of internal and external conflicts. Although they are not a part of the standard diagnostic nomenclature, these types of anxiety are easy to recognize, especially in medical and surgical patients.

A. Situational anxiety. Severe stress, such as **adjustment disorders** (acute reactions to stress) or **post-traumatic stress disorders** (delayed reactions), may overwhelm anyone's ability to cope temporarily.

1. **Symptoms.** When current stress reminds the patient of previous and unresolved conflicts, a relatively minor situation may feel overwhelming because it recalls other situations in which the patient was unable to cope. The intensity and nature of anxiety that evolves from a stressful situation depends upon the patient's previous level of adjustment. A relatively well-adjusted patient may experience only transient symptoms, while an underlying psychosis may be precipitated in a more marginally compensated patient.

2. **Management.** When the patient must contend with acute, ongoing stress, antianxiety medication, when appropriate, and support should be offered. In addition, the patient should be encouraged to talk about what the stress means to him or her.

B. Anxiety about death. Even a nonfatal illness may remind a patient of his or her mortality. Persistent fear of death, even in the terminally ill patient, symbolizes concern about loss of control, pain, isolation, helplessness, and the prospect of losing important relationships. Reassurance that the patient will not be left alone and in pain often decreases the apparent fear of death.

C. **Anxiety about mutilation, loss of prowess, and loss of attractiveness** is especially common in a patient who feels that love, approval, and self-esteem are dependent upon his or her strength or beauty.

   1. **Symptoms.** The patient becomes frightened if an illness threatens appearance or prowess and expresses excessive fear of side effects and aftereffects of the illness, complains continuously, or fails to improve as expected. The patient may also attempt self-reassurance by demonstrating attractiveness (e.g., by behaving seductively) or strength (e.g., by exercising conspicuously) in inappropriate or even dangerous ways.

   2. **Management.** The patient should be reassured that he or she still possesses valued traits, and the family's reaction to the patient's illness or surgery should be evaluated.

D. **Anxiety about loss of self-esteem.** A patient whose self-esteem is fragile is especially vulnerable to experiencing illness as imperfection, weakness, or failure, which can lead to attempts to bolster a sense of self-worth by boasting about importance and superiority.

   1. **Symptoms.** The patient may adopt a self-important air, insisting on being treated only by the most senior or well-known physician and treating others as worthless inferiors. Attempts to convince the patient that he or she is not as important as he or she thinks only increases insecurity, which the patient attempts to cover up with greater protestations of importance and, by comparison, the unimportance of others.

   2. **Management.** The patient should be approached with appropriate deference and should be reassured that he or she is still important. Reasonable requests should be granted.

E. **Separation anxiety.** Children and regressed adults (i.e., those who function psychologically more as children than as adults, a condition that is seen in hospitalized, overly dependent, and some psychotic individuals) may become frightened when they are separated from important caretakers.

   1. **Symptoms.** The patient signals distress by becoming anxious, by complaining (e.g., of pain), or by ringing for the nurse whenever he or she is left alone. He or she often fears that, once out of sight, the caretaker will never return.

   2. **Management.** Family and close friends should be encouraged to be with the patient as much as possible; the nursing staff should be encouraged to visit the patient frequently for brief periods of time; and a roommate should be provided.

F. **Stranger anxiety**

   1. **Symptoms.** A patient who suffers from separation anxiety also may react adversely to unfamiliar people, including new physicians, nurses, and visitors. In a hospitalized adult this can lead to distress at changes of shift or in other situations in which there are new caretakers.

   2. **Management.** As much continuity in personnel as possible should be provided (e.g., the same nurse should be assigned to the patient each day). Unrestricted visiting by those familiar to the patient should be allowed, and unfamiliar visitors should be limited. Changes in roommates should be minimized

G. **Anxiety about loss of control**

   1. **Symptoms.** Because others must make decisions for him or her, illness and hospitalization may be threatening to a patient with a strong need to feel in complete control of his or her life and environment. The patient may attempt to regain control by refusing to comply with the physician's advice, by becoming excessively demanding, by making the physician feel helpless, or by otherwise asserting control over the physician, whom the patient feels is in control.

   2. **Management.** The patient should be allowed as much control as possible over his or her own care. For example, the patient's opinion about therapeutic decisions should be solicited or he or she could be consulted about medication schedules.

H. **Anxiety about dependency.** A patient who fears loss of control also commonly has anxiety about dependency. Often normal dependency needs were not met in childhood (e.g., because of parental illness or unavailability).

1. **Symptoms.** Extremely strong wishes to be cared for, which have been unchanged since childhood, threaten to break through when the patient is put in a dependent position (e.g., as a result of becoming ill). Because the patient is afraid that he or she will not be able to control dependency needs, the attempts of others to be helpful are rejected and the patient becomes hostile toward potential caretakers. The patient also may be noncompliant, may fail to keep appointments, or otherwise may attempt to indicate that he or she does not need care.

2. **Management.** When possible, the patient should be reassured that the illness and the dependency required by it are temporary. He or she should be helped to maintain as much independent function as possible.

I. Anxiety about closeness

1. **Symptoms.** A patient with concern about dependency also may be afraid of becoming too close emotionally to caretakers or loved ones, which leads to maintenance of greater than normal emotional distance, attempts to ward off (e.g., through hostility) people who are nice or express concern, and distress at expressions of friendliness or intimacy.

2. **Management.** Intimacy must not be forced on the patient, who should be allowed to determine interpersonal distance.

J. Anxiety about being punished

1. **Symptoms.** A patient with an underlying sense of guilt about real or imagined transgressions may have a conscious or unconscious expectation of punishment. The patient may attempt to relieve this anxiety by self-inflicting punishment (e.g., through an unhappy marriage, repeated accidents, and alcoholism).

2. **Management.** The patient's suffering should be acknowledged, and an attempt to uncover the source of the patient's guilt should be made. A patient with some insight may benefit from psychotherapy.

K. Signal anxiety

1. **Symptoms.** When awareness of a previously unconscious, unresolved psychological conflict is stimulated by some external occurrence (e.g., the patient's age is the same as that of a parent at the time of death), anxiety may signal the emergence of the conflict. This anxiety may call forth **psychological defenses,** which tend to be unconscious and keep the conflict out of the patient's awareness.
   a. **Repression** (forgetting) is an automatic process by which memories, thoughts, and feelings are excluded from the patient's awareness.
   b. **Rationalization** is explaining away a psychological symptom in order to remain unaware of its cause.
   c. **Reaction formation** is feeling the opposite of an affect in order to avoid an awareness of it (e.g., experiencing excessive affection toward someone who actually elicits hostility).
   d. **Isolation of affect** is experiencing the content of a thought without its associated emotions.

2. **Management.** When it is possible and practical, an attempt to resolve the underlying conflict should be undertaken. Behavioral and adjunctive measures that are useful for control of exogenous anxiety may help to ameliorate signal anxiety.

L. Anxiety about the emergence of another affect. A problem related to signal anxiety occurs when the patient is threatened by the awareness of an unconscious affect (e.g., anger or depression) that he or she considers bad or intolerable.

1. **Symptoms.** The patient may experience anxiety without a specific cause—mimicking endogenous anxiety. When the underlying affect is intense or psychotic, defenses that tend to distort reality may be necessary for the patient to control it.
   a. **Denial** is remaining unaware of some aspect of reality (e.g., feeling that one does not have to be afraid of the consequences of an illness because one is not really sick).
   b. **Projection** is attributing one's own motives to someone else.
   c. **Projective identification** is incompletely projecting an intense emotional state, which is usually anger, onto another individual while inducing the emotion in the object of the projection through provoking behavior. The patient also experiences the original emotion but feels that this is only because he or she is attempting to protect him- or herself from the other individual's affect.

2. **Management.** An attempt to uncover the underlying affect must be made. When the patient

cannot tolerate an awareness of his or his own motives, he or she should be helped to develop less disabling defenses against them (e.g., isolation of the affect rather than denial of it).

VII. TREATMENT

A. Psychotherapy is most effective for the treatment of exogenous anxiety and anxiety due to identifiable intrapsychic conflict. It is not clearly effective for panic attacks and phobias. It may be facilitated by medication and behavior techniques.

1. **Supportive therapy.** Psychotherapy that is primarily supportive is useful to acutely ill patients, patients under severe stress, and patients with limited emotional and psychosocial resources (e.g., because of organic brain disease or personality disorders).
   a. The principal therapeutic approach involves encouraging the **development of defenses** that are as adaptive as possible. For example:
      (1) A patient with an acute myocardial infarction should be helped to minimize the immediate danger since intense fear may contribute to the onset of lethal arrhythmias. When symptoms begin, however, denial may lead to a fatal delay in seeking medical attention.
      (2) A marginally compensated schizophrenic patient might be encouraged not to pay too much attention to psychotic thoughts that cannot be dealt with constructively by directing his or her attention to problems in everyday living that can be solved.
   b. A patient who tends to distort reality should be helped by encouraging **reality testing,** which is a continuous assessment of reality through objective evaluation of the world and one's relationship to it.
   c. **Advice** should be given, especially when the patient attempts to avoid anxiety through destructive or self-destructive behavior. For example, he or she might be advised to stop attempting to relieve anxiety by arguing with a spouse and to learn relaxation techniques instead.
   d. Adaptive behavior by the patient should be **reinforced** (encouraged).

2. **Insight psychotherapy.** A patient whose anxiety reflects intrapsychic conflicts and who is able to and is interested in understanding him- or herself may gain more control of the symptoms by learning more about the psychological meaning of the anxiety. Before applying insight psychotherapy, it is important that the patient's ability to be aware of emotions without acting on them and to handle frustration as well as his or her willingness and ability to look into him- or herself be assessed. Components of insight psychotherapy include:
   a. **Clarification** of the patient's statements in order to make them more comprehensible.
   b. **Confrontation** of aspects of reality or the patient's emotions that he or she is ignoring (e.g., "You say that you are not anxious, but you look very nervous").
   c. **Interpretation** of unconscious thoughts and feeling in order to bring them into the patient's awareness (e.g., "Do you think that you are anxious around your boss because he is so much like your father?").

B. Behavior therapy is very effective for phobias, especially those that develop after a frightening experience (exogenous phobic avoidance).

1. In **systematic desensitization,** the patient is taught deep muscular relaxation, which is incompatible with anxiety. Situations that cause anxiety are imagined by the patient while relaxed in this way. When the patient can imagine the most anxiety-provoking scene while still feeling relaxed, he or she will experience much less anxiety in the corresponding real-life situation. In vivo exposure is usually necessary to solidify these gains.

2. **Graduated in vivo exposure** gradually involves the patient, usually with a family member, friend, or physician for reassurance, in situations in which he or she has become increasingly phobic. Systematic desensitization may be necessary first if the patient is too frightened to face phobic situations.

3. **Adjunctive behavioral techniques** may be useful to patients who suffer from any type of anxiety.
   a. **Relaxation techniques.** Since an individual cannot feel tense and relaxed at the same time, any method that decreases tension tends to relieve anxiety.
   b. **Hypnosis** is an altered state in which the patient is helped in focusing intense concentration on calming thoughts and away from those that provoke anxiety. A patient with excessive fear of loss of control or with an organic brain syndrome often cannot be hypnotized.
   c. **Biofeedback** is a technique that is useful for a patient who prefers to learn to relax with a machine or alone. It also has been used to treat migraine and tension headaches and mild

essential hypertension. The level of muscular tension, usually in the forearm or frontalis muscles, is "fed back" through a visual or auditory stimulus to help the patient learn to decrease tension and, with it, anxiety.

C. **Psychopharmacology. Medication** is indicated for treatment of endogenous anxiety and endogenous phobic avoidance (i.e., anxiety and phobias that arise spontaneously, not in response to specific trauma or conflict). It is also indicated if a 3-month trial of psychotherapy and behavior therapy for treatment of exogenous anxiety is unsuccessful. Adjunctive use of antianxiety medication may facilitate psychotherapy and behavior therapy in a patient with acute stress reactions or chronic anxiety. Conversely, if endogenous anxiety or phobic avoidance are still present after primary drug therapy, behavior therapy should be added to the drug regimen. If complete recovery does not follow appropriate drug therapy, the diagnosis may be incorrect (e.g., the patient may be psychotic or have an organic brain syndrome).

1. **Benzodiazepines** are the safest and generally most effective antianxiety drugs. They are most useful for acute situational anxiety, anticipatory anxiety associated with panic attacks, and chronic anxiety that is unresponsive to other forms of treatment or that afflicts a patient who is unable to resolve the cause of anxiety.
   a. **Uses**
      (1) For the treatment of **endogenous anxiety,** some clinicians prefer to begin alprazolam (Xanax), a triazolobenzodiazepine. Recovery should be apparent after 2 weeks of treatment with an average dose of up to 6 mg/day. If the patient recovers, the medication should be continued for 6 to 12 months and then gradually be discontinued for a drug-free trial. If recovery is not complete after 2 weeks, another medication should be tried (see section VII C 2).
      (2) Benzodiazepines commonly prescribed for **exogenous anxiety** include diazepam (Valium), chlordiazepoxide (Librium), lorazepam (Ativan), chlorazepate (Tranxene), and oxazepam (Serax).
      (3) Benzodiazepines such as flurazepam (Dalmane), temazepam (Restoril), and triazolam (Halcion) are the preferred medications for **insomnia.**
   b. **Administration.** Benzodiazepines generally should not be prescribed for acute exogenous anxiety for more than 6 to 8 weeks. The best results are obtained with treatment of time-limited anxiety that occurs in response to clear-cut stress. Occasionally, the chronically anxious patient or a patient with limited intrapsychic or external resources needs long-term therapy.
   c. **Addiction** to benzodiazepines is rare in medical patients. Individuals with a history of alcohol or drug abuse, physician shopping, and antisocial behavior as well as those who request a specific drug are at higher risk.
   d. **Abstinence syndromes** (withdrawal symptoms) may appear up to 10 days after abrupt discontinuation of moderate doses of benzodiazepines that have been taken for more than 1 month. Signs and symptoms of withdrawal include anxiety, insomnia, irritability, and, at times, delirium and seizures.

2. **Tricyclic and tetracyclic antidepressant drugs.** Imipramine, maprotiline, and trazodone have been found to be most effective in the treatment of endogenous forms of anxiety and phobias. At optimal dose (i.e., 150 mg/day to 300 mg/day of imipramine or its equivalent), tricyclic and tetracyclic antidepressant drugs may improve endogenous anxiety after 6 to 8 weeks. If effective, antidepressants should be continued for 4 to 6 months before an attempt is made to stop them.

3. **MAOIs** are medications that are used to treat atypical depression, depression that does not respond to other drugs, and post-traumatic stress disorder; they may be effective when standard antidepressants do not work. They may also be effective in relieving endogenous forms of anxiety and phobias when the other medications discussed above are ineffective. Phenelzine (45 mg/day to 60 mg/day) and tranylcypromine (20 mg/day to 80 mg/day) are used most frequently in the United States. If a MAOI is effective, it should be continued for 6 to 12 months, followed by a drug-free trial. MAOIs may produce hypertensive crises when given with a variety of foods and medications.

4. **Barbiturates** (e.g., phenobarbital and secobarbital) and related compounds (e.g., meprobamate and glutethimide) cause addiction and severe abstinence syndromes and are extremely dangerous if they are taken in overdose. They should **not** be prescribed for anxiety or insomnia except for the rare patient who has been taking them for years and cannot be withdrawn.

5. **Antihistamines** (e.g., hydroxyzine and diphenhydramine) are especially useful as antianxiety drugs and hypnotics for elderly patients and for those in whom addiction may be a problem. They are not as predictably effective as other antianxiety drugs.

6. **Neuroleptics** (antipsychotic drugs). Although usually indicated for schizophrenia, mania, and some forms of psychotic depression, low doses of nonsedating neuroleptics such as trifluoperazine and haloperidol may help to relieve anxiety in the patient who becomes more anxious upon sedation with standard antianxiety drugs. The anticholinergic side effects may help some patients with functional bowel disorders. The danger of long-term **side effects,** especially tardive dyskinesia, precludes long-term administration to nonpsychotic patients.

7. **Beta-blocking agents** (e.g., propranolol) are indicated for anxiety that is accompanied by signs of adrenergic stimulation. They are not as predictably effective in relieving anxiety as benzodiazepines, however. High doses can diminish assaultiveness in the brain-injured patient. One dose may be useful in relieving stage fright.

STUDY QUESTIONS

Directions: Each question below contains five suggested answers. Choose the **one best** response to each question.

1. All of the following statements characterize both post-traumatic stress disorder and adjustment disorder with anxious mood EXCEPT

(A) the disorders can be seen in veterans
(B) impairment of social functioning can occur
(C) the disorders may persist long after the stress has abated
(D) obsessive rumination about the stress by patients is common
(E) the disorders may be accompanied by depression

2. All of the following treatment modalities are usually helpful for post-traumatic stress disorder EXCEPT

(A) patient discussion of the precipitating event
(B) relaxation techniques
(C) biofeedback techniques
(D) use of antianxiety drugs
(E) use of monoamine oxidase inhibitors (MAOIs)

3. A 25-year-old man who recently had an extramarital affairs feels that his physician disapproves strongly of his behavior. This probably represents

(A) denial
(B) repression
(C) reaction formation
(D) isolation
(E) projection

4. Correct statements about diazepam include all of the following EXCEPT

(A) addiction is rare
(B) it is an effective treatment for endogenous anxiety
(C) it generally should not be prescribed for more than 6 to 8 weeks
(D) it is an effective hypnotic
(E) it is an effective sedative

5. Before a diagnosis of endogenous anxiety can be made, all of the following conditions must exist EXCEPT

(A) the occurrence of at least three discrete episodes in a 3-week period
(B) the presence of symptoms for at least 1 month
(C) identification of an environmental stressor
(D) another psychiatric illness
(E) the occurrence of spontaneous anxiety attacks

Directions: Each question below contains four suggested answers of which **one or more** is correct. Choose the answer

    A if **1, 2, and 3** are correct
    B if **1 and 3** are correct
    C if **2 and 4** are correct
    D if **4** is correct
    E if **1, 2, 3, and 4** are correct

6. A few days after a mastectomy, an attractive 35-year-old woman is heavily made-up, wearing a flimsy negligee, and is making seductive comments to her 25-year-old intern. She had been remarried 1 year previously after divorcing her first husband for seeing a younger woman. She has no previous psychiatric history. Factors attributable to her behavior that should be considered first include

(1) anxiety that her new husband may no longer find her attractive
(2) acute schizophrenic psychosis
(3) acute organic brain syndrome
(4) stranger anxiety

7. Soon after his admission to the coronary care unit after experiencing his first myocardial infarction, a 45-year old businessman refuses to be examined by the house officers and demands to see the most senior cardiologist in the hospital immediately. He then insists that his secretary be permitted unrestricted visiting privileges because he has many important business deals that require prompt attention. He adopts a condescending attitude toward the physicians and nurses working with him. Reasonable management approaches might include

(1) telling the patient that he is very ill and must cooperate with his physicians or risk serious consequences
(2) restricting visiting by the secretary until the patient has recovered
(3) discussing with the patient the impact of his illness on his self-esteem
(4) agreeing that the patient is an important person who needs good care from all concerned

8. A middle-aged man complains of chest pain and palpitations for which careful examination and follow-up reveal no apparent cause. Which of the following symptoms might suggest that his condition is related to anxiety?

(1) Constipation
(2) Feelings of unreality
(3) A conviction of having cancer
(4) Circumoral paresthesias

9. True statements concerning anxiety that arises in the context of an obviously stressful situation include

(1) it may result from the stimulation of previously unresolved conflicts
(2) it may respond to antianxiety drugs
(3) it may be of mild to psychotic intensity
(4) exogenous anxiety is present

10. Management of a hospitalized patient who becomes hostile whenever his feelings about his illness are questioned or other attempts to get to know him are made might include which of the following approaches?

(1) Telling the patient that his hostility is interfering with the physician-patient relationship
(2) Helping the patient to see that his anger is really due to anxiety
(3) Attempting to behave in a more friendly manner
(4) Allowing the patient to determine the degree of interpersonal distance

11. A 25-year-old man becomes anxious whenever he must work closely with an authority figure. Which of the following factors would indicate his candidacy for insight psychotherapy?

(1) Frustration tolerance
(2) Social class
(3) Interest in self-awareness
(4) The nature of the conflict

12. Of the following techniques, those appropriate for the management of phobias include

(1) systematic desensitization
(2) insight psychotherapy
(3) monoamine oxidase inhibitor (MAOI) therapy
(4) biofeedback

---

13. Correct statements about the use of medication in the treatment of the anxious patient include

(1) it may improve most forms of endogenous anxiety
(2) it may be adjunctive to the treatment of post-traumatic stress disorder
(3) it may ameliorate phobias
(4) it may undo the effectiveness of psychotherapy

14. A 30-year-old man complains of panic attacks and anticipatory anxiety. Which of the following drugs would be effective treatment?

(1) Haloperidol
(2) Imipramine
(3) Meprobamate
(4) Diazepam

15. Appropriate indications for propranolol in the treatment of anxiety include

(1) stage fright
(2) panic attacks
(3) sympathetic arousal
(4) phobias

Directions: The groups of questions below consist of lettered choices followed by several numbered items. For each numbered item select the **one** lettered choice with which it is **most** closely associated. Each lettered choice may be used once, more than once, or not at all.

Questions 16–20

Match each clinical situation listed below with the medication most likely to be associated with it.

(A) Benzodiazepines
(B) Tricyclic and tetracyclic antidepressant drugs
(C) Monoamine oxidase inhibitors (MAOIs)
(D) Barbiturates
(E) Antihistamines

16. They may be used as a hypnotic (sleeping pill) in the elderly

17. They tend to produce addiction and tolerance

18. They rarely cause addiction

19. They may cause late abstinence syndromes

20. They may be effective treatment for phobias and endogenous anxiety

Questions 21–25

Match each statement below with the type of anxiety that it describes.

(A) Signal anxiety
(B) Situational anxiety
(C) Separation anxiety
(D) Anxiety about dependency
(E) Anxiety about loss of self-esteem

21. It may be associated with fear of loss of control

22. It results in distress when the patient is alone

23. It is manifested in part by condescending treatment of others

24. It results from rising awareness of an unconscious conflict

25. It may occur immediately or at a later time

ANSWERS AND EXPLANATIONS

1. The answer is C. *(I D 4, 6 d)* Post-traumatic stress disorder tends to have a delayed onset and may persist for years after the stress has abated. Although the clinical significance of this syndrome was initially appreciated in veterans, it may develop after any severe stress. A soldier, under the stress of battle, may develop the more acute adjustment disorder, which resolves when the stressful situation ceases. Many patients who become anxious immediately or long after a severe stress tend to become preoccupied with the event in an attempt to master it in their minds.

2. The answer is D. *(I B 4)* Monamine oxidase inhibitors (MAOIs) have been found to ameliorate symptoms in some patients with post-traumatic stress disorder. Antianxiety drugs are generally useful only if the patient is reacting to an acute, short-lived stress. Discussion of the patient's feelings about the stress and its psychological significance is a cornerstone of the treatment of all situational anxieties, including both post-traumatic stress disorder and adjustment disorder. Biofeedback, meditation, and related relaxation techniques may be useful; however, behavior therapy such as systematic desensitization is more appropriate to the treatment of phobias. It is extremely important to differentiate post-traumatic stress disorder from schizophrenia since symptoms may become chronic if the patient is approached as a schizophrenic and if specific treatment for post-traumatic stress disorder is not instituted.

3. The answer is E. *(V K 1, L 3)* Projection is attributing to others one's own feelings, thoughts, or impulses that are personally unacceptable. Denial involves ignoring some elements of external reality, while repression involves forgetting memories, thoughts, and feelings that cause internal conflict. Reaction formation (adopting the opposite attitude or interest of an unconscious psychological state) and isolation (repressing the affect that is associated with the mental state) are defenses that help support repression.

4. The answer is B. *(VII C 1)* Alprazolam and antidepressants are more effective treatment for endogenous anxiety than diazepam, which is indicated for the short-term treatment of exogenous anxiety. Diazepam is safe when prescribed appropriately for anxiety and insomina, although the resulting sedation may bother some patients.

5. The answer is C. *(I A 1)* Endogenous anxiety (panic disorder) occurs spontaneously without a precipitating event and tends to acquire a life of its own independent of psychosocial stressors. Diagnosis of this condition requires that symptoms be present for at least 1 month and that at least three anxiety attacks occur within a 3-week period.

6. The answer is B (1, 3). *(V C)* A mastectomy may be a threat to a woman who values her beauty and whose first husband found another woman to be more attractive. However, one must also consider the possibility that a complication of surgery, a drug effect, an action of the illness (e.g., brain metastasis), or a new intercurrent illness is causing an organic brain syndrome. It is unlikely that schizophrenia would appear suddenly for the first time when an individual is in his or her thirties, and signs of psychosis would be expected. Since the patient is exhibiting anxiety in the presence of a familiar caretaker rather than in the presence of someone with whom she is unfamiliar, stranger anxiety is unlikely.

7. The answer is D (4). *(V D)* An attempt to frighten the patient into submission is likely to increase his fear that his illness will have disastrous consequences, and his attempt to reassure himself through protestations of his importance may increase. Since the patient seems to need his secretary both as an indicator of his importance and possibly as a familiar, reassuring person, restricting his access to her also may increase his panic. Unless the patient gives a clear indication that he wishes to discuss his underlying fears, attempts to uncover his insecurities may further threaten his fragile sense of self-worth. Support of the patient's attempts to increase his self-esteem, especially while he is acutely ill, is more likely to ensure his compliance and decrease the possible adverse physiologic effects of anxiety on the heart.

8. The answer is C (2, 4). *(II A, B, C; III A)* Anxious patients may experience feelings of unreality in two different forms: depersonalization (the patient has changed) and derealization (reality has changed). When hyperventilation occurs, light-headedness, paresthesias, and carpopedal spasm may occur. Diarrhea is more common than constipation in anxiety. While preoccupation with heart disease might be understandable in a patient with chest pain, an unrealistic fear of having cancer is more likely to indicate a delusion.

9. The answer is E (all). *(I A 2; V A; VII C 1)* Although most individuals might suffer in a situation that evokes exogenous anxiety, the subjective meaning of the stress, the way in which the individual has handled similar circumstances in the past, and overall adjustment (i.e., whether the individual has an underlying psychosis or is fundamentally healthy psychologically) determine the extent of the anxiety. Antianxiety drugs are most appropriately used during short-term stresses.

10. The answer is D (4). *(V I)* Although a few acutely ill patients who fear closeness may benefit from understanding the reasons for their reactions, most are made more anxious by attempts to decrease interpersonal distance, which include greater friendliness, attempts to understand them too deeply, or attempts by the physician to force him- or herself on the patient.

11. The answer is B (1, 3). *(VII A 2)* Insight psychotherapy may be helpful to the patient whose unresolved conflicts are stimulated by an external event if the patient can keep him- or herself from acting on impulses and strong emotions that can be stimulated by this form of treatment and who is interested in gaining self-awareness. Although the patient must be willing to make a commitment to treatment, social class and the nature of the conflict (as opposed to the personality of the patient) do not determine response to therapy.

12. The answer is B (1, 3). *(VII B, C)* Systematic desensitization helps the phobic patient feel comfortable in anxiety-provoking situations. Monoamine oxidase inhibitors (MAOIs) may be effective drug therapy when alprazolam and tricyclic antidepressants have failed. Biofeedback is a useful nonspecific technique for reducing anxiety, but it is not particularly helpful in treatment of phobias. Insight psychotherapy has not been shown to be effective in the phobic patient.

13. The answer is A (1, 2, 3). *(VII C)* Alprazolam, antidepressant drugs, and occasionally monoamine oxidase inhibitors (MAOIs) may ameliorate endogenous anxiety and phobias, while MAOIs have been used successfully to treat some patients with post-traumatic stress disorder. When used appropriately, medication facilitates rather than interferes with psychotherapy.

14. The answer is C (2, 4). *(VII C 1, 2)* Imipramine and similar antidepressant drugs may abort spontaneous panic attacks, while diazepam and related benzodiazepines are helpful for treatment of the associated anticipatory anxiety. Haloperidol is occasionally helpful to the patient who fears sedation, but it should not be prescribed as the first drug or on a long-term basis. The dangers of addiction and withdrawal preclude the use of meprobamate as an antianxiety drug.

15. The answer is B (1, 3). *(VII C 7)* Treatment with propranolol may be helpful when anxiety is accompanied by marked arousal, and it may ameliorate stage fright when it is taken shortly before a performance. Panic attacks and phobias should be treated with alprazolam, antidepressants, or monoamine oxidase inhibitors (MAOIs).

16–20. The answers are: 16-E, 17-D, 18-A, 19-A, 20-C. *(VII C)* Antihistamines may be used effectively and safely as sleeping pills in the elderly, although they are not always as effective as other drugs. While addiction to benzodiazepines is rare when they are prescribed properly, they may produce abstinence syndromes if they are withdrawn too suddenly. Barbiturates, on the other hand, cause addiction and severe abstinence syndromes. Monoamine oxidase inhibitors (MAOIs) may be useful in treatment of phobias and endogenous anxiety, but their numerous adverse interactions preclude their use as a first drug.

21–25. The answers are: 21-D, 22-C, 23-E, 24-A, 25-B. *(V A, D, E, H, K)* A patient who is afraid of becoming too dependent upon or emotionally close to others may also be anxious about losing control. On the other hand, a patient who becomes overly dependent may regress (i.e., adopt a psychological posture more appropriate to that of a child) and exhibit distress when he or she is left alone. A patient with vulnerable self-esteem may attempt to make him- or herself seem more important by treating others as though they are less important. Signal anxiety indicates (signals) that a conflict of which the patient previously has been able to remain unaware is rising to the patient's consciousness; the anxiety may cause repression and other defenses to remove the conflict from the patient's conscious mind. Anxiety that develops in a stressful situation may occur either while the stress is still ongoing or long after the external stress has abated.

6

Somatoform Disorders

James H. Scully

I. PSYCHOLOGICAL FACTORS AFFECTING PHYSICAL CONDITIONS

A. Introduction. The extent to which psychological factors are judged to contribute to medical disorders, which is not a diagnosis per se, is indicated by the term "psychological factors affecting physical conditions." This term is preferred to the terms "psychosomatic" and "psychophysiologic" disorders, which are no longer felt to be accurate. Disorders with a demonstrable organic pathology are differentiated from somatoform disorders, which present with physical symptoms with no known physiologic abnormalities. One-third of all patients seen by physicians have a mixture of psychological and physical distress; whereas all patients have some psychological reaction to their illnesses, this group has psychological problems that are thought to contribute in some causal way.

1. **Specificity theory.** The theory of emotional specificity (physiologic expression of blocked emotions) has lead to personality studies of patients with peptic ulcers, coronary artery disease, and cancer. Although these studies have lent some support to the theory, it has, in general, lost favor as a comprehensive explanation. Freud and his followers studied somatic involvement in psychological conflict and were particularly interested in **conversion reactions,** in which a psychological problem is symbolically manifested physically, although physiologic tissue damage cannot be demonstrated. Dunbar suggested that **specific conscious personality traits** cause specific psychosomatic diseases. Alexander theorized that **specific unconscious conflicts** cause specific illnesses in organs innervated by the autonomic nervous system. This occurs because prolonged tension can produce physiologic disorders, leading to eventual pathology. He also believed that there are constitutional predisposing factors involved. Alexander's theory led to the concept of the classic psychosomatic diseases:
   a. Bronchial asthma
   b. Rheumatoid arthritis
   c. Ulcerative colitis
   d. Essential hypertension
   e. Neurodermatitis
   f. Thyrotoxicosis
   g. Duodenal peptic ulcer

2. **Nonspecificity theory.** Whatever event is perceived by the patient as stressful can produce **stress,** whether this event is the death of a loved one, divorce, financial loss, or illness. Psychological reactions to stress can lead to a failure of adaptive physiologic responses, which can lead to a **nonspecific cause of disease. Hormones,** especially cortisol, are released in response to stress and act on different organs to produce a variety of changes. There is a **neurophysiologic** reaction to stress, which activates the pituitary-adrenal axis.
   a. This reaction is known as the **general adaptation syndrome.** The nonspecific systemic reactions of the body to stress include:
      (1) Alarm reaction (shock)
      (2) Resistance (adaptation to stress)
      (3) Exhaustion (resistance to prolonged stress cannot be maintained)
   b. The **physiologic reactions** to stress include the following.
      (1) Fight-flight response is arousal of the sympathetic nervous system, resulting in increased production of epinephrine and norepinephrine with an increase in pulse and muscle tension. When an affected individual can neither fight nor flee, this state of arousal can lead to organic dysfunction.
      (2) Withdrawal-conservation. Engel and coworkers showed that when an individual is threatened with loss (real or imagined), there can be a decrease in metabolism. The in-

dividual withdraws into him- or herself to conserve energy. Pulse and body temperature decrease, and the individual may become susceptible to illness, particularly infection. Studies on the psychophysiologic effects of bereavement support this hypothesis: Morbidity and mortality rates are higher during the first year after death of a spouse in a bereaved group compared to those rates in an age-controlled nonbereaved group. The theory of withdrawal-conservation may also explain sudden death from hexes and curses.

B. Major illnesses with psychological factors

1. Gastrointestinal disorders. Emotional states have long been known to cause a reaction in the gastrointestinal tract. Vague complaints of nausea, indigestion, diarrhea, constipation, and abdominal pain are common.

a. Peptic ulcers

(1) Etiology. Gastric, duodenal, and acute post-traumatic stress ulcers all have different etiologies. The Mirsky study of army recruits showed that several factors are necessary for the development of ulcers, including high stress, the constitutional factor of high pepsinogen secretion, and psychological (dependency) conflict. Although conflicts involving dependency are noticeable in ulcer patients, not all individuals affected by these conflicts either develop ulcers or are prone to developing ulcers.

(2) Treatment. Patients who are complying with good medical management do not usually require psychotherapy. The physician should help the patient identify those areas of his or her life that seem to cause stress. Also, it may be useful to teach the patient relaxation techniques, in which an individual tenses all of his or her muscles and then relaxes them in groups (e.g., arms, hands, legs, and feet), notices the resultant feeling, and practices the technique. Antianxiety agents are occasionally indicated along with antispasmodics.

b. Ulcerative colitis

(1) Etiology. A large proportion of familial occurrence of ulcerative colitis would suggest a genetic cause; however, the exact etiology is unknown. It has been demonstrated clearly that exacerbation of ulcerative colitis is associated with psychological stress and remission is associated with psychological support. Stress, such as unresolved grief on the anniversary of a death, can precipitate the disorder. Associated psychological factors include immaturity, indecisiveness, conscientiousness, a covertly demanding behavior, and fear of loss of an important individual.

(2) Treatment. Although psychotherapy cannot guarantee that the condition will not recur, it is useful when it is focused on helping the patient to develop mature ways of expressing needs as well as helping him or her to deal with any unresolved losses.

c. Irritable bowel syndrome (also termed spastic colon and nervous diarrhea) is disordered bowel motility, including both hyper- and hypomotility.

(1) Etiology. Although the syndrome is usually associated with environmental stress, patients tend to have other psychological symptoms, such as anxiety and depression.

(2) Treatment. Brief psychotherapy to help the patient identify environmental stress and to effect changes where possible usually aids in decreasing symptoms.

2. Cardiovascular disorders. There is much evidence that the cardiovascular system reacts to the emotional state of the patient.

a. Coronary artery disease is by far the most common cause of death in the United States.

(1) Etiology. Multiple nonpsychiatric elements are implicated in the development of coronary artery disease, including genetics, diet, smoking, high blood pressure, obesity, and amount of physical activity. A personality type has also been implicated. The **type A behavior pattern** is only one risk factor out of many, and its exact role in the development of coronary artery disease is unclear, although men who fall into this type of behavior pattern are at twice the risk for coronary artery disease as those who do not. Characteristics of the type A personality include:

(a) Competitiveness
(b) Ambition
(c) Drive for success
(d) Impatience
(e) A sense of time urgency
(f) Abruptness of speech and gesture
(g) Hostility

(2) Treatment. Behavioral methods designed to decrease environmental stress and modify life-style when mutable are increasingly common.

b. Essential hypertension

(1) Etiology. The causes of essential hypertension are unknown, but psychological factors were initially thought to involve conflicts between passive-dependent and aggressive tendencies in patients who repressed their hostility. Unfortunately, there is no reliable evidence to support this theory. On the other hand, a common reaction to stress is an elevation of blood pressure. Patients who have a biologic susceptibility to essential hypertension may react to a stressful situation by exacerbating that hypertension rather than, for instance, increasing gastrointestinal motility.

(2) **Treatment** of hypertension most commonly involves either relaxation therapy or biofeedback, in which the patient is attached to a machine that provides information about ordinarily unnoticed biologic parameters (e.g., a tone sounds when the patient's blood pressure goes up; the patient can learn to relax to decrease the tone as well as his or her blood pressure). Biofeedback therapy, however, does not tend to be long lasting and must be repeated to maintain the effect.

c. Arrhythmias

(1) **Etiology.** Even in the absence of heart disease, psychological factors can influence the normal rhythm of the heart beat. **Stress** may cause arrhythmias by arousal of the sympathetic nervous system (as is evident in the fight-flight reaction). Sinus tachycardia, a paroxysmal atrial tachycardia (PAT), and ventricular ectopic beats are the most common arrhythmias to arise in reaction to stress. These reactions may be more common in patients who are already fearful of heart disease.

(2) **Treatment** involves questioning the patient about unreasonable fears of heart disease and helping the patient identify environmental stresses that precipitated the reaction. The condition may be part of an anxiety disorder, which should be treated. Benzodiazepines may be useful for a limited time as may blocking agents such as propranolol.

3. Respiratory disorders. Changes in respiration in the normal individual may correspond to an emotional state (e.g., the sigh of boredom and the gasp of surprise). The strongest psychological reactions associated with respiratory disease, however, are those that develop secondary to the illness. The panic associated with shortness of breath can be quite disabling.

a. Hyperventilation syndrome

(1) **Etiology.** This disorder is often associated with **anxiety** (see Chapter 5, "Anxiety"), which may cause an increased depth or rate of breathing. In turn, this leads to **respiratory alkalosis** and then to lightheadedness, paresthesias, and carpopedal spasms. These symptoms increase the anxiety in the patient, resulting in a vicious circle of increased hyperventilation and respiratory alkalosis.

(2) **Treatment.** Educating the patient about the syndrome once the acute event is past may be sufficient treatment; however, if underlying anxieties continue to provoke the syndrome, psychotherapy is indicated.

b. Bronchial asthma

(1) **Etiology.** Once thought to be caused by psychological factors, asthma attacks now are believed rarely to be the result of only these factors. A genetic determinant, allergies, and infections are more likely to be the cause of the disorder. Nevertheless, stress and an ambivalent relationship between the asthmatic child and an overly protective mother may be a factor in the onset. Both overly dependent patients who react to any slight changes of symptoms and overly independent patients who deny symptoms are at greater risk for hospitalization than are psychologically normal patients.

(2) **Treatment.** Psychotherapy is usually indicated only when anxiety is not relieved by the supportive care of a physician. Family therapy may be helpful in separation issues.

4. Migraine headache

a. Etiology. Over 90% of chronic, recurrent headaches are either migraine, tension, or mixed migraine-tension. Although anxiety and stress commonly precipitate all three types of headache, the theory that specific psychological dynamics such as repressed hostility lead to migraine headaches has not been proven. Depression should be ruled out as a cause and treated if present.

b. Treatment of migraine headache includes:

(1) **Drug therapy**
   (a) Ergotamine
   (b) Propranolol
(2) **Biofeedback**
(3) **Psychotherapy** in cases where psychological stresses are chronic

5. Immune disorders. Psychological states affect immune response in complex, not yet fully understood, ways. Stress may depress cell-mediated (via T lymphocytes) immune response. It also affects neuroendocrine systems [e.g., some depressed patients have increased levels of corticosteroids and do not suppress production of these when challenged with dexamethasone (cortisol levels are normally lower following dexamethasone administration)]. Disorders of immune response may involve susceptibility to the following.

      a. Autoimmune diseases including:
        (1) Systemic lupus erythematosus
        (2) Rheumatoid arthritis
        (3) Pernicious anemia
      b. Allergic disorders
      c. Cancer. (Studies show that the patient who reacts to stress with feelings of hopelessness or depression is at higher risk for cancer.)

Table 6-1. The Five S's of Conversion Disorder

Stress
The formation of a symptom helps the patient deal with a psychological stress or an acute conflict.

Sensory-Motor Symptoms (Special Senses)
The symptoms that develop are, by definition, pseudoneurologic. These include such symptoms as blindness, paralysis, paresthesias, and seizures.

Significant Other
The patient identifies with someone who has a similar symptom, which is due to an organic neurologic illness.

Secondary Gains
Most illnesses have secondary gains (the patient is cared for by others and may avoid unpleasant duties).

Symbolic Nature of the Symptom
Although the symptom may be symbolic (e.g., because the patient has an unconscious wish to strike out, an arm becomes paralyzed), symbolism may be difficult to uncover.

II. SOMATOFORM DISORDERS, including somatization, conversion, and psychogenic pain disorders and hypochondriasis, present with physical symptoms; however, no known physiologic factors can be demonstrated. Somatoform disorders are not under the voluntary control of the patient, nor is the motivation for developing the symptoms known to the patient (Table 6-2).

    A. Somatization disorder

      1. Clinical presentation. The patient, who is usually a woman, presents with a history of recurrent multiple physical complaints of several years' duration. The disorder begins before the age of 30 years, generally in adolescence. Whereas the description of the symptoms may often be vague, the presentation is dramatic. The *Diagnostic and Statistical Manual of Mental Disorders,* third edition, (*DSM III*) requires complaints of at least 14 of the 37 listed symptoms for women and 12 of the 37 for men for diagnosis. These symptoms involve complaints in many organ systems and include the following.

        a. Conversion symptoms such as:
          (1) Paralysis or weakness
          (2) Seizures
          (3) Urine retention and difficulty in urinating
          (4) Difficulty in swallowing
          (5) Blurred vision and double vision
          (6) Blindness

Table 6-2. Patient Control of Symptoms

Illness	Control of Symptoms	Motive
Somatization disorder	Involuntary	Unconscious
Conversion disorder	Involuntary	Unconscious
Psychogenic pain disorder	Involuntary	Unconscious
Hypochondriasis	Involuntary	Unconscious
Factitious disorder	Voluntary	Unconscious
Malingering	Voluntary	Conscious

        (7) Fainting or other loss of consciousness
        (8) Loss of voice
        (9) Stiffness
     b. Menstrual symptoms (pain, irregularity, and excessive bleeding)
     c. Gastrointestinal symptoms such as:
        (1) Nausea and vomiting
        (2) Abdominal pain
        (3) Diarrhea
        (4) Bloating
        (5) Food intolerance
     d. Pain (usually ill-defined in various joints, the back, extremities, and in urination)
     e. Psychosexual symptoms (lack of sexual drive, lack of pleasure during intercourse, and pain during intercourse)
     f. Cardiopulmonary symptoms (shortness of breath, palpitations, chest pains, and dizziness)

2. **Incidence and prevalence.** Approximately 2% of women have this disorder, and it is thought to be less common in individuals with higher education.

3. **Etiology** is unknown but is assumed to be psychological. Patients with this disorder have an increased incidence of conversion disorder. There is an association with a histrionic personality style of dramatic, exaggerated complaints. Somatization disorder is linked to a relatively high incidence of alcoholism and sociopathy in first-degree male relatives and somatization disorder in first-degree female relatives.

4. **Complications** include many medical evaluations due to constant consultation with various physicians and, frequently, unnecessary surgery. Anxiety and depressive symptoms are common. There is a wide range of interpersonal difficulties, including marital problems. Substance abuse, largely due to involvement with various prescribed medications, is a high risk, and patients who have a problem with substance abuse are also at risk for suicide.

5. **Differential diagnosis** of all of the somatoform disorders is discussed in section II E of this chapter.

6. **Treatment** of somatization disorder is difficult and frustrating. As described, the illness is a lifelong pattern of multiple somatic complaints that fluctuate depending upon stress in the patient's life. There is no specific treatment for the illness. Instead of medication and diagnostic workups, the physician should offer a supportive relationship that focuses on the patient's functioning rather than symptoms. The physician should expect feelings of frustration and anger in the management of this problem and not overreact when they appear. General principles of treatment include the following.
     a. Unnecessary surgery should be avoided, and whenever a surgical procedure is considered, the physician should think twice about the expected gains in comparison to potential complications.
     b. Patients with somatization disorder are still at **risk for organic illness.** New symptoms must be evaluated when they occur, and the physician must weigh the amount of workup to be done.
     c. Habit-forming medications should be avoided. Antianxiety medications can be helpful for periods of up to 2 weeks or less during times of high stress. In general, however, since most of the antianxiety medications are eventually addicting, they are not useful in the chronic management of somatization disorder.

B. Conversion disorder (also called hysterical neurosis, conversion type)

1. **Clinical presentation**
     a. Associated features. Conversion disorder involves the "conversion" of psychological conflict into a loss of physical functioning, which suggests a neurologic disease. It is seen in a wide range of psychiatric illnesses from schizophrenia to personality disorders, but it is also seen in cases in which there is real organic physical illness (e.g., the occurrence of conversion seizures in conjunction with a true seizure disorder). An additional psychiatric diagnosis can be made in 30% to 50% of patients; for instance, a histrionic personality type is a common finding in patients with conversion disorder. "La belle indifference," in which the patient exhibits little concern over the symptoms, is sometimes present; however, it is not a reliable sign of conversion disorder alone since a patient with a physical illness may be stoic about his or her condition. Modeling is common—the patient unconsciously imitates the symptoms observed in an important individual in his or her life.
     b. Symptoms may be inconsistent with known pathophysiology (e.g., a "paralyzed" patient may protect him- or herself upon falling). The patient classically presents with an acute loss

of function, which suggests neurologic disease. Symptoms, which may be bizarre or unusual, include:

(1) Paresthesias
(2) Gait disturbances (e.g., astasia and abasia)
(3) Loss of consciousness and seizures
(4) Aphonia
(5) Vomiting
(6) Fainting
(7) Visual disturbances (e.g., blindness and tunnel vision)

2. **Incidence and prevalence** are not known with certainty; however, conversion disorder seems to be less common now than in the past. It may present with less classic symptomatology than was seen previously. For instance, psychogenic pain disorder (see section II C) is the diagnosis when pain, which is a neurologic phenomenon, is psychogenic in origin. Psychogenic pain disorder may fulfill some of the same unconscious roles for patients that conversion disorder did in the past. Conversion disorder is seen more frequently in low socioeconomic classes, and most cases are found on neurology wards and in military settings. Although the disorder occurs more commonly in women, it is seen in men. Usually onset is in adolescence to the twenties; however, it can occur initially in middle age.

3. **Etiology** is thought to be psychological.
   a. Two mechanisms have been described that explain the gains experienced by the patient in conversion disorder.
      (1) The **primary gain** is that internal conflict is kept from consciousness. Stress from the external environment stimulates internal conflict, and the symptoms of the disorder symbolize this conflict (e.g., paralysis of the arm stops the patient from striking out).
      (2) The **secondary gains** are both that the patient is taken care of by others and he or she may avoid unpleasant duties because of the symptoms. Some secondary gain is seen in almost all illnesses, however.
   b. Other etiologies that are postulated include the following.
      (1) The less powerful individual gains control over his or her environment by the elaboration of symptoms (i.e., the concern and attention of others are focused on the patient).
      (2) The symptoms are learned and are then reinforced by the reaction of those around the patient.
      (3) The theory of a physiologic basis may be supported by the fact that the symptoms are seen more frequently in patients with brain injuries and other neurologic defects.

4. **Differential diagnosis.** It is important to note that 15% to 30% of patients diagnosed as having conversion disorder have an undiagnosed physical illness.

5. **Prognosis.** A good prognosis is associated with good premorbid functioning, acute onset, an obvious stressful precipitant, and the absence of other forms of psychopathology.

6. **Treatment.** The patient should not be confronted with the psychological cause of his or her symptoms. When a supportive physician-patient relationship has been established, it is possible that the patient may be helped to see the symbolic aspects of the symptoms, and thus future occurrences may be prevented. The stressful aspects of the patient's life should be focused upon, and the patient must be helped to deal with the environment and significant individuals more directly.
   a. **Suggestion** can be useful in that the physician suggests that the patient's condition will resolve over time, which allows the patient to let go of symptoms without losing face. Occasionally a "dramatic cure" can be obtained with hypnosis and other forms of suggestion.
   b. **Psychoanalytic therapy** is helpful to some patients in whom there is an actual life-style of the disorder; however, there is a large investment of time and money.
   c. **Pharmacologic therapy** for an associated illness, such as depression, anxiety, and schizophrenia, may be indicated.
   d. The results of **behavior therapy** are unclear.

C. **Psychogenic pain disorder**

1. **Clinical presentation.** The patient complains of severe and unrelenting pain for which there is no demonstrable physical cause. The patient is unable to see any connection between his or her psychological state and the pain: A high degree of stress is present for which the symptoms are a solution. Commonly, the patient has some minor physical ailment but exaggerates the symptoms all out of proportion. The issues of secondary gain are prominent and may involve monetary compensation, the avoidance of objectionable work, and may enable the patient to control the significant others in his or her life. Psychogenic pain disorder can lead to one of the following:

a. Problems with the physician-patient relationship
b. Multiple physical examinations
c. Unnecessary surgery
d. Substance abuse

2. Incidence and prevalence are unknown; however, it is a common condition in a primary care setting. The disorder occurs more frequently in women than in men.

3. Etiology
   a. Psychological mechanisms associated with the disorder are not fully known.
      (1) One theory suggests that, as a child, the patient learned to express emotions not verbally but physically.
      (2) A painful childhood illness may be causative.
   b. Physical theory suggests endogenous opiate-like substances in the brain, which raise the pain threshold, to be causative. The presence of these **endorphins** implies the possibility of biochemical differences among individuals that affect their perceptions of pain (i.e., individuals with low levels of endorphins may be prone to symptoms of pain under stress).

4. Differential diagnosis is discussed in section II E; however, particular issues for psychogenic pain disorder include the necessity of a complete diagnostic workup to rule out **organic pathology.** A patient may exaggerate the symptoms of insignificant physical findings because of personality traits (e.g., histrionic) or because of culturally learned styles of communication. In addition, **depressive disorders** may be present along with psychogenic pain disorder. Pain may be the presenting complaint in a patient who also has depressive symptoms that come to light when the history is taken.

5. Treatment. The patient with psychogenic pain is difficult and frustrating to treat. The patient is notoriously unwilling to consider any psychological cause for the pain and is unresponsive to traditional psychotherapy. The physician should allow the patient to talk about the pain, but aspects of life (e.g., family and work) and how the pain affects them should be stressed and discussion of symptoms limited. The patient may be resistant to examining stress as a cause of pain but may be able to examine pain as a cause of stress, and thus make a connection. Physicians should avoid the use of narcotics for the treatment of chronic pain as well as any other habit-forming drugs such as sedatives.

D. Hypochondriasis

1. Clinical presentation. The patient is preoccupied by fear that he or she has an illness rather than being affected by a specific symptom or loss of function. The patient sees him- or herself as a sick individual and is not especially reassured by being told that nothing is wrong; he or she refuses to consider an emotional cause for the symptoms. Normal physical sensations such as sweating and bowel movements are misinterpreted, and minor ailments such as a cough or backache can be exaggerated until the condition becomes disabling. Physician shopping is common.

2. Incidence and prevalence. As many as 1% of all patients may be hypochondriacal. Hypochondriasis is very common in primary care practice and is seen in both men and women, beginning at any age but commonly in the fourth and fifth decades of life.

3. Etiology. Although the patient complains of somatic problems, the nature of the disorder is psychological. For whatever reason, the patient may elaborate a minor physical ailment until it becomes a disabling condition.
   a. Some researchers have speculated that due to problems in early development the patient may be unable to express emotions other than in physical terms. This called **alexithymia.**
   b. Others have suggested that in our culture when an individual is unable to cope with the demands of life, one of the only acceptable excuses is to be ill. Being ill is also a way in which dependency needs can be met. If the overt request for caring is not tolerable to an individual, it may be allowed when that individual is "sick."

4. Treatment
   a. Physician reaction to hypochondriacal patients is often negative. If the physician is unaware of such feelings, he or she may act on them in an antitherapeutic way, such as overprescribing medication or performing unnecessary diagnostic procedures.
   b. It is not helpful to tell the patient that his or her problems are psychologically caused. The reality of the patient's symptoms should be acknowledged early in treatment. Regular follow-up appointments legitimize the patient's need to be sick.
   c. It may be necessary to prescribe medication; however, the patient should be told that it will only help and not "cure" the ailment. Narcotics and other habit-forming drugs should not be prescribed in order to preclude addiction.

E. Differential diagnosis of the somatoform disorders. The possibility exists in all of the somatoform disorders that the patient may have an undiagnosed physical disorder with inconsistent, vague, or confusing symptoms. Several illnesses should be considered.

1. Systemic lupus erythematosus is associated with multiple organ systems and is characterized by exacerbation and remissions. The illness begins in late adolescence or the early twenties, and women are nine times more likely to have systemic lupus erythematosus than men. The onset may be vague, and psychiatric symptoms such as mood disorders and even schizophreniform disorder may be present.

2. Endocrine disorders
  a. Hyperthyroidism may be present with complaints of fatigue, palpitations, dyspnea, and anxiety.
  b. Hypothyroidism also may present with fatigue and anxiety. Mood disorders, including depression, are possible. Menstrual problems are commonly seen and may be dismissed as a somatization problem.
  c. Hyperparathyroidism may present with severe anxiety, gastrointestinal symptoms, polyuria, and some pain.

3. Neurologic disorders. Any physical illness that begins early in life and that is associated with an insidious or intermittent onset of symptoms should be considered in the differential diagnosis of a somatoform disorder.
  a. Multiple sclerosis may have transient, remitting neurologic symptoms associated with dysphoric mood and anxiety and often is misdiagnosed as a psychiatric illness early in its course.
  b. Temporal lobe or **complex partial seizures** may cause a distorted body image as well as mood disorders and changes in personality.
  c. Acute intermittent porphyria is rare, but it may mimic somatization disorder with its gastrointestinal pain and neurologic complaints.

4. Psychiatric disorders
  a. Schizophrenia occasionally presents with multiple somatic complaints or somatic delusions as well as affective illness, particularly depression.
  b. Symptoms of **depression** and **anxiety** commonly occur in the somatoform disorders and do not have to be diagnosed separately. However, major depression may also be present and mimic some of these disorders, or the symptoms of somatoform disorders may be part of the presentation of the depression. Somatic concerns of patients with psychotic depression include delusions about dying, rotting inside, and other morbid apprehensions about health.

III. FACTITIOUS DISORDER

A. Clinical presentation. The patient is in voluntary control of his or her symptoms of physical illness in that, although his or her behavior is deliberate, what precipitates this behavior is not.

1. Symptoms may range from complaints of pain when the patient feels no pain to self-inflicted infection, such as that arising from self-injection with feces or saliva, which can develop into life-threatening illness. The medical knowledge of the patient is often highly sophisticated, and, by complaining of bizarre or unusual symptoms, he or she may encourage invasive diagnostic procedures, such as laparotomy and angiography. The patient may lie about any aspect of his or her history with dramatic flair (**pseudologia fantastica**). Narcotic abuse and addiction are associated findings in about one-half of these patients.

2. History. Upon hospital admission, patient behavior is disruptive and demanding. Symptoms change as workups prove negative. Eventually the patient is confronted with evidence of faking, and he or she usually reacts angrily and leaves against medical advice. This pattern of behavior can become chronic and involve multiple admissions to different hospitals, and it is then called **Munchausen syndrome**. Other names for factitious disorder with physical symptoms include the following.
  a. Polysurgical addiction
  b. Hospital hoboes
  c. Hospital addiction

B. Incidence and prevalence. The disorder may seem to be more common than it actually is because a single patient may interact with many physicians in different hospitals. It seems to be more common in men than in women, and it usually begins in adult life and is a lifelong condition.

C. Etiology. Although an illness or operation in early childhood may be a contributing factor, the disorder is considered to be entirely psychological. There may have been an experience with a physician in early life either through a family relationship or through illness. A significant proportion of these patients are employed in the health care field as paraprofessionals. Masochism has been considered to be an important feature in a patient who seeks out unnecessary surgery. The illness has also been conceptualized as a variant of the borderline syndrome in that the physician becomes the perpetual object of transference: The patient continually reenacts with the physician the disordered relationship with his or her parents.

D. Differential diagnosis

1. **Physical illness.** A patient with a true physical disorder may present symptoms with an unusual or dramatic flair, which makes the physician suspicious of faking and which is more likely to occur if the patient also has a personality disorder, including one of the following types:
   a. Histrionic
   b. Borderline
   c. Schizotypal

2. **Somatization disorder.** The symptoms are not under the patient's voluntary control, and the patient does not usually insist on hospitalization. Conversion disorder is often also present.

3. **Hypochondriasis.** The essential feature of this disorder is the patient's preoccupation with illness in general rather than symptoms. The symptoms are not under the voluntary control of the patient. Hypochondriasis starts later in life than factitious disorder, and the patient is less likely to insist on hospital admission or submit to dangerous diagnostic procedures.

4. **Malingering.** Although it is difficult to differentiate malingering from factitious disorder, the goals in malingering are clear to both patient and physician, and the symptoms can be stopped when they no longer serve an end (see Table 6-2).

E. Treatment. A patient with factitious disorder with physical symptoms rarely receives psychiatric treatment. The physician's reactions are usually strongly negative, which also prevents psychiatric evaluation. Until the patient is willing to face the fact that he or she has a psychiatric illness and agrees to psychiatric hospitalization or treatment, the prognosis is likely to be poor. The approach to the patient is one of management rather than cure, and unnecessary diagnostic procedures should be avoided. The patient should be confronted in a calm, noncondemning manner, and the cost of the illness emotionally as well as financially should be pointed out.

IV. MALINGERING

A. Clinical presentation. Malingering is not considered to be a mental disorder. The malingering individual willfully and deliberately fakes or exaggerates an illness with the conscious intent to deceive others. His or her reasons for faking the illness (e.g., monetary and legal concerns) can be understood by examining the circumstances affecting the individual rather than his or her psychological makeup. The individual is often evasive and uncooperative upon examination, and there is a marked discrepancy between his or her claimed disability and the physical findings. An individual who malingers may have an antisocial personality disorder (see Chapter 11, "Personality Disorders").

B. Incidence and prevalence. True malingering is rarely seen. A physician is more likely to diagnose this condition incorrectly in a patient with one of the somatoform disorders because of a negative reaction to the patient and the inability to see that a disorder such as hypochondriasis is not consciously faked by the patient.

C. Differential diagnosis. In **factitious disorder** with physical symptoms, the goals of the patient cannot be clearly understood, as they can in the case of malingering, even though the patient is voluntarily causing the symptoms of illness.

D. Treatment. Since **malingering is not an illness,** there is no medical or psychiatric treatment.

V. PLACEBO RESPONSE has been defined as any effect attributable to a medication, procedure, or other form of therapy but not to the specific pharmacologic property of that therapy. For instance, 30% to 40% of patients in pain respond equally well to placebos as to morphine. There is no particular personality type that responds to a placebo (e.g., a histrionic patient is no more likely to have a placebo response than is any other patient).

   Physicians use the placebo response (mistakenly) to help differentiate "real" from "psychological" symptoms in their patients. The placebo response is a powerful aspect of most medical care. It operates commonly, even when the physician is unaware of it. However, it does not differentiate physical from psychological symptoms.

   Recent findings suggest that the placebo response to pain is a **physiologic phenomenon.** Placebo response can be blocked by a narcotic antagonist, naloxone, which suggests that the analgesic effect of a placebo may be based upon the action of endorphins, the naturally occurring opioid substances in the brain, which raise the pain threshold.

BIBLIOGRAPHY

American Psychiatric Association: *Diagnostic and Statistical Manual of Mental Disorders*, 3rd ed. Washington, D.C., American Psychiatric Association, 1980

Mirsky IA: Physiologic, psychologic and social determinants in the etiology of duodenal ulcer. *Am J Dig Dis* 3:285, 1958

STUDY QUESTIONS

Directions: Each question below contains five suggested answers. Choose the **one best** response to each question.

1. Antianxiety medications, which may be indicated for the treatment of somatization disorder, are characterized best by which of the following statements?

(A) They may help the patient accept the emotional cause of symptoms
(B) They may be useful for short periods of time
(C) They may mask a physical illness
(D) They may precipitate more symptoms
(E) They may interfere with the physician-patient relationship

2. All of the following statements about conversion disorder are true EXCEPT

(A) concurrent psychiatric diagnoses are frequent
(B) the symptoms are involuntary
(C) incidence is decreasing
(D) the symptoms are consistent with pathophysiology
(E) it is seen more commonly in women

3. The term alexithymia refers to inability to

(A) control emotions
(B) control motor activity
(C) control language
(D) trust physicians
(E) put feelings into words

4. Preoccupation with the idea or fear of having an illness is termed

(A) hypochondriasis
(B) phobia
(C) conversion disorder
(D) somatization disorder
(E) factitious disorder

5. All of the following are characteristics of hypochondriasis EXCEPT

(A) physician shopping
(B) higher occurrence in women than in men
(C) increased complaints with reassurance
(D) exaggeration of minor ailments
(E) onset in the third and fourth decades of life

6. The most common associated finding in patients with factitious disorder is

(A) relatives in health-care professions
(B) narcotic abuse and addiction
(C) depressive disorder
(D) poor health in childhood
(E) a criminal record

7. The classic psychosomatic illnesses include all of the following EXCEPT

(A) essential hypertension
(B) rheumatoid arthritis
(C) hyperventilation
(D) thyrotoxicosis
(E) neurodermatitis

8. All of the following physiologic changes are a result of the withdrawal-conservation reaction to stress EXCEPT

(A) decrease in heart rate
(B) decrease in body temperature
(C) decrease in immunologic suppression
(D) decrease in metabolism
(E) none of the above

9. Patients with psychological factors contributing directly to their medical problems are the most common patients seen by physicians. They represent at least what percentage of all patients?

(A) 90%
(B) 25%
(C) 50%
(D) 33%
(E) 10%

Directions: Each question below contains four suggested answers of which **one or more** is correct. Choose the answer

A   if **1, 2, and 3** are correct
B   if **1 and 3** are correct
C   if **2 and 4** are correct
D   if **4** is correct
E   if **1, 2, 3, and 4** are correct

10. Symptoms that are commonly present in patients with somatization disorder include

(1) painful menstruation
(2) heart palpitations
(3) anxiety
(4) nausea

11. Complications that are likely to be associated with somatization disorder include

(1) psychiatric hospitalization
(2) unnecessary surgery
(3) factitious disorder
(4) substance abuse

12. Malingering differs from somatoform disorders in which of the following ways?

(1) It occurs rarely
(2) Patient gains are obvious
(3) It is not a mental disorder
(4) It involves multiple organ systems

13. The five S's of conversion reaction include

(1) symbolic nature of symptoms
(2) somatization
(3) stress
(4) sterotyped behavior

Directions: The group of questions below consists of lettered choices followed by several numbered items. For each numbered item select the **one** lettered choice with which it is **most** closely associated. Each lettered choice may be used once, more than once, or not at all.

Questions 14–19

Match the statements below with the physical disorder that they describe.

(A) Ulcerative colitis
(B) Cardiovascular disease
(C) Migraine headache
(D) Immune disorder
(E) Bronchial asthma

14. Psychological factors of the disorder include immaturity, covertly demanding behavior, and sensitivity to the threat of loss.

15. Overly independent as well as overly dependent patients are at higher risk for hospitalization than are those who are psychologically "normal."

16. Some studies have shown that patients who react to stress with feelings of hopelessness or depression are at higher risk for this disorder.

17. A behavior pattern that features competitiveness, ambition, and impatience is considered to be predisposing.

18. Unresolved grief on the anniversary of the death of a loved one can be a precipitating event.

19. The theory that specific psychological conflicts such as repressed hostility are causal has not been proven.

ANSWERS AND EXPLANATIONS

1. The answer is B. *(II A 6 c)* Antianxiety medications may be useful in a somatization disorder in cases in which there is a great deal of anxiety present. Symptoms may be acutely relieved, even though the patient remains unaware of the psychogenic cause of these symptoms. Since there is a risk for substance abuse, the physician should only prescribe antianxiety medications for a short period of time. They will not generally mask the more serious physical illness and do not tend to precipitate more symptoms, although patients with somatization disorders tend to have more side effects from any medication. Rather than interfering with the physician-patient relationship, antianxiety therapy may aid it.

2. The answer is D. *(II B 1 b)* Often symptoms in a conversion disorder are inconsistent with the normal anatomy of the nervous system (e.g., a stocking-glove type of anesthesia). Concurrent psychiatric diagnoses are common, and the patient may be unaware that the symptoms are caused by psychological conflict. Incidences of conversion disorder seem to be decreasing rather than increasing, particularly as our population becomes more psychologically sophisticated. Although conversion disorder tends to be more common in women than in men, this predomination is not exclusive.

3. The answer is E. *(II D 3 a)* "Thymia" comes from the Greek root for feelings; "lex" for words; therefore, not to have words for feelings is referred to as alexithymia. This concept does not refer to the inability to control emotions, language, or motor activity, and it does not involve trusting physicians. It is thought to be a problem in early development, and it is considered to be a possible etiology for hypochondriasis.

4. The answer is A. *(II D 1)* Hypochondriasis is defined as the preoccupation with the idea of or fear of illness. Phobias, which are also fears, involve specific reactions to external stimuli rather than preoccupation with ideas. Conversion disorder involves a loss of function, and somatization disorder is associated with multiple symptoms rather than a fear of illness. Factitious disorder involves voluntary production of symptoms.

5. The answer is B. *(II D 2)* Hypochondriasis is seen in both sexes, but the specific ratios are unknown. Women are more commonly diagnosed as having other somatoform disorders than are men. Physician shopping results often from a patient's reaction to being told in reassurance that there is nothing wrong. Exaggeration of minor ailments is a hallmark of the illness and, unlike many other psychiatric illnesses, hypochondriasis is more likely to begin in the fourth and fifth decades of life.

6. The answer is B. *(III A 1)* Although associated findings in a patient with factitious disorder may include relatives in health-care professions, depression, and poor health in childhood, the most common complication is narcotic abuse, occurring in over one-half of patients.

7. The answer is C. *(I A 1)* Although essential hypertension, rheumatoid arthritis, hyperventilation, thyrotoxicosis, and neurodermatitis all have psychological factors involved, hyperventilation is generally not considered to be a disease but more of a syndrome that is associated with anxiety. The other distractors (hypertension, rheumatoid arthritis, thyrotoxicosis, and neurodermatitis) were all originally felt to be the result, at least in part, of psychological conflicts of the patient. These conflicts either were believed to cause or significantly to affect the development and course of these illnesses.

8. The answer is C. *[I A 2 b (2)]* When heart rate, body temperature, and metabolism in general decrease, it has been noted that the immune system is less reactive and that patients may be more susceptible to illness, particularly infections, in a generalized state of withdrawal-conservation. They also may be susceptible to bradycardia and arrhythmias, which develop secondary to this, so that susceptibility to illness increases rather than decreases.

9. The answer is D. *(I A)* While many physicians feel that all of their patients have a major psychological component to their illnesses, others feel that none of their patients do. Clearly all patients have a psychological reaction to their illnesses, but here we are considering those patients whose psychological conflicts are more than a reaction to the illnesses and actually contribute to them. In many cases it is believed, at least partially, that psychological conflicts are involved in the pathophysiology of an illness even if the mechanisms are not fully understood; this represents by most estimates about one-third of all patients.

10. The answer is E (all). *(II A 1)* Painful menstruation, palpitations, and nausea all may be present in patients with somatization disorder, which is more common in women; multiple somatic symptoms are the hallmark of the disorder. Anxiety, while not a somatic symptom, is a commonly associated finding in this disorder. Patients may also complain of the somatic aspects of anxiety, including rapid pulse, sweating, and shortness of breath.

11. The answer is C (2, 4). *(II A 4)* Patients with chronic physical complaints for which there are no clear diagnoses commonly elicit strong feelings of frustration and helplessness in their physicians. If the physician is unaware of these strong reactions, he or she is likely to prescribe unnecessary procedures such as surgery as well as stronger and stronger drugs, leading to iatrogenic substance abuse. While these patients may require psychiatric hospitalization, this is less likely to occur than unnecessary surgery or substance abuse. Factitious illness, in which the patient is faking the illness for an unknown reason, is a separately diagnosed disorder.

12. The answer is A (1, 2, 3). *(IV A, B)* Malingering is rarer than physicians usually realize. They often diagnose malingering in patients with somatoform disorders because they have difficulty accepting that a patient's production of symptoms when there is no organic illness is not voluntary. Physicians should discover obvious patient gains from the production of a faked symptom. Malingering is not a mental disorder since it is under the control of the individual and is done for felonious or other reasons. Malingering may involve more than one system; it may involve as many systems as the malingerer feels are necessary to fool the examiner.

13. The answer is B (1, 3). *(Table 6-1)* While it may be difficult to discover at first, the majority of the symptoms that a patient presents with in a conversion reaction tend to have some symbolic meaning. For example, an individual with an angry, aggressive impulse may find his or her arm paralyzed. Conversion reactions are always reactions to acute stress and are a way of dealing with the stress. Although it is not somatization of a conflict, this process occurs in all of the other somatoform disorders and not specifically in a conversion reaction. Stereotypic behavior is not a feature of a conversion reaction, but it is seen in other disorders such as schizophrenia.

14–19. The answers are: 14-A, 15-E, 16-D, 17-B, 18-A, 19-C. *(I B 1 b, 2 a, 3 b, 4, 5)* A significant number of patients with ulcerative colitis have concerns of unresolved grief and fears about the threat of future loss. They also tend to have more image or personality developmental problems. Whether this a causative factor of the illness is unclear.

It has been shown that individuals who are overly independent or overly dependent may be, for the most part, the same kind of asthma patient. In the case of the overly independent patient, there is a denial of the early symptoms of illness, which leads to improper care and the need for hospitalization as a last resort, whereas symptoms in the overly dependent patient are overattended, which leads to early hospitalization. In both cases there is more hospitalization than occurs in a psychologically normal patient.

There seems to be a connection between affective states of depression, in particular those associated with feelings of hopelessness, and the immune function. Where there is depression of the emotional state there may also be depression of the immune state. This may be a factor in the development of cancer.

Individuals with a type A behavior pattern with competitiveness, ambition, and particularly time pressure and impatience seem to show a risk two times greater for coronary artery disease than those who do not exhibit this behavior. This increased risk exists even taking into account other important causative factors such as smoking, lack of exercise, the state of blood lipids, and so forth.

As previously noted, many ulcerative colitis patients suffer from issues concerning the threatened, imagined, or real loss of a significant individual. The death of a loved one can be a precipitating event of the disease. The physician should attend to this in terms of treatment.

The understanding of migraine headaches has been changing in recent years. It is questioned now whether or not there is a spectrum disorder involving a combination of both tension and migraine headaches. Other factors such as allergies and chemical factors may be more important than issues of psychological conflict.

7
Sexual Issues
James H. Scully

I. NORMAL SEXUAL RESPONSE

A. General issues. Sexuality is a part of the human condition and involves all aspects of the biologic, psychological, and social framework. It concerns not only the mental and physical aspects of an individual's life but the cultural, social, and religious aspects as well.

1. An **assessment of sexual functioning** by the physician ought to be a part of every complete medical evaluation and often is not, more because of the physician's attitude and anxiety than because of the patient's needs or concerns.

2. In order to understand sexual disorders, **the physician must understand normal sexual function**. The **stages of sexual response** in both men and women include desire, excitement, plateau, orgasm, and resolution. Physiologic studies in recent decades have produced much data about sexual response and have greatly increased the understanding of both healthy and impaired sexual functioning.

3. **Sexual arousal can be produced by either physical or psychic stimuli.** Physical stimulation of the genitals, bowel, and bladder may produce an involuntary sexual response via spinal reflex. Psychic stimuli are mediated through the limbic system, the hypothalamus, and the lateral spinal cord. Erection and lubrication depend on parasympathetic response. Arousal of the sympathetic nervous system inhibits this response. This usually occurs in situations of fear and anxiety.

B. Excitement stage

1. **Male.** Erection of the penis begins about 20 to 30 seconds following stimulation due to increased blood flow into the erectile tissue. The urethral meatus dilates, the testes elevate slightly, the heart rate increases to 100 to 180 beats per minute, and diastolic pressure increases by 20 to 40 mm Hg.

2. **Female.** The breasts increase in size, and the nipples stand out. The labia majora and minora engorge with blood and spread. The clitoris lengthens. Heart rate and blood pressure increase.

C. Plateau stage

1. **Male.** The testicles elevate and become engorged with blood. Secretions from Cowper's gland appear on the glans of the penis. The scrotum thickens and looses all the folds. There is general muscle tension and hyperventilation.

2. **Female.** The clitoris becomes very sensitive and retracts. The labia deepen in color. The orgasmic platform develops, in which the outer one-third of the vagina narrows due to swelling and muscle tension and the inner two-thirds lengthens and widens. The vagina becomes lubricated. General muscle tension increases, and there is hyperventilation.

D. Orgasm stage

1. **Male.** The sensation of ejaculating inevitably occurs before orgasm. The muscles of the perineum contract rhythmically, and the prostate gland, seminal vesicles, and urethra also contract, causing the emission of semen.

2. **Female.** There may be a variety of experiences in women. The orgasmic platform contracts rhythmically, and the rectal and urethral sphincters close.

E. Resolution stage

    1. Male. Detumescence of the penis occurs. There is general muscle relaxation. The testes become uncongested and descend. There is a refractory period during which the male cannot have an erection. The length of the refractory period increases from a minute or so in adolescents to hours in older men.

    2. Female. There is a general relaxation. Vasocongestion is lost, and the labia return to their original size and shape. The inner vagina remains distended for several minutes. Women do not have a refractory period and may be able to achieve another orgasm immediately.

II. NORMAL SEXUAL FUNCTION

A. Gender identity

    1. Gender identity is one's **sense** of being masculine or feminine rather than the biologic state of being masculine or feminine. An infant is assigned a sex, usually on the basis of genitalia, and is reared with all of the parents' and society's attitudes regarding that sex. By about 3 years of age, gender identity appears to be set.

    2. The early embryo is undifferentiated sexually (i.e., it is bisexual). The Y chromosome is necessary for the development of male genitalia. Androgens are produced by the fetal testicles. The androgens influence the organization of the developing brain, which later produces "male" behavior. This behavior is not totally fixed, however, because human beings are the most sensitive of all animals to environmental forces.

B. Sexual identity or sex role. Behavior that is masculine or feminine appears to be determined much more by learning and culture than by biology. The theories described below, especially those with respect to girls, have been seriously challenged by more current research on psychosexual development.

    1. Freud described sexual behavior as beginning in early childhood. His theory of psychosexual development follows.
        a. The **oral phase** occurs in the first year of life. Pleasurable sensations are focused around the mouth and lips: Feeding, sucking, and tasting are the expressions of sexuality in this phase.
        b. The **anal phase** occurs in the second and third years of life when the child begins to obtain control over bodily functions. Control over defecation and urination appears to give pleasure in this phase of development.
        c. The **phallic phase** occurs in the third and fourth years. There is increased awareness of the genitals in children of both sexes.
            (1) Fears of bodily injury are common during this phase.
            (2) Masturbation becomes obviously pleasurable.
            (3) There is awareness in boys of the father's sexual as well as physical superiority.
            (4) In girls, according to Freud, there is awareness of the lack of a penis and the need to give up the primary relationship with the mother.
            (5) Fear of genital penetration and mutilation develops in girls.
        d. The **oedipal phase** occurs in the fifth and sixth years of life. Boys resolve their fear of the father by identification with him, and they become "masculine." Girls resolve conflict by giving up desire for a penis and by supposedly adopting a passive role.

    2. There is a theory that the early mother-infant relationship is **symbiotic**, that is, the infant experiences him- or herself and the mother as merged. There is no clear difference between masculine and feminine behavior prior to 1 year of age.

    3. Separation and **individuation** occur in part due to development of masculine behavior in boys. Failure of separation may lead to problems of gender identity and sexual perversions.

    4. It has been suggested that the quality of "masculinity" is more fragile and susceptible to traumatic disruption than that of "femininity." Males are at a much higher risk for gender identity disorders than are females.

III. TRANSSEXUALISM is a gender identity disorder.

There is a persistent belief on the part of the affected individual that, despite being normal, he or she belongs to the opposite sex. The individual wishes to be rid of his or her own genitals and live as a member of the other sex. This disorder usually begins in childhood.

A. In males there is a history of crossdressing in 75% of individuals with this disorder before the age of 4 years. The transsexual boy believes that he will grow up to be a woman and lose his penis and testicles.

B. **Females tend to be masculine in appearance and behavior.** The transsexual girl believes that she will grow up to be a man with a penis and will not develop breasts.

C. **The etiology of transsexualism is not known for certain.**

1. **Males** who develop this condition often have excessively close physical and emotional ties to their mothers and fathers who were absent during childhood. Their mothers crossdressed them and treated them as girls.

2. **Females** with this disorder have a history of mothers who were distant and unavailable either physically or emotionally during childhood. These girls apparently identified with their fathers.

D. **Treatment**

1. **Primary transsexualism**
   a. **Surgical.** Primary transsexualism in men, in which the patient has always felt that inside he has been a woman, has been treated by **sexual reassignment surgery**. When surgery is successful, patients describe a good readjustment to life. Female-to-male sexual reassignment has been less successful.
   b. There is **no effective psychological treatment** to help patients give up the gender identity problem and become comfortable with their anatomical sex when the disorder is primary.

2. **Secondary transsexualism** is the development of a gender identity problem later in life, after there have been periods of apparently normal sexual identity. This may be the most common kind of gender identity disturbance seen. In these cases, the transsexual identity may result from problems of separation from the mother. It may also develop as a reaction to awareness of homosexual feelings that are unacceptable to the patient.
   a. These patients do not adjust as well with sexual reassignment surgery as patients with primary transsexualism.
   b. **Extended psychotherapy** to explore the meanings of the wish to change sex is indicated.

IV. PARAPHILIAS

A. **General issues.** Previously referred to as **sexual deviations**, these disorders consist of marked and repetitive behavior that involves nonhuman objects for sexual arousal, human beings in activities that are humiliating or involve suffering, and human beings who do not consent to the sexual activity (as occurs in rape). Paraphilic imagery is necessary for masturbation in these disturbances.

   The patient is usually unable of becoming sexually aroused in normal ways and is unable to control the deviant impulses. Although the affected individual may be distressed by the impulses, he or she often does not see him- or herself as "sick" and may only come to medical attention after legal difficulties. The patient may feel shame or guilt about this behavior, and depression is common, especially when the patient's interpersonal relationships suffer because of his or her sexual problem.

B. **Etiology.** Although not fully understood, **the paraphilias are thought to result from problems in early development** rather than from genetic or biologic factors. Males are almost exclusively at risk for these disorders. An exception is sadomasochism, which often involves women.

   It is speculated that problems in the mother-child relationship lead to a poor body image, especially with regard to the genitals. The child becomes unsure and anxious about his penis and its function. "Normal" sexual desire and behavior is too threatening, and this leads to "abnormal" choices for the expression of sexuality.

C. **Specific disorders**

1. **Fetishism. The patient needs a nonliving object such as women's clothing for sexual arousal.** This does not include objects designed for sexual stimulation such as vibrators.

2. **Transvestism. The patient**, who is generally heterosexual and not transsexual, **must dress in women's clothes in order to become sexually aroused.** The crossdressing may range from wearing underwear alone to full feminine regalia and assuming full feminine behavior. The crossdressing is compulsive, and the patient feels intensely frustrated when he cannot do it.

3. **Zoophilia. The patient prefers animals for sexual activity or fantasy.** The occasional sexual use of animals that occurs when there are no humans available or in experimentation by adolescents who live around animals is **not** considered a paraphilia.

4. **Pedophilia**
   a. In this disorder, **the sexual activity or fantasy involves prepubertal children of either sex.**

By definition, the adult is at least 10 years older than the child. If the patient is a late adolescent, diagnosis requires clinical judgment as to the relative maturity of both the patient and the child.

    b. This disorder should be distinguished from an organic brain syndrome in which an impaired individual with a problem in impulse control has some sexual activity with a child. In these cases, the sexual behavior is not prominent but is a part of a picture of overall disability.

    c. Sexual abuse of children may be a great deal more common than has been appreciated in the past. Incest as a specific issue is covered in Chapter 10, "Child Psychiatry."

5. Exhibitionism

    a. In this disorder, **the affected individual exposes his genitals in order to obtain sexual gratification**. The "victims" of this behavior are almost always women or girls, and the disorder only occurs in males.

    b. Exhibitionists are psychologically immature men. They become sexually aroused only when exposing themselves, either during or after the event. Sometimes they masturbate while exhibiting themselves.

    c. Hostility is usually present. The person wishes to shock the stranger. The act usually occurs in socially inappropriate places. However, despite the wish to frighten, most of these individuals are not dangerous nor do they take further action.

    d. Occasionally exhibitionism is part of a more pervasive personality disorder, which also includes pedophilia.

6. Voyeurism involves the achievement of sexual excitement by observing naked bodies, especially the genitals. It is usually heterosexual in nature. The voyeur does not seek contact with the observed person and achieves orgasm by masturbating while looking. The excitement is heightened by the idea that the victim would feel humiliated knowing that someone is watching. The "Peeping Tom" is usually male. This disorder is differentiated from watching pornography or normal sexual play in which the individuals being watched are willing. Exhibitionism often occurs with voyeurism.

7. Masochism

    a. This disorder, which commonly coexists with sadism, **involves the achievement of sexual pleasure only through physical pain or suffering**. Fantasies of being bound, raped, or hurt that lead to sexual excitement are not sufficient for the diagnosis. Moral masochism, in which a person takes on the martyr's role of psychological suffering and sacrifice in ongoing interpersonal relationships, is also a different disorder.

    b. In the sexual disorder of masochism, the individual prefers or requires bondage, beatings, humiliation, or other physical suffering to achieve sexual excitement. If the person has intentionally participated in even a single episode in which he or she was physically harmed or his or her life was threatened in order to achieve sexual excitement, the diagnosis can be made.

8. Sadism. Like masochists, **individuals with this disorder need pain and suffering to achieve sexual gratification**. In sadism the pain is inflicted on another. Repeated and intentional physical or psychological pain has been inflicted on a nonconsenting partner, humiliation combined with simulated or mild injury has been used with a consenting partner, or extensive, permanent, or possibly fatal injury has been used with a consenting partner to achieve sexual excitement. Rape can sometimes result from this disorder, but not all rapists are sadists and vice versa.

D. Treatment

    1. The physician should assess all areas of the patient's level of functioning. Many of these patients have other psychological deficits as well, and they should be referred for treatment to qualified specialists.

        a. Long-term psychotherapy, including psychoanalysis, has been effective for some patients, but it is expensive, time-consuming, and limited to patients with a relatively high level of functioning.

        b. Behavior modification has also been successful in the treatment of severe and driven perversions.

        c. Antiandrogen drugs such as medroxyprogesterone have been used with some success in male patients with severe antisocial paraphilias.

    2. Patient motivation is extremely important. Paraphilias involve sexual gratification, and it is difficult for anyone to give up an area of sexual pleasure, even when there is legal risk involved. Recidivism rates remain high, even in cases of pedophilia in which the affected individual has been sent to jail.

V. PSYCHOSEXUAL DISORDERS

A. General issues. Most types of psychosexual disorders, whether affecting men or women, have certain features in common. **The disorder may be primary**, that is, lifelong, **or secondary**, acquired after a period of normal functioning. **The disorder may be generalized or situational**, that is, it exists only in certain situations or with specific partners. Finally, **the disorder may be either total or partial**, that is, to a degree or frequency that is less than total.

In order to diagnose sexual dysfunction, the physician must consider:

1. Subjective distress

2. Frequency of occurrence

3. Effect of the condition on other areas of the patient's functioning

B. Inhibited sexual desire

1. The criterion for diagnosis of inhibited sexual desire in the *Diagnostic and Statistical Manual of Mental Disorders*, third edition, (*DSM III*) is **persistent and pervasive inhibition**. The clinician must take into account many factors that can affect sexual desire, such as age, health, intensity and frequency of sexual desire, and the norms of sexual behavior in the context of the patient's life. The diagnosis only applies if there is distress from this lack of desire on the part of either partner. This diagnosis is not used if the cause is organic.

2. In one study of stable marriages, 2% of couples reported never having intercourse and 8% had intercourse less than once a month. Another study of young married couples found that one-third had definable periods of no sex starting around 8 weeks after marriage. Multiple reasons were given to explain the cessation of sexual activity, but the most common reason was **marital discord**.

C. Inhibited sexual excitement used to be termed **impotence** in men and **frigidity** in women. The word impotence implies a weakness and powerlessness that goes beyond a sexual disorder; frigidity implies a coldness and reserve of personality. The negative connotation of these words in the description of inhibited sexual excitement is not only unfortunate, it is inaccurate. Women with inhibited sexual excitement can be warm in other areas of their lives; men with failure of erection may be aggressive and powerful in other areas of their lives.

1. **Diagnosis** is not made if the condition is caused by organic factors. Before diagnosing inhibited sexual excitement, the physician must determine that the sexual activity in question is adequate in focus, intensity, and duration.

   a. In **men** there is recurrent and persistent partial or complete failure to attain or maintain an erection through completion of the sex act.

   b. In **women** there is partial or complete failure to attain or maintain the lubrication and swelling response to sexual excitement until completion of the sex act.

2. **Erectile dysfunction**

   a. Primary erectile dysfunction is a condition in which the man has never been able to have an erection sufficient to allow penetration of the vagina. It is not common and is usually associated with an overly rigid upbringing in which any expression of sexuality was punished. Occasionally it is associated with homosexuality.

   b. Secondary erectile dysfunction involves the failure to achieve an erection for intercourse, having been successful on previous occasions. The failure must be a persistent event (i.e., it must occur in 20% to 30% of all attempts). As is true in orgasmic dysfunction in women, the problem may be present in only certain situations or with certain partners.

   c. Causes

      (1) Anxiety from whatever source inhibits sexual arousal. The sympathetic nervous system is stimulated, thus inhibiting the parasympathetic nervous system, and erections depend upon parasympathetic innervation. Anxiety about sexual performance is the most common psychological cause of inhibited sexual excitement.

      (2) Overindulgence in alcohol often precipitates failure of erection. The patient subsequently becomes overly concerned and anxious about his sexual performance, and a vicious circle begins. Anxiety leads to failure, which increases the anxiety.

   d. Failure of erection due to organic causes becomes increasingly common with age.

      (1) In ruling out organic causes, it is important to question early morning erections, nocturnal emissions, and erection with self-stimulation and fantasy.

(2) Erections occur normally during rapid eye movement (REM) sleep. Plethysmography can be used to measure nocturnal tumescence: It measures the strength of an erection while the patient sleeps. The presence of erections at night indicates that the problem is less likely to be organic in origin.

D. Inhibited female orgasm is defined in the *DSM III* as **recurrent and persistent inhibition of orgasm after a sexual excitement phase** that ought to be adequate in focus, intensity, and duration. Some women experience difficulty in both the excitement and orgasm stages. Other women may be able to have an orgasm during noncoital clitoral stimulation but not during coitus, which, although probably a normal variation, concerns some patients.

1. **Primary orgasmic dysfunction.** Women who have never had an orgasm may have never learned what to expect physically. Primary orgasmic dysfunction may be easier to treat than secondary orgasmic dysfunction because the problem can be solved through education: The patient can be taught how to achieve orgasm. The physician must also help the patient cope with psychological inhibitions, which often involves ''giving permission'' for sexual pleasure. These women have often been taught that sex is ''dirty.''

2. **Secondary orgasmic dysfunction** involves a history of successful achievement of orgasm with the subsequent failure to achieve orgasm in all or some situations, either with particular partners or in particular settings.

3. **Causes.** Inhibited female orgasm is thought to be common but is not always indicative of psychopathology. Women with this problem may function quite well in all other areas of their lives.
   a. **Cultural restrictions** of women's sexuality probably account for some inhibition.
   b. **Financial concerns, alcohol abuse, and extramarital affairs** add tension to the relationship, making it more difficult to relax and achieve orgasm.
   c. **Psychological issues are the most common cause of secondary inhibition of orgasm.** Problems of passivity versus assertiveness, issues of control, and guilt feelings can all interfere with sexual pleasure. **Lack of communication** of needs and desires between partners is common. The man may lack sensitivity to his partner's needs, and she may be unable to tell him because of perceived role expectations, anger, or guilt.

4. **Symptoms.** Some women who do not have orgasms are nonsymptomatic and report satisfactory sex lives. Others may develop symptoms of pelvic pain, vaginal discharge, tiredness, and irritability.

E. Inhibited male orgasm. In this relatively rare condition, **there is recurrent and persistent delay or absence of ejaculation following an adequate phase of sexual excitement**. The diagnosis is not made when the cause is organic.

1. **The most common causes of delayed ejaculation are side effects due to medication**, particularly phenothiazines.

2. **Psychological causes include overly strict attitudes about sex** imposed during development and **discord in the adult relationship**.

F. Vaginismus

1. **Involuntary tightening of the paravaginal muscles to prevent penile penetration** can occur in all sexual encounters or only in specific situations. This problem is sometimes seen in the physician's office during a pelvic examination, preventing insertion of the speculum.

2. Patients often have backgrounds where sex was considered to be sinful and parents were overly controlling. Intercourse is experienced as painful and traumatic.

3. Vaginismus occasionally develops secondary to vaginal infections, especially if intercourse during the infection is painful.

G. Functional dyspareunia is recurrent and persistent pain in intercourse, which is **not due to physical causes.**

1. **In women** most of the time, however, painful intercourse **is** due to physical causes such as:
   a. Infections
   b. Endometriosis
   c. Lack of lubrication in postmenopausal women

2. **In men** painful intercourse is occasionally associated with neuroleptic medications, particularly thioridazine.

H. Premature ejaculation is the most common sexual dysfunction reported by men. The diagnosis requires a judgment by the physician that there is recurrent and persistent lack of control over ejaculation.

   1. Previously, premature ejaculation was defined as the inability of the man to delay ejaculation during intercourse until his partner achieved orgasm in more than 50% of the attempts. This definition, however, did not take into account the possibility of sexual dysfunction in the partner. Some men complain if they cannot sustain intercourse for 30 minutes or more. Although this may be a problem to the patient, the diagnosis of premature ejaculation should not be made. More commonly, the man ejaculates one or two strokes after insertion or even before insertion.

   2. Causes
   a. The causes of premature ejaculation are **usually psychological.** Often the man has "learned" to ejaculate rapidly from early sexual experiences in which anxiety was high because of fear of getting caught in the act by parents or other authorities.
   b. Other causes include guilt about sex or hostility on the part of the man towards his partner.
   c. Arousal of the sympathetic nervous system due to anxiety from whatever source can cause premature ejaculation as well as failure of erection.

I. Premenstrual syndrome has been defined as a complex of physical and psychological symptoms that begin during the week prior to menstruation and usually disappear shortly after the onset of the menstrual flow. The two primary elements in the diagnosis are a number of **typical symptoms** and their **time of occurrence** in the menstrual cycle.

   1. Typical symptoms
   a. Pain cluster
   (1) Abdominal cramps
   (2) Headache
   (3) Backache
   (4) Muscle spasms
   b. Psychological cluster
   (1) Tension
   (2) Irritability
   (3) Depression
   (4) Anxiety
   (5) Mood swings
   c. Edema/water-retention cluster
   (1) Breast tenderness
   (2) Weight gain
   (3) Swelling of joints or extremities
   (4) Bloating
   (5) Abdominal heaviness
   (6) Pelvic pressure
   d. Other symptoms
   (1) Food cravings
   (2) Dizziness
   (3) Clumsiness
   (4) Insomnia

   2. Timing. The cyclic nature of the symptoms is crucial for the diagnosis. Symptoms usually begin 1 to 10 days prior to menstruation and continue through the beginning of menses. Occasionally the symptoms begin after ovulation and continue through most of the menstrual period. There is always a symptom-free period of at least 1 week during the cycle.

   3. Etiology. The cause of premenstrual syndrome is not well established, and a number of theories have been proposed. These include the following.
   a. There is an imbalance in the ratio of estrogen to progesterone after ovulation.
   b. Estrogen increases aldosterone levels, causing water retention.
   c. Alterations in neurotransmitters such as dopamine and acetylcholine affect neurohormones.
   d. Prostaglandins are elevated, causing water retention.
   e. Psychologically, women who expect to have premenstrual symptoms will have them.

   4. Treatment
   a. Education. The patient should be taught to understand her cycle and to anticipate problems.

    b. Diet. Many symptoms can be controlled by a low-sodium, low-sugar, and low-caffeine diet along with regular meals.

    c. Exercise. Regular physical exercise helps to reduce tension and stress.

    d. Medication may be useful in relieving symptoms. Medications include:

        (1) Bromocriptine (for breast symptoms)

        (2) Diuretics

        (3) Prostaglandin inhibitors

        (4) Progestins

        (5) Oral contraceptives

        (6) Antianxiety medication

VI. HOMOSEXUALITY

A. General issues. Homosexuality per se is no longer considered to be an illness. Over 33% of males and over 10% of females have had orgasm with a partner of the same sex at least once in their lives. Approximately 4% of male adults and 2% of female adults in the United States are exclusively homosexual in behavior.

    1. The incidence and prevalence of mental illness is about the same in homosexuals as in heterosexuals.

    2. Some homosexuals may have many sexual partners. This leads to an increased risk for medical illnesses such as acquired immune deficiency syndrome (AIDS), hepatitis, and venereal disease, especially in men.

    3. The physician must be aware of his or her attitudes about homosexuality so that they do not interfere with establishing a good physician-patient relationship.

B. Ego-dystonic homosexuality

    1. This is a psychosexual disorder diagnosed when the patient reports being persistently distressed by his or her homosexual orientation. The patient wishes to change sexual orientation despite weak or absent heterosexual arousal. There is often a wish for marriage and children. The patient is usually lonely and feels guilty. Shame, anxiety, and depression may be present.

    2. Treatment aimed at changing sexual preference is difficult.

        a. Behavior modification has been tried using painful stimuli to make homosexual arousal noxious. Success with this treatment has been generally lacking.

        b. It is more useful to help the patient come to terms with his or her homosexual orientation.

VII. SEXUAL DYSFUNCTION

A. Sexual history. All patients deserve a routine review of their sexual functioning. However, a thorough discussion of sexual functioning is necessary for many patients in whom dysfunction may be related to medical problems such as diabetes, heart disease, and surgery.

    1. A sexual history should be taken at the time of the complete patient history and physical examination. It should not be delayed until the physician is comfortable discussing sex because that time rarely comes. **The physician's discomfort is the primary reason why an adequate history of sexual functioning usually is not obtained**.

    2. While discussing the history of the presenting illness, the physician should ask, "How has your sexual functioning been affected by the illness?" or "Many patients experience changes in sexual functioning as a result of this problem—how has it affected you?" **More important than how the physician asks the question is how the physician listens**. He or she should convey openness and a willingness to discuss the subject of sex.

    3. During the review of systems a more complete sexual history can be taken.

        a. Pathology involving the genital organs such as venereal disease, pain, and discharge should be evaluated.

        b. Sexual development questions can also be asked at this point in the examination. These include:

            (1) First childhood awareness of sexuality, including attitudes and punishment

            (2) Problems with gender identity

            (3) First sexual experience, including masturbation

            (4) Age of and reaction to puberty, including menarche in women

            (5) History of sexual abuse

            (6) Patient knowledge about sex and where it was acquired

            (7) First experience with a sexual partner, including intercourse

(8) Homosexual experiences and interest. Does the patient see these as problems?
(9) Current sexual functioning, including frequency and satisfaction
(10) Questions about extramarital partners if the patient is married
c. **Problems that may be uncovered in the sexual history include:**
(1) Concern about normal sexuality or sexual development secondary to the patient's lack of knowledge or misinformation
(2) Sexual aspects of a pervasive problem in the relationship with the sexual partner
(3) Sexual problems that result from the presenting medical or surgical problem
(4) Primary sexual dysfunction that needs further evaluation and treatment

B. **Treatment of sexual dysfunction.** Most physicians can use the **P-LI-SS-IT model** developed by Annon in the treatment of sexual dysfunction.

1. **P stands for permission.** The physician is in a position of authority and conveys a sense of approval for both discussing and enjoying sexuality.

2. **LI stands for limited information.** Many cases of sexual dysfunction result from lack of information or misinformation about sex. The physician can reassure as well as educate the patient about "normality."

3. **SS stands for specific suggestion.** This type of intervention requires more skill on the part of the physician, and the level of intervention depends upon the complexity of the problem. Masters and Johnson, among others, have developed therapy programs for couples, which employ short-term behavior approaches. After an extensive history is taken and physical and laboratory examinations are conducted, the couple is taught **sensate focusing**. The couple learns to "pleasure" each other without the demand of intercourse. Further treatment depends upon the specific problem.
a. **Premature ejaculation** is treated by either the **squeeze technique** or the **stop-and-go technique**. The man is stimulated to the point just before ejaculatory inevitability. Ejaculation is then prevented by squeezing the penis at the frenulum and coronal ridge or simply by stopping stimulation. This treatment has been very successful in most cases.
b. **Male or female orgasmic dysfunction.** Sensate focusing is used until erection or vaginal lubrication occurs. At first there is no vaginal penetration, then only containment followed by minor thrusting. Sexual position is also arranged to relieve the dysfunctional partner of performance demands. The exercises are gradually increased towards orgasm.

4. **IT stands for intensive therapy.** Patients who do not respond to the basic therapy described above may require psychotherapy and should be referred. In these cases, there are usually more complex problems in the relationship or associated psychopathology.

VIII. SEX AND PHYSICAL ILLNESS

A. **General issues.** Illness, whether medical or surgical, is a threat to self-esteem. The patient's physical appearance may be altered by either the illness or the treatment for the illness. The patient's self-image and sense of sexual attractiveness is also likely to be altered.

Pain, malaise, and anxiety tend to decrease interest in sex markedly. Occasionally, however, as a compensatory reaction to the fear of loss of attractiveness, there is an increase in libido and sexual behavior. In acute illness, the disturbance in sexuality usually resolves with the illness. In chronic illness, however, the physician should explore the patient's adaptation with respect to sexual functioning as a part of ongoing medical care.

B. **Specific conditions**

1. **Cardiovascular disease**
a. **Coronary artery disease.** Almost all patients with angina and those who have suffered a myocardial infarction are concerned that sex will affect their heart conditions. It is important to discuss the resumption of sex after a myocardial infarction with both partners since the spouse may also have concerns.
(1) The patient may cease all sexual activity for fear of precipitating another myocardial infarction unless the physician intervenes. In general, if the patient can walk up two flights of stairs without symptoms, sexual intercourse should not present a problem. The position of the partners does not seem to make a difference in terms of cardiac stress.
(2) The patient can be counseled to have sex in the morning after a good night's sleep rather than after a hard day's work or a party when he or she is tired and possibly intoxicated.
(3) Occasionally a patient may need to use nitroglycerine prophylactically prior to sex to prevent angina.

b. Hypertension. The major sexual problems associated with hypertension are usually secondary to antihypertensive medication. These drugs can interfere with both erection and ejaculation. Reserpine and guanethidine cause the worst problems. Methyldopa is less likely to interfere, and propranolol and clonidine cause the fewest side effects.

c. Other cardiovascular diseases, such as valvular disease of the heart, which interfere with cardiac output, may affect the patient's ability to sustain sex.

2. Neurologic illness

a. Spinal cord lesions. The support of the physician is crucial in facilitating a frank discussion of sexuality following injury to the spinal cord. Although these rates do not apply to married women who are injured, divorce rates increase following spinal cord injury in men. Exploration of alternative means of sexual expression, such as oral and manual stimulation, is necessary. Control of bowel and bladder function is an important aspect of sex. Avoiding stimulants such as caffeine may help prevent spasms.

(1) The level of injury is crucial to whether the male patient is able to obtain an erection. Upper motor neuron lesions, especially those higher up in the spinal cord, may not affect reflexogenic erections, which occur either secondary to a full bladder or from direct stimulation of the penis. Loss of both ejaculation and the experience of orgasm occurs if the upper motor neuron lesion is complete.

(2) Female sexual responses, such as vaginal lubrication and orgasm, are also affected by the level of the injury, but the pathophysiology is less well-known.

b. Diabetes mellitus. The possibility of adult-onset diabetes should always be considered in men over 50 years old who develop erectile failure. Approximately 50% of men with diabetes fail to have erections secondary to diabetic neuropathy. However, the sexual drive tends to remain strong in these men regardless of success or failure in the treatment of the diabetes. Penile implants, which allow the patient to maintain an erection artificially, can be surgically inserted to allow continuation of an active sex life. The surgery usually involves removing some penile tissue, and thus the patient can never again have a natural erection.

c. Multiple sclerosis can also cause erectile failure, which can be treated by a penile implant.

d. Other illnesses causing neurologic impairment of sexual functioning include tumors, syphilis, and pernicious anemia.

3. Surgical procedures

a. Prostatectomy. Removal of the prostate gland secondary to benign hypertrophy is a relatively common procedure in elderly men. Impotence frequently occurs but is often due to the patient's expectation rather than to any surgical interruption of the sympathetic plexis of nerves around the abdominal aorta. Retrograde ejaculation into the bladder following surgery is also common.

b. Orchiectomy. Because of the risk of cancer, surgical removal of the testes may be necessary upon failure of one of the testicles to descend. Testicular carcinoma also requires removal of one or both testes. Erectile failure should not develop even with bilateral orchiectomy in adult men, but it often occurs when the testicles are removed in boys. Reassurance and counseling are required to avoid unnecessary psychological and sexual dysfunction.

c. Hysterectomy is now the most common surgical procedure in the United States. The psychological associations of the uterus for the patient affect the psychological outcome of the surgery. Most women report no change in sexual functioning following hysterectomy. Because the fear of pregnancy is eliminated, some women derive more enjoyment from sex after surgery. When the surgery is performed for cancer, damage may be extensive and the psychological stress is greater. This can lead both to increased organic and psychological impairment of sexual functioning.

d. Mastectomy. The breasts are an obvious aspect of a woman's sexual identity. Disfiguring loss of a breast due to mastectomy can have a major effect on a woman's self-image and thus her sexual functioning, even if there is no direct effect on sexual physiology.

The patient may feel that she is no longer attractive to her husband and that he will shun her. The husband may feel guilty or simply be afraid to touch or even look at his wife's body. He may think she wishes to be left alone. This withdrawal confirms the patient's fears that she is deformed and repulsive, leading to further isolation and a breakdown in the relationship. The physician must initiate open communication between the couple about the fears and misconceptions that both may have.

e. Ostomy. An ostomy usually causes concern in the patient about sex. There are worries about pain, damage to the stoma, as well as about odors of elimination during sexual activity. A single patient who wants a sexual relationship is uncertain when and how a prospective sexual partner should be told about the ostomy. There are no simple or easy answers. It is crucial that the physician be willing and able to listen to the patient and offer support and understanding.

4. Drugs and alcohol
   a. Prescribed medications that can interfere with sex include:
      (1) Antihypertensives and other blocking agents, which can cause erectile failure
      (2) Antipsychotics and antidepressants, which may cause retrograde ejaculation as well as erectile failure
   b. Alcohol is the most common cause of sexual dysfunction. It increases sexual desire but decreases performance. Chronic alcoholism also may affect sexual function via liver disease. Cirrhotic livers are unable to detoxify estrogens in men, leading to testicular atrophy and decreased sexual performance.
   c. Narcotics decrease libido. Drug addiction of all sorts generally leads to decreased interest in sex.

BIBLIOGRAPHY

American Psychiatric Association: *Diagnostic and Statistical Manual of Mental Disorders*, 3rd ed. Washington, D.C., American Psychiatric Association, 1980

Annon JS, Robinson CH: The use of vicarious learning in the treatment of sexual concerns. In *Handbook of Sex Therapy*. Edited by Piccolo JL, Piccolo LL. New York, Plenum Press, 1978, pp 35–56

STUDY QUESTIONS

Directions: Each question below contains five suggested answers. Choose the **one best** response to each question.

1. What is the most common reason that adequate sexual histories are not obtained from patients?

(A) The patient is embarrassed about the subject of sex
(B) The patient has religious or moral qualms about the subject of sex
(C) The physician does not think that sex is as important as other medical issues
(D) There is not enough time to cover the subject adequately in taking a routine history
(E) The physician is uncomfortable with the subject of sex

2. All of the following statements about gender identity are true EXCEPT

(A) gender identity is set by 1 year of age
(B) the early embryo is undifferentiated sexually (i.e., it is bisexual)
(C) gender identity refers to one's sense of being masculine or feminine
(D) an infant is assigned a gender identity on the basis of genitalia
(E) the Y chromosome is necessary for the development of male genitalia

3. According to Freud's theory of psychosexual development, which of the following statements is most characteristic of the phallic phase?

(A) Control over urination gives pleasure
(B) Fears of bodily injury are common
(C) Girls adopt a passive role
(D) Boys identify with the father
(E) The symbiotic relationship with the mother stops

4. All of the following statements about transsexualism are true EXCEPT

(A) the disorder usually begins in childhood
(B) transsexual boys believe that they will lose their penises and testicles when they grow up
(C) transsexual girls usually have been dressed like boys by their mothers
(D) the etiology of transsexualism is not known for certain
(E) the transsexual wishes to live as a member of the opposite sex

5. All of the following statements about pedophilia are true EXCEPT

(A) it is often caused by an organic brain syndrome
(B) the adult perpetrator must be at least 10 years older than the victim
(C) the disorder involves prepubertal children of either sex
(D) the diagnosis can be made when sexual stimulation is achieved by fantasy
(E) sexual abuse of children may be more common than has been thought

6. Lubrication of the vagina is a prominent feature of which of the following stages of normal sexual response in women?

(A) Desire
(B) Excitement
(C) Plateau
(D) Orgasm
(E) Resolution

7. All of the following statements about secondary failure of erection are true EXCEPT

(A) it may be present in only certain situations
(B) it must occur in 20% to 30% of attempts at intercourse for diagnosis
(C) it becomes increasingly common with age
(D) overindulgence in alcohol is often the precipitating factor
(E) it usually is associated with an overly rigid upbringing

8. Which of the following statements most accurately defines premature ejaculation?

(A) The cause is usually psychological, and the disorder has been "learned" by the patient
(B) The disorder has become relatively uncommon
(C) It is the inability of the partner to achieve orgasm more than 50% of the time
(D) It can be diagnosed if the man cannot sustain intercourse for more than 30 minutes
(E) It is generally associated with arousal of the parasympathetic nervous system

9. All of the following statements regarding homosexuality are true EXCEPT

(A) approximately 4% of men in the United States are exclusively homosexual
(B) over one-third of males have had an orgasm with a partner of the same sex at least once
(C) there is a higher incidence of some mental illnesses, such as affective disorders, in homosexuals than in heterosexuals
(D) there is a higher incidence of some physical illnesses, such as hepatitis, in homosexuals than in heterosexuals
(E) treatment aimed at changing homosexual to heterosexual preference is generally unsuccessful

10. When a sexual history must be taken from a patient, it is **most** important that the physician

(A) find out about family attitudes towards sex
(B) evaluate the status of the patient's relationship with his or her spouse
(C) diagnose any medical condition that might interfere with sex
(D) overcome nervousness and embarrassment
(E) take an open, nonjudgmental stance in listening to the patient

11. What physical impairment is most responsible for sexual dysfunction in men?

(A) Spinal cord injury
(B) Diabetes mellitus
(C) Benign prostatic hypertrophy
(D) Testicular carcinoma
(E) Multiple sclerosis

Directions: Each question below contains four suggested answers of which **one or more** is correct. Choose the answer

A   if **1, 2, and 3** are correct
B   if **1 and 3** are correct
C   if **2 and 4** are correct
D   if **4** is correct
E   if **1, 2, 3, and 4** are correct

12. To obtain a thorough sexual history, it is necessary for the physician to inquire about

(1) familial attitudes about sex
(2) any history of sexual abuse
(3) the first sexual experience
(4) current sexual functioning

13. Vaginismus involves tightening of the paravaginal muscles to prevent penile penetration. Characteristics of the disorder include

(1) occasional occurrence during pelvic examinations
(2) occasional development secondary to vaginal infections
(3) occurrence in all or only some sexual encounters
(4) a history of sexual abuse in childhood

14. True statements concerning inhibited female orgasm include

(1) inhibited female orgasm is common and usually does not indicate psychopathology
(2) primary orgasmic dysfunction is more difficult to treat than secondary orgasmic dysfunction
(3) associated symptoms include pelvic pain and vaginal discharge
(4) physiologic impairment is the most likely cause of secondary orgasmic dysfunction

SUMMARY OF DIRECTIONS

A	B	C	D	E
1, 2, 3 only	1, 3 only	2, 4 only	4 only	All are correct

15. True statements concerning the sexual disorder of masochism include

(1) fantasies of being bound or hurt that lead to sexual excitement are sufficient to make the diagnosis
(2) the patient takes on the martyr's role of suffering and sacrifice in interpersonal relationships
(3) the patient is not likely to achieve sexual gratification by inflicting pain on another, only by receiving it
(4) a single episode in which the patient was physically harmed in order to achieve sexual excitement is sufficient to make the diagnosis

16. The psychosexual disorder of inhibited sexual desire can be diagnosed in patients with which of the following findings?

(1) Inhibition of sexual desire lasting more than 6 months
(2) Lack of sexual desire following major surgery
(3) Distress reported by the sexual partner rather than by the patient
(4) Lack of sexual desire with the marriage partner but not with other partners

ANSWERS AND EXPLANATIONS

1. The answer is E. (*VII A 1*) The most common reason that physicians do not ask adequate questions concerning sexuality is their own anxiety about the subject. Patients are certainly embarrassed as well, but, if there is a problem, they usually hope that their physicians will take the lead in discussing it. Religious and moral objections to talking about sex are not very common. Physicians' impressions that sex is not as important as other medical issues is usually only a cover for their anxiety. It only takes a moment to ask screening questions about sexuality, and, if there are difficulties, the subject can be dealt with later when there is adequate time.

2. The answer is A. (*II A*) Gender identity, which is set by about the age of 3 years, is one's sense of being masculine or feminine rather than a biologic state of being. The early embryo is bisexual and requires a Y chromosome for the development of male genitalia. Infants are assigned a sex usually on the basis of their external genitalia and are reared as that sex with the parents' and society's attitudes regarding it.

3. The answer is B. (*II B 1 c*) According to Freud's theory of psychosexual development, during the phallic phase there is an increased awareness of the genitals in children of both sexes, and it is during this period that fears of bodily injury are common. Control over urination, while involving the genitals, gives pleasure during the anal phase, when children begin to obtain control over several bodily functions. That girls adopt a passive role is a theory proposed by Freud, who suggested that this passivity evolved in the resolution of the oedipal phase. During the oedipal phase, boys supposedly identify with their fathers as a way of dealing with their competitive feelings. The developmental theory of the symbiotic relationship with the mother is not freudian.

4. The answer is C. (*III*) Although the etiology of transsexualism is not known for certain, boys have histories of being crossdressed by their mothers as well as having overly close physical and emotional ties to them; their fathers generally have been absent. Girls tend to have distant relationships with their mothers, who are seen as unavailable physically or emotionally during formative years. The disorder begins in childhood, and boys believe that they will lose their penises and testicles when they grow up. This is not a homosexual condition; patients wish to live as members of the opposite sex.

5. The answer is A. (*IV C 4*) When an individual with an organic brain syndrome engages in sexual activity with a child, pedophilia is not diagnosed; inappropriate sexual activity can be characteristic of brain damage. By definition, an adult with pedophilia must be at least 10 years older than the victim. When the perpetrator is a late adolescent, the age difference is less clear and clinical judgment must be used. The disorder involves prepubertal children of either sex, and the diagnosis can be made when the sexual stimulation is achieved by fantasy alone. The incidence of sexual abuse of children appears to be much higher than had been previously thought, and statistics are changing as the general population becomes more aware of the problem.

6. The answer is C. (*I C 2*) During the plateau stage of normal sexual response in women, the clitoris becomes sensitive and retracts, the labia deepen in color, and the vagina becomes lubricated. During the excitement phase, breast size increases, nipples stand out, the clitoris lengthens, and the heart rate and blood pressure increase. During the orgasm stage, there is a rhythmic contraction of the orgasmic platform. During resolution, vasocongestion is lost.

7. The answer is E. (*V C 2*) Primary erectile dysfunction is usually associated with an overly rigid upbringing in which any expression of sexuality was punished. Secondary erectile dysfunction usually results from anxiety about sexual performance. It may be present in only certain situations or with certain partners. Diagnosis is not made when it is a rare or occasional event but when it occurs in about 25% or more of attempts at intercourse. It becomes increasingly common with age and is often precipitated by a bout of drinking, which leads to increased anxiety about performance.

8. The answer is A. (*V H*) Premature ejaculation is the most common sexual dysfunction reported by men. Causes are usually psychological. Often the man has "learned" to ejaculate rapidly from early sexual experiences in which anxiety was high because of fear of getting caught in the act by parents or other authority figures. Defining the disorder is difficult because definitions must take into account the patient's idea about what is the proper duration of sexual intercourse: It is not diagnosed when intercourse lasts less than 30 minutes, although sometimes this is a complaint. It is not defined by the inability of the partner to achieve orgasm more than 50% of the time because this does not take into account the possibility of sexual dysfunction in the partner. Arousal of the sympathetic nervous system, rather than arousal of the parasympathetic nervous system, is associated with the dysfunction.

9. The answer is C. (*VI A*) One of the reasons that homosexuality is no longer considered to be a mental illness is because the incidence and prevalence of mental illness in homosexuals are no higher than in heterosexuals. According to several surveys, conservatively, 4% of the adult male population in the United States is exclusively homosexual, but a much higher percentage (i.e., approximately 33%) of males have had orgasm with an individual of the same sex at least once, which does not indicate homosexuality. There is a higher incidence of some illnesses such as acquired immune deficiency syndrome (AIDS), hepatitis, and venereal disease in homosexuals who have many sexual partners. Treatment aimed at changing homosexual preference has been generally unsuccessful.

10. The answer is E. (*VII A 2*) The most important aspect in obtaining a complete sexual history is an attitude of openness and impartiality on the part of the physician. Specific questions concerning sexuality are not as important. Family attitudes about sex and the status of the sexual relationship are easier for the patient to talk about if he or she feels that the physician is nonjudgmental. Medical conditions that interfere with sex should be diagnosed but, again, are easier to discuss once the basic relationship with the physician has been established.

11. The answer is B. (*VIII B 2 b*) Diabetes mellitus is a very common cause of sexual impairment in men, and it should always be considered as a possible cause of erectile failure in men over 50 years of age. Approximately one-half of men with adult-onset diabetes develop erectile failure secondary to diabetic neuropathy. Spinal cord injury is a far less common cause of sexual impairment, but certainly issues of sexuality need to be discussed with these patients. Benign prostatic hypertrophy should not cause sexual impairment; occasionally the surgery for the condition does. In comparison to diabetes, testicular carcinoma is a rare cause of dysfunction as is multiple sclerosis.

12. The answer is E (all). (*VII A*) A discussion lead by the physician with the patient concerning the attitudes of the patient's family concerning sex is important in obtaining a thorough sexual history. Was sex seen as dirty and was discussion prohibited, or was there an openness about sexuality? In addition, it is increasingly important that discussion with the patient include any history of sexual abuse; this is particularly important with women patients. Questioning the patient about his or her first sexual experience is also important, particularly whether it was a pleasant or frightening event. Even the most basic screening questions should evaluate the patient's current sexual functioning.

13. The answer is A (1, 2, 3). (*V F*) Patients with vaginismus often come from backgrounds in which sex was considered sinful and behavior by the parents was overcontrolling; however, there is no known increased incidence of sexual abuse in the background of these patients. The paravaginal muscles are tightened involuntarily, thus preventing penile penetration. Occasionally this condition occurs in the physician's office during a pelvic examination; sometimes it develops secondary to vaginal infections and irritation. By definition, it can occur in all sexual encounters or only in some.

14. The answer is B (1, 3). (*V D*) While some women who do not have orgasms are nonsymptomatic, others may develop symptoms of pelvic pain, vaginal discharge, and feelings of tiredness and irritability. The disorder is common, but its presence does not always indicate psychopathology because there are often cultural restrictions regarding women's sexuality. These women have a normal excitement phase, but it does not lead to orgasm. Primary orgasmic dysfunction may be more easily treated because women may not have "learned" to have an orgasm and can be taught once inhibitions about sexuality have resolved. When secondary orgasmic dysfunction develops, it is almost always as a result of psychological issues in the sexual relationship.

15. The answer is D (4). (*IV C 7*) If the patient even once allows him- or herself to be harmed in order to achieve sexual excitement, the diagnosis of the sexual disorder of masochism can be made. Fantasies about being bound or hurt alone are not sufficient to make the diagnosis. The martyr's role of suffering and sacrifice in an interpersonal relationship is moral masochism; it is not the sexual disorder of masochism. Whereas the other paraphilias are almost exclusively seen in men, masochism can also be seen in women, although not commonly. Sadism, the achievement of sexual gratification by inflicting pain on others, is often seen in conjunction with masochism, hence the disorder, sadomasochism.

16. The answer is B (1, 3). (*V B*) The diagnostic criterion of inhibited sexual desire is persistent and pervasive inhibition. The clinician must take into account factors that affect sexual desire, such as health. Generally, the disorder is not diagnosed if the patient has a normal lack of sexual desire immediately following major surgery or if there are marital problems such that one partner lacks sexual desire for the spouse but not for other partners. If the patient's sexual desire has been inhibited for more than 6 months, the diagnosis can be made. A diagnosis is also valid upon report of distress from the partner rather than the patient.

8

Eating Disorders
William V. Good

I. ANOREXIA NERVOSA

A. Introduction. Anorexia nervosa is a disorder exemplified by obsessional weight loss without an identifiable organic cause.

  1. The **diagnostic findings** include the following (information is taken from the *Diagnostic and Statistical Manual of Mental Disorders*, third edition, *(DSM III)*.

    a. Except in unusual cases, the age of the onset is before 25 years.
    b. Weight loss is at least 25% of the original body weight or of the ideal body weight.
    c. Fear of becoming obese (and of eating) is paramount in the clinical picture.
    d. The body image of the patient is disturbed (i.e., the patient feels fat despite emaciation). This perception may not be limited to anorectics, however, and is sometimes found in normal-sized adolescents.
    e. The patient refuses to maintain her weight and involves herself in weight-losing activities.

  2. There are a variety of **associated findings,** which may precede or accompany the onset of illness.
    a. Amenorrhea
    b. Lanugo hair development
    c. Bradycardia
    d. Heightened activity level
    e. Vomiting and purging
    f. Laxative abuse

B. Epidemiology

  1. The **prevalence** of anorexia nervosa is approximately 1 in 200 girls at puberty. The disorder occurs in girls much more commonly than in boys at a ratio of between 10 and 20 to 1.

  2. The **incidence** of the disorder is increasing, probably due to altered social attitudes and changing roles for women.

  3. Anorexia nervosa appears to be more common in Western civilization, and Caucasians have the highest rate of this disorder, particularly girls of Jewish and Italian families. Middle- and upper-class families are at the greatest risk.

  4. The average age of onset of the illness is 13 to 14 years; the onset often is preceded by a period of mild obesity or mild dieting. It is interesting to note that a relatively high percentage of anorectics lose a parent within the year preceding the onset of the illness.

  5. Anorexia nervosa is associated with Turner's syndrome, with absence of the second X chromosome (XO). There may be a slight increased risk of anorexia nervosa developing in mentally retarded children.

  6. An association exists of subsequent affective disorders in anorectic patients. Anorectic patients are at greater risk than is the general population of developing either unipolar or bipolar affective disturbances. These disturbances tend to occur later in life and probably are not the underlying cause of anorexia nervosa. The risk for suicide is increased.

C. Etiology

1. One **psychological theory** holds that anorectic patients have a deep fear of impregnation and an accompanying fantasy that impregnation occurs through the oral route. They defend themselves against pregnancy by not eating. A corollary to this theory is that affected adolescents fear sexuality, menarche, and pregnancy and starve themselves to remain prepubertal.

2. The **transactional theory** accomodates the interactions between parent and child. A series of particular interactions may cause slight changes in the family system, which in turn may lead to a new and more deviated set of interactions. This pertains to anorexia nervosa in that the child's request not to eat or refusal to eat is overridden by the parent's need to feed the child. Eventually, the child loses the ability to regulate her own eating and becomes dependent on her environment in a pervasive way for cues concerning this and other areas of self-regulation. For example, anorectic girls are unable to maintain weight at a norm. Lacking the ability to follow internal cues (e.g., satiety and hunger), such girls rely on strict diet, observations of parents, and careful calorie counts to guide eating behavior. They may depend on parental approval to guide social activity rather than feeling a sense of who *they* are and what *they* want to do with themselves.

3. The **mother-daughter relationship** could play a role in the etiology. Mothers of anorectic girls are often controlling, allowing their daughters little autonomy. The child's developing and maintaining control over eating and weight could be a method for counteracting such maternal effects.

4. The **fathers** of anorectics can be obsessive-compulsive. They may participate in quasi weight-control activities such as distance running. They may transmit their attitudes about weight to their daughters.

5. **Endocrinologic disorders** have been proposed as etiologic.
   a. An increase in catecholamine activity at various central nervous system sites could account for some of the stigmata of this illness.
   b. A variety of endocrine abnormalities (listed in section I D), which may signify some alteration in normal hypothalamic-pituitary functioning, occur in this disease.

D. Differential diagnosis

1. **Medical**
   a. **Addison's disease** may present with weight loss, anorexia, vomiting, and electrolyte abnormalities. It differs from anorexia nervosa in that listlessness and depression are frequent concomitants (in contrast to the hyperactivity of anorexia nervosa). Sodium concentration is low, potassium concentration is high, and serum cortisol levels should be suppressed in Addison's disease.
   b. **Hypothyroidism** may present with cold intolerance, constipation, bradycardia, low blood pressure, and skin changes similar to those seen in anorexia nervosa (i.e., dry, scaling skin). Obsessional food handling, weight loss (and accompanying fear of weight gain), and hyperactivity are not usual, however.
   c. **Hyperthyroidism** presents with elevated vital signs, hyperactivity, and, sometimes, weight loss. However, hyperthyroid patients usually are not obsessive about food.
   d. **Any chronic illness** (e.g., Crohn's disease, ulcerative colitis, rheumatoid arthritis, collagen-vascular disease, and tuberculosis) can cause progressive weight loss but should be readily identifiable as a physical disorder.
   e. **Central nervous system tumors** can cause endocrine malfunction. Visual disturbances or panhypopituitarism secondary to the tumor should be evident.
   f. **Superior mesenteric artery syndrome** can cause vomiting and anorexia. The mechanism is thought to involve compression of the duodenum by the superior mesenteric artery, particularly when the patient is supine and especially in individuals who are already thin.

2. **Psychiatric**
   a. **Schizophrenia.** Although schizophrenics may be delusional about food, the delusions are much more bizarre than those seen in anorectics (e.g., "there's poison in this" versus "this will make me fat"). Other stigmata of schizophrenia should be present.
   b. **Bulimia** involves binge eating followed by some form of purging in a patient who otherwise maintains her weight.
   c. **Depression** is often accompanied by anorexia. In this case, the anorexia is a so-called vegetative sign of depression, and a depressed mood is usually pronounced.
   d. **Hysterical noneating** is distinguishable by absence of a morbid concern with weight and calories.

3. **Anorexia nervosa as a syndrome.** Recent research suggests that anorexia nervosa is a syndrome that can be subclassified. Such subclassification is useful both prognostically and (perhaps) in treatment.
   a. Patients with bulimia may form a distinct subgroup. As such, these patients seem to be more extroverted, present with the disorder later in life, and have a worse prognosis than patients who indulge only in persistent self-starvation.
   b. The anorexia nervosa subgroup is characterized by strict self-starvation.
   c. Vomiters may form another subgroup.
   d. Male anorectics may form yet another distinct subgroup.

E. **Associated findings**

1. Normal thyroid-stimulating hormone (TSH) levels; possible low triiodothyronine (T_3) levels

2. Normal or overstimulated adrenal axis; possibly a loss of normal diurnal variation in cortisol secretion.

3. Amenorrhea, which may occur before, during, or after weight loss; menses do not necessarily resume with weight gain versus amenorrhea secondary to simple malnutrition (the reason that menstruation is not necessarily tied to weight loss in anorexia nervosa is unknown)

4. Characteristically normal serum protein and albumin concentrations

5. Increased serum carotene, which is rare in other causes of weight loss

6. Partial development of diabetes insipidus

7. Possible increase in growth hormone levels

8. Dehydration and serious electrolyte abnormalities

9. Abdominal pain

10. Three personality styles, which are classically cited as preceding the onset of anorexia nervosa:
    a. Obsessive-compulsive [perfectionistic]. (A girl who is perfectionistic about other areas of her life may focus her compulsivity on her eating.)
    b. Hysterical. (A hysteric overly sexualizes his or her relationships because of conflicts about sexuality. Such conflicts can also play a role in the etiology of anorexia nervosa.)
    c. Schizoid [schizotypal]. (Because a schizoid individual is prone to odd behavior, he or she is more likely to have unusual eating behavior.)

F. **Treatment**

1. **Medication**
   a. Antidepressant drugs are generally of no value, but they may be useful in rare, individual cases.
   b. Cyproheptadine may be of some value because it has appetite-stimulating properties.
   c. Antipsychotic medication should be used only when the patient suffers from preschizophrenic illness.

2. **Psychotherapy**
   a. Psychotherapy is nearly always a useful adjunct to other treatment modalities, but it is rarely effective alone. Psychoanalysis is usually particularly ineffective in anorexia nervosa if it is the only treatment intervention. Both can foster a regression in patients, which, in treatment, is only useful when the patient has the ability and strength to pull out of the regression at the end of the session. Neither of these treatments provides enough structure for the patient (e.g., anorectics may need to be watched and to be told what to do through most of the day).
   b. **Contraindications**
      (1) The patient steadfastly refuses to work with the therapist.
      (2) If the patient suffers from a severe borderline personality disorder, psychotherapy may worsen her condition because anorectics may be intolerant of regression. This is usually not predictable, however, until a trial of psychotherapy has been instituted.
   c. **Mechanism and approach**
      (1) Initially the therapeutic work should be aimed at forming an alliance with the patient to work on particular problems.
      (2) Gaps in the patient's ego should be clarified (e.g., when the patient is obviously angry about something but is unaware of this, her affect can be pointed out to her).

(3) Transference reactions should be interpreted if and when they interfere with the patient's ability to work on and talk about her problems.

(4) An empathic stance should be maintained with the patient.

3. Hospitalization

a. Indications

(1) The patient loses weight despite outpatient intervention.

(2) The patient is suicidal.

(3) Vomiting and purging are causing acid-base or electrolyte problems.

(4) The family cannot tolerate having the child at home any longer.

b. Contraindications.
There are no contraindications. If the patient refuses hospitalization and is in danger either medically or psychiatrically (if she is suicidal), she should be held against her will.

c. Treatment approach

(1) **Medical management** should include monitoring the electrolyte and hydration status of the patient. Thyroid supplementation is usually unnecessary. The patient should be weighed every other day. If the patient steadfastly refuses to eat, alimentation should be provided by a nasogastric tube; if the food is vomited, it should be readministered. In the extremely unlikely event that this fails, intravenous hyperalimentation through a central line may be required.

(2) **Behavior modification** usually must be implemented. The patient's privileges (e.g., confinement in a locked unit versus freedom to leave the ward) should be tied to the behavioral approach and be commensurate with the patient's ability to regulate her own activity and eating. **Splitting** (putting one staff member against another) **and manipulations concerning eating are common,** should be acknowledged, and should be dealt with at staff meetings and with the patient. Flexibility is important. These patients can be extraordinarily manipulative. Peer interaction and feedback should be sought and emphasized since adolescents often pay more attention to their peers than to adults.

(a) Either failure of psychotherapy or not enough time to await the results of psychotherapy are **indications for behavior modification.**

(b) The **methods of implementation** are geared to the following. The patient's weight should be the target symptom, not the eating behavior, amount of exercise, or vomiting, and reinforcers should be tied to weight fluctuation. Once the patient is stable medically and has some weight reserve, urine can be monitored for ketones before each meal. This checks starvation states, provides the patient with immediate feedback, and offers her the opportunity to alter her starvation state immediately. If she is spilling ketones, her activities and privileges should be completely restricted until her urine reverts to normal.

4. Family therapy

a. Some form of **family intervention is nearly always indicated,** especially for adolescents.

b. There are no **contraindications.**

c. **Approach.** Styles of family interaction should be clarified, and projections and vicarious pleasures that family members derive from the patient's symptoms should be interpreted. The family should be allied with the staff, working toward the patient's betterment, and not with patient to her detriment.

G. Prognosis

1. **The earlier the onset of the disease, the better the prognosis**, and the longer the disease course, the worse the prognosis. Decreased denial of a problem and admitting to feeling hungry are good prognostic signs, as is gainful employment. A schizoid personality disorder bodes a bad prognosis.

2. On the average, 30% to 40% of patients have a relatively complete recovery; 30% or more may undergo a period of obesity; and 40% continue to demonstrate bizarre eating habits, weight loss, and a severe disease course.

3. The mortality rates are reported to be 5% to 15%. Death, when it occurs, is due to electrolyte abnormalities, suicide, or possibly to too rapid a rehydration and weight gain.

II. BULIMIA

A. Definition.
As a distinct diagnostic entity, bulimia consists of ravenous overeating followed by guilt, depression, and anger at oneself for doing so. Although there usually is some accompanying feeling of loss of control of eating, there is no significant loss of weight below the normal for age and size. Other findings include the following.

1. High-calorie food is usually ingested.

2. Individuals with bulimia usually hide their eating.

3. Weight may fluctuate.

4. There may be attempts to lose weight (e.g., dieting, use of cathartics, and exercise).

5. Eating episodes may be terminated by sleep, abdominal pain, social interruption, or self-induced vomiting.

B. Epidemiology. Primarily a disorder of adolescent girls, the disorder is probably very common, existing in gradations from mild (perhaps a variant of normal) to severe.

C. Etiology. Very little is known about the cause of the disorder; the following etiologies remain tentative.

   1. Psychiatric.

   a. Bulimia could be caused by a need to take in something orally—perhaps as a substitution for some degree of maternal deprivation.

   b. Some children of short stature fantasize that eating ravenously can help them grow.

   c. Bulimia has been described in children with psychogenic dwarfism (retarded growth due to emotional neglect).

   2. Medical. A lesion of the satiety center in the hypothalamus could contribute to bulimia, but such a lesion has not been defined or discovered.

D. Differential diagnosis

   1. Prader-Willi syndrome: Continuous overeating is accompanied by mental retardation, hypogonadism, hypotonia, and diabetes mellitus.

   2. Klüver-Bucy syndrome: Objects are examined by mouth, there is altered sexual behavior, and hyperphagia is characteristic.

   3. Kleine-Levin syndrome manifests as hyperphagia and hypersomnia; both occur in spurts of 2 to 3 weeks. This disorder is more common in boys.

   4. Hypothalamic lesions should be considered.

   5. Anorexia nervosa. A component to anorexia nervosa may be binge eating, but simple bulimia does not include significant weight loss.

III. RUMINATION

A. Definition. This is a rare disorder of infancy consisting of purposive expulsion of previously ingested food, followed by rechewing the food. This usually occurs while the infant is alone.

B. Epidemiology. The disorder is very rare and may be decreasing in incidence.

C. Etiology. Although theories abound, the disorder often occurs in families where the parents are psychosexually immature and distant. Food and chewing may take on a transitional quality for the child and sooth the infant when alone, much in the way of a special doll or blanket.

D. Treatment

   1. Dyad (mother-child) interactions should be observed. Cues that the parent gives the child that encourage regurgitation should be interpreted and eradicated.

   2. Indepth psychotherapy of one or both parents is often needed.

   3. The infant's nutritional status should be followed closely.

IV. PICA

A. Pica is a disorder involving the eating of nonfood products. Mouthing inanimate objects is normal between 6 and 12 months of age.

B. Epidemiology. This problem may be more common in lower socioeconomic groups.

C. Etiology

   1. Mentally retarded children mouth objects more than normal children.

2. Iron deficiency can cause a craving for ice and nonfood items.

3. Mother-child problems (especially where repeated, traumatic separations are involved) are etiologic in some cases.

4. A variety of rare neurologic conditions can cause children to mouth nonfood items (e.g., Klüver-Bucy syndrome).

D. Complications

1. Bezoars

2. Lead poisoning can present with a variety of neurologic and psychiatric manifestations. It is extremely dangerous, more common in areas of older homes with lead-based paint, and should be suspected in any child with an encephalopathy or unusual behavior.

E. Treatment

1. Dangerous objects should be removed from the child's environment.

2. Increasing the amount of stimulation to a child can be helpful. (Most cities offer infant-stimulation programs.)

3. Psychotherapy for the child and parents may be needed.

V. FAILURE TO THRIVE

A. Definition. Failure to thrive is diagnosed when a child fails to maintain weight above the third percentile for his or her age group. Failure to grow in height sometimes accompanies this, but failure of head circumference growth occurs only in severe cases.

B. Etiology

1. Failure to thrive as a **psychiatric condition** has protean causes and manifestations. The following list divides these causes by developmental phase, but it is not meant to be complete.
  a. Early infancy: Prior to 8 or 9 months of life, a child is inactive and relies on parental feeding. Failure to thrive in this age range may mean poor parenting or troubled parent-child interactions.
  b. Late infancy: After 8 months, failure to thrive may be secondary to anaclitic depression, poor parenting, or childhood psychosis.
  c. Toddler stage: The negativism associated with the terrible twos can also apply to eating. Children may refuse to eat in the service of autonomy. Sometimes this negativism may develop earlier, as when parents frantically force food on a 1-year-old child.

2. A variety of **medical conditions** can cause failure to thrive and should be evaluated. These include juvenile-onset diabetes mellitus, other endocrine disorders, and malabsorption syndromes.

C. Treatment. Any organic cause must be ruled out, and parent-child interactions should be evaluated carefully. The child should be hospitalized in some cases to observe if he or she can gain weight in a new environment. Underlying disorders should be treated.

BIBLIOGRAPHY

American Psychiatric Association: *Diagnostic and Statistical Manual of Mental Disorders,* 3rd ed. Washington, D.C., American Psychiatric Association, 1980

Halmi KA, Falk JR: Anorexia nervosa: a study of outcome discriminators in exclusive dieters and bulimics. *J Am Acad Child Psychiatry* 21:369, 1982

Lesser LI, Ashenden BJ, Debuskey M, et al: Anorexia nervosa in children. *Am J Orthopsychiatry* 30:572, 1960

Sameroff AJ, Chandler M: Reproductive risk and the continuum of caretaking casualty. In *Review of Child Development Research,* vol 4. Edited by Horowitz F. Chicago, The University of Chicago Press, pp 187–244, 1975

STUDY QUESTIONS

Directions: Each question below contains five suggested answers. Choose the **one best** response to each question.

1. A 15-year-old girl presents to the emergency room with severe weight loss. On physical examination, she is cachectic with a weight of 68 lbs; her heart rate is 36, and her blood pressure is 72/50. The first intervention should be

(A) evaluation of the family to determine the family dynamics
(B) immediate administration of a high-protein and carbohydrate diet via a nasogastric tube
(C) drawing blood for serum electrolyte determination and then starting intravenous (IV) feeding
(D) arrangements to have the patient admitted to the psychiatric service
(E) arrangements for electroconvulsive therapy

2. Psychotherapy is contraindicated in the treatment of anorexia nervosa when

(A) the patient gets angry at the therapist
(B) the patient's weight drops below 80 lbs
(C) the patient starts abusing laxatives
(D) the patient says she no longer wants to be in psychotherapy
(E) none of the above

3. Which of the following statements concerning the use of a nasogastric tube in the treatment of anorexia nervosa is true?

(A) It is contraindicated because the tube may remind the patient of a penis; therefore, hyperalimentation through a central intravenous (IV) catheter should be used
(B) It is contraindicated because of the pain involved in passing the tube
(C) It is contraindicated because not enough calories can be provided to the patient by a nasogastric tube
(D) It is indicated in cases where the patient is at risk of starving to death
(E) It is indicated as a form of punishment when the patient refuses to eat

4. Failure to thrive is most often caused by

(A) psychological factors
(B) hypothyroidism
(C) fetal alcohol syndrome
(D) constitutional factors
(E) Addison's syndrome

5. In a family therapy session for a patient with anorexia nervosa, the father reveals that he has sexually molested the 13-year-old patient. You should

(A) let the family know that this is inappropriate behavior that must be stopped and follow up on the family's compliance within 1 week
(B) immediately leave the session to report the abuse to the child protective service agency
(C) recommend individual psychiatric treatment for the father
(D) tell the family that you and they should continue discussing the problem, reporting it only if it persists
(E) none of the above

6. A patient with anorexia nervosa is at risk of serious medical complications from starvation. She is 14 years old and refuses hospitalization. Your next step should be to

(A) continue the efforts at outpatient treatment
(B) place a hold on the patient and force her to come into the hospital against her will
(C) refer the patient to a colleague with the hope that he or she will have more success
(D) have the parents sign a release absolving you of responsibility for the case
(E) trick the patient into being admitted by telling her that you will not say anything about food or weight while she is an inpatient

7. Which of the following prognoses is most accurate for anorexia nervosa?

(A) Most patients recover
(B) Most girls recover, but very few boys recover
(C) The earlier the onset in life, the better the outcome of the disease
(D) Thirty to forty percent of patients die by the age of 30 years
(E) None of the above

8. Failure to thrive usually presents with

(A) weight loss
(B) reduced height or length
(C) reduced head circumference
(D) vomiting
(E) regurgitation

9. The Prader-Willi syndrome is characterized by which constellation of symptoms?

(A) Overeating, mental retardation, and stealing food
(B) Hypersexuality, overeating, and mouthing objects
(C) Wide fluctuations of weight with lengthy phases of normal eating
(D) Overeating and hypersomnia
(E) None of the above

Directions: Each question below contains four suggested answers of which **one or more** is correct. Choose the answer

A if **1, 2, and 3** are correct
B if **1 and 3** are correct
C if **2 and 4** are correct
D if **4** is correct
E if **1, 2, 3, and 4** are correct

10. True statements concerning the presentation of anorexia nervosa include

(1) age of onset is 13 to 14 years
(2) boys are affected at an older age than girls
(3) onset is often preceded by a period of normal dieting
(4) a suicide attempt is a frequent indication of onset

11. Factors associated with anorexia nervosa include which of the following?

(1) Mental retardation
(2) Turner's syndrome
(3) Above-average intelligence
(4) High socioeconomic status

12. The typical serum electrolyte pattern in Addison's disease is

(1) an elevated serum sodium and normal or decreased serum potassium
(2) an elevated serum sodium and serum potassium
(3) low sodium and low potassium
(4) low sodium and elevated potassium

13. Which of the following factors may be etiologic in the development of anorexia nervosa?

(1) Cultural influences
(2) Hypothalamic-pituitary abnormalities
(3) Controlling parents
(4) Dysthymic disorder (depression)

Directions: The group of questions below consists of lettered choices followed by several numbered items. For each numbered item select the **one** lettered choice with which it is **most** closely associated. Each lettered choice may be used once, more than once, or not at all.

Questions 14–17

Match each disorder listed below with its typical complication.

(A) Bezoars
(B) Hypercarotenemia
(C) Spurts of overeating
(D) Extreme guilt
(E) Urticaria

14. Pica
15. Anorexia nervosa
16. Kleine-Levin syndrome
17. Bulimia

ANSWERS AND EXPLANATIONS

1. The answer is C. *(I F 2, 3 c)* Although family dynamics and psychiatric intervention are important in the long-term management of anorectics, they should not take priority over medical intervention. Five to fifteen percent of anorectic patients die, usually of fluid and electrolyte problems. Electrolytes should be checked first and corrected based on whether and how abnormal they are. Immediate naso-gastric administration of a high-protein and carbohydrate diet would not solve any fluid and electrolyte problems quickly. Electroconvulsive therapy does not correct electrolyte problems and is ineffective treatment of anorexia nervosa.

2. The answer is E. *[I F 2 b (1), (2)]* Many patients in the course of treatment indicate that they are angry or fed up with psychotherapy. This is usually not an indication for stopping the therapy. In the course of treating a patient for anorexia nervosa, the therapist can expect considerable negative feelings. These children have never been able to vent their anger.

3. The answer is D. *(I F 3 c)* A nasogastric tube probably is the treatment of choice when an anorectic patient suffers from severe inanition. Its use is simple, safe, and can provide the patient with sufficient calories. Although there may be negative connotations in association with the use of a nasogastric tube, these should not prevent appropriate medical management of the patient. Such negative con-notations include the concern that the tube hurts, is too forceful, or is too messy. The tube does hurt some, but probably no more than an intravenous (IV) catheter; it is much safer than a central IV catheter.

4. The answer is A. *(V B 1)* Although hypothyroidism, fetal alcohol syndrome, constitutional factors, and Addison's syndrome all can cause failure to thrive, psychological causes are most common. Ironically, most children who are admitted to a pediatric hospital for failure to thrive get a full medical workup before anyone considers psychological factors. By leaving psychological etiologies for last, pediatric care providers prolong hospitalization, shorten the amount of time that a psychiatrist can work with the problem, and (subtly) cause psychological factors to seem less important to the family.

5. The answer is E. *(I C 1)* The protective service agency should be notified within 24 hours of any inci-dent of sexual or physical abuse of a child. A problem of this sort should be reported in every situation. However, leaving the session immediately to report it is not necessary and may indicate to the family that the therapist is extremely anxious about the situation and cannot handle it. Discussing the inap-propriateness of the behavior can be helpful, but it is not enough. The family's treatment need not end with the reporting of an incident of child abuse. Continued work on the problem is indicated after abuse has been reported.

6. The answer is B. *(I F 2 b, 3 b)* Parents do not have the right to allow their child to starve to death, nor does a child have the right to starve herself to death. In such cases, even when the child is underage, a hold should be placed and the patient should be forced to come to the hospital against her will. This should always be done upfront, and the patient should never be tricked into hospitalization. Outpa-tient therapy for anorexia nervosa cannot effectively control all of the weight-losing behavior of the child when she gets to the point of starvation. Consultation with a colleague is recommended for dif-ficult cases but should not replace the appropriate intervention of hospitalizing the patient to save her life. The physician probably remains legally liable for the patient even if the parents sign a release of responsibility. The parents and child who refuse hospitalization in these circumstances have faulty judgment; the child should be protected and treated.

7. The answer is C. *(I G 1, 2, 3)* Curiously, the earlier the onset in life, the better the prognosis of anorexia nervosa. The death rate of the disease is listed as 5% to 15%; death is usually due to metabolic or electrolyte abnormalities or suicide. Most of these girls actually continue to cycle through phases of weight gain and weight loss. The prognosis for recovery for boys may be worse than it is for girls, but most girls do not fully recover.

8. The answer is A. *(V A)* Loss of weight (or failure to gain weight) is usually the first symptom of failure to thrive, followed by loss of length and then a drop in growth and head circumference. Failure to thrive can be caused by medical conditions (e.g., endocrine disorders and infectious diseases). How-ever, it usually is the result of psychological problems between parents and child. Understanding child development helps to sort out possible psychological etiologies. For example, a 2-year-old child may refuse to eat because he or she wants to control his or her own life. In this case the treatment would be to help the mother give her child more control over what he or she eats (or whatever). A 5-month-old infant could develop failure to thrive due to neglect. At this age, a child cannot feed him- or herself and so is vulnerable to poor parenting. This can be diagnosed by putting the child in the hospital; if he or she grows there, a serious parenting problem is indicated.

9. The answer is A. *(II D 1, 2, 3, 4)* Prader-Willi syndrome consists of ravenous overeating; it is probably due to a hypothalamic lesion. Examining objects by mouth, altered sexual behavior, and hyperphagia are attributed to the Klüver-Bucy syndrome. Kleine-Levin syndrome causes overeating and hypersomnia. (It should be remembered that overeating is not always due to bulimia.)

10. The answer is B (1, 3). *(I B 2, 4)* The average age of onset of anorexia is 13½ years, and the onset is usually preceded by a period of normal dieting. The disease rarely occurs in boys. Suicide attempts, although increased in incidence, are infrequent.

11. The answer is E (all). *(I B 3, 5)* Anorexia nervosa is associated with all of the distractors (i.e., mental retardation, Turner's syndrome, above-average intelligence, and a high socioeconomic status); however, these are associations only and do not imply cause or effect. Anorexia nervosa is more common in Jewish and Italian families, Caucasians, and in Western countries, and the incidence of the disease is increasing. The increased incidence is probably due to cultural factors (i.e., thin is beautiful).

12. The answer is D (4). *(I D 1 a, F 3 c)* Addison's disease causes low serum sodium and high potassium levels. It can mimic anorexia nervosa because it can cause nausea, vomiting, and weight loss. It can also cause depression and an organic brain syndrome. Anorexia nervosa may result in fluid and electrolyte problems; the electrolyte abnormalities vary. In addition, anorectics who vomit may develop a metabolic alkalosis; those who abuse laxatives could become acidotic.

13. The answer is A (1, 2, 3). *(I C 3, 5; D 2 c)* In America, the association of thinness with beauty is strong, which may account for the increase in anorexia nervosa in this country. A variety of endocrine abnormalities occur in anorectics, and controlling parents are often found in the families. Parental control may cause the child to fight for autonomy by controlling her eating. Although depression may follow anorexia nervosa, it is not part of the etiology. Personality styles that precede the illness are schizoid, hysterical, and obsessive-compulsive.

14–17. The answers are: 14-A, 15-B, 16-C, 17-D. *(I E 6; II A, D 3; IV D 1)* Pica is the eating of nonfood substances, and bezoars can form as the result of ingesting nondigestible material. Trichobezoars are hair balls in the stomach; phytobezoars are masses of vegetable matter. All can cause intestinal obstruction, necessitating surgery.

Hypercarotenemia is caused by ingesting too many carrots, and the result is an orange skin discoloration. Otherwise, hypercarotenemia is clinically insignificant. Because anorectics mainly subsist on fruit, vegetables, and cheese, the skin discoloration would not be unusual in those patients who favor carrots.

Kleine-Levin syndrome causes overeating and hypersomnia. These symptoms are periodic, lasting several weeks. The disorder begins in adolescence and is more common in boys. Other symptoms include memory impairment, withdrawal, and negativism. The etiology is unknown.

Bulimia is accompanied by guilt. Other symptoms are ingestion of high-calorie foods, secretiveness about eating, weight fluctuation, and purging. Purging usually is by vomiting. Bulimia can accompany anorexia nervosa; however, with this condition, serious weight loss also occurs.

9

Psychiatric Emergencies
Eugene V. Friedrich

I. OVERVIEW. A **psychiatric emergency** or crisis **is a stress-induced pathologic response** that physically endangers the affected individual or others or that significantly disrupts the functional equilibrium of the individual or his or her environment. The pathologic response may be manifested by an acute alteration in the individual's thought, mood, or behavior. Either the **individual,** the **environment,** or **both** may experience or react to the situation as emergent.

A. Evolution of a crisis

1. A **stressor** from any source presents an individual with a situation or problem to resolve; however, in a crisis the usual **coping mechanisms** of the individual are insufficient and are overwhelmed.

2. **Increased anxiety and disorganization** may follow, which can further impair the individual's functional integrity and problem-solving capacity.

3. An adaptive reorganization or response may resolve the crisis; however, **failure of adaptation** may result in an increasing sense of helplessness, accompanied by panic, depression, or both and then in further disorganization.

4. In this spiraling situation there is an increased likelihood of impulsive, maladaptive, and even desperate attempts by the person to regain **any** equilibrium. The new equilibrium may reorganize the individual and reduce dysphoria but still be maladaptive in the limitations in function of the individual or disruption of the environment required to maintain it. For example, an individual may diminish the anxiety and reduce the nightmares following a traumatic event by using alcohol but eventually may develop medical, social, and occupational complications from excessive use.

5. An individual may request or be brought for help at any time during this cycle depending on his or her response and current social context. A person with any psychiatric diagnosis or a person without any preexisting psychopathology can present with a psychiatric emergency. A diagnosis of a major mental disorder may be the result of an individual's maladaptive responses.

B. Components of stress-induced responses. There is a dynamic **interplay among the stressor, the affected individual, and the social matrix** that influences the response of the individual. It is the **severity of the psychopathologic response** that creates a psychiatric emergency out of a particular crisis.

1. **Stressors** always depend on the interplay of individual and social factors, but they may be considered predominantly either internal or external.
   a. An **internal stress** may result when a person faces a normal developmental task for which he or she is ill-equipped or ill-prepared. A seemingly minor environmental event may have massive personal psychological meaning for the individual. The result may be that the individual experiences a disruptive increase in needs, a loss, or a conflict. Examples include an anxious adolescent who becomes disorganized upon leaving his or her family for college and an aging, lonely woman who becomes suicidal following the death of her cat.
   b. An **external stress** is a life event that would readily be recognized objectively as a source of stress, independent of subjective meaning. Examples include the death of a family member, a divorce, and a major illness. (A major illness may be an endogenous psychiatric illness such as mania; this can be an external stressor.)

2. The affected **individual** is a crucial determinant of whether the stress is major or minor and whether the response is adaptive or maladaptive.

   a. At one end of the spectrum is a healthy individual who resolves the crisis in an adaptive, growth-promoting fashion.
   b. In the middle is a person who may have been relatively healthy but who is so overwhelmed by massive trauma as to manage only a pathologic adaptation, which leaves him or her more vulnerable to future stress.
   c. At the other extreme is an individual with significant psychopathology who decompensates with even minor environmental stress.

3. The **social matrix** in which the individual lives is the third crucial component of stress-induced responses. Each individual varies in his or her need for external support and structure and in his or her capacity to accept them. Both the type of stress and kind of response influence the amount of environmental support that can be recruited.
   a. The individual may have multiple supportive resources that facilitate finding an adaptive resolution to the crisis.
   b. In the middle is the individual who may have a couple of primary sources of support that are reliable but that are not sufficient in the face of severe stress.
   c. At the other extreme, the individual may have a few supports that are easily overwhelmed and withdrawn or are even actively intolerant of his or her attempts at reconstitution. Rather than being a source of support, the external environment becomes another source of stress.

II. GENERAL PRINCIPLES OF EVALUATION

A. Immediate assessment of the condition and the dangerousness of the patient's behavior is essential. Such an assessment can be made on the basis of the following.

1. The patient's behavior. Loud, pressured, agitated, angry, and threatening behavior requires limit-setting and control before further evaluation.

2. The circumstances surrounding the patient's arrival in the emergency department. A patient who is brought in handcuffed or otherwise restrained requires cautious assessment despite calm or withdrawn behavior. The patient may have calmed as a result of external control, and to withdraw this control prematurely may result in escalation of agitated behavior.

3. The reports of others. Reports of dangerousness from family members and others must be given credence and must be investigated in spite of apparent inconsistencies with the patient's history or behavior.

B. A situation conducive to a more extended evaluation is necessary. This situation should be secure and provide for the safety and comfort of both the evaluator and patient. The first and second steps outlined below should be routine. The remaining three may not be immediately necessary with a cooperative patient. However, if indicated by history or by escalation of the patient's behavior, the remaining steps should be initiated before the evaluation can proceed safely.

1. The physical setting should be quiet, open, and sparsely furnished (there should be a minimum of objects that could be used as weapons). Both interviewer and patient should have an unobstructed exit from the room. A call button to summon immediate help must be easily accessible to the interviewer.

2. Sufficient trained help, who provide a show of force and can subdue an agitated patient, should be readily available. (It may be necessary to have help in or just outside of the interview room.)

3. A search for weapons may be indicated by history or the patient's behavior before further evaluation takes place.

4. Verbal and nonverbal expression of expectation of the patient to control him- or herself and to be responsible for his or her behavior may help the patient cooperate with the task at hand. The patient may need to be reminded that external control is also available.

5. Physical restraint in the form of 2- or 4-point leather restraints is indicated if the patient cannot respond to verbal limit-setting and reassurance. The need for safety for all concerned must supercede the patient's requests, but the clinician must recognize the patient's vulnerability and helplessness if restrained and treat him or her with respect and compassion.
   a. If the patient arrives in restraints or handcuffs, adequate evaluation must take place before any change in status is permitted.
   b. If previous interventions are not sufficient to control an unrestrained patient and provide for the safety of the patient and others, he or she should be placed in leather restraints until the evaluation is completed. A patient should not be restrained supine; rather he or she should be restrained on the side or with the head elevated to prevent aspiration if vomiting occurs. In addition, a patient in restraints requires constant monitoring.

C. Identification of a crisis situation

1. **Overt.** Evidence of a crisis may be immediately apparent from the patient's behavior or the circumstances surrounding his or her arrival in the emergency department.

2. **Covert.** The patient may be quite calm and superficially cooperative; he or she may present with relatively minor somatic complaints and deny any serious emotional disturbances. Nevertheless, the patient may be potentially lethal to him- or herself or others. Empathic, detailed history-taking in the context of a high level of suspicion often reveals the true nature of the emergency. The following factors should raise the index of suspicion.

   a. **Risk factors.** Certain historic data and mental status findings increase the probabilities of particular emergencies occurring and should serve as red flags to guide assessment.

   b. **Unanswered questions.** Vague, evasive, and qualified answers to questions in crucial areas such as suicide, homicide, and impulse control must be vigorously pursued. A patient's attempt to minimize or ignore consequences of observed or reported behavior should not be accepted without investigation. Discrepancies between the patient's history and the reports of reliable others must be explored, which may involve meeting with the other parties apart from the patient in order to ascertain their true concerns.

   c. **Feelings of unease or discomfort** on the part of the physician should not be ignored but should be examined and used to the extent that they are reflective of the patient. An intuitive, experienced physician may read between the lines of a patient's communication, detect subtle discrepancies between affect and content, and accurately uncover a latent but emergent situation.

D. Chief complaint and present illness

1. **Patient.** Rapport is facilitated by allowing the patient to tell his or her own story as much as possible. The examiner should listen for information gained from the following questions and inquire further if indicated.

   a. What are the symptoms or problems that led the patient to seek help?

   b. Why is the patient requesting help now?

   c. Why are these symptoms a problem at this particular time?

   d. What are the person's normal coping mechanisms in times of stress?

   e. What is his or her level of functioning in general?

   f. How did he or she cope previously with similar stresses?

   g. What attempts is he or she presently making to resolve the problem?

2. **Others.** Family members, friends, employers, and coworkers may be able to answer many of these questions if the patient will not or cannot answer them accurately. Different individuals may accurately describe a particular aspect of the patient's situation or level of function; it is up to the physician to compose an integrated picture.

E. Patient history

1. **Past history.** The more detailed the history available, the more complete is the picture of the patient. In a crisis situation detailed history-taking may not be feasible; however, the two following areas must be explored in all patients.

   a. **Previous psychiatric illnesses.** The symptoms, circumstances, treatment, and response to treatment of previous illnesses should be outlined.

   b. **Dangerous behavior.** Previous episodes of self-destructive or assaultive behavior must be carefully explored as they have significant predictive value.

2. **Medical history**

   a. **Significant medical illnesses** may have direct bearing on the current crisis, may color the presentation, or may produce chronic vulnerability to stress.

   b. **Drugs.** Prescribed medication, alcohol, and illicit drugs can profoundly affect thinking, feeling, and behavior. They may cause the crisis or significantly impair the patient's adaptive capacity.

F. Mental status examination

1. **Observed mental status.** This is a complete description of the patient's appearance, manner, and behavior throughout the entire interaction. The following areas should be specifically addressed:

   a. Quantity and quality of speech

   b. Organization and goal direction of thought processes

   c. Predominant themes and preoccupations in the content of the communication, including delusions and obsessions

   d. Perceptual disturbances, including illusions and hallucinations.

    e. Range and quality of affective responses
    f. Overall mood
    g. Manner of relating to the interviewer

  2. Formal mental status. This is a more systematic evaluation of the patient's intellectual and cognitive functioning. It is a screening examination and cannot rule out subtle disturbances in cognitive function; positive findings should be investigated and explained. It is important to recall that significant impairment in the level of consciousness or attention precludes an accurate assessment of the other intellectual functions that are dependent on the relative intactness of these. The following areas should be routinely evaluated:

    a. Level of consciousness, including evidence of fluctuation
    b. Attention and concentration, which can be tested by means of digit repetition and serial subtractions
    c. Orientation to person, place, time, and situation
    d. Memory
       (1) Immediate recall, which is tested by digit repetition
       (2) Short-term memory and the ability to learn new information, which are tested by having the patient learn four unrelated words and repeat them in 5 minutes
       (3) Recent and remote memory, which is assessed by the patient's recollection of historic events and dates and by his or her answers to inquiries concerning some historic facts.
    e. Fund of knowledge, which is dependent on educational background and which can be assessed by asking general information questions of varying difficulty
    f. Calculating ability, which can be tested by serial subtractions, other calculations of varying complexity, or having the patient make change for a hypothetical purchase
    g. Abstracting ability, which can be assessed by the patient's interpretation of similarities and proverbs, with attention paid to bizarre and idiosyncratic responses as well as to concrete ones
    h. Judgment and insight, which are usually apparent in the way the patient discusses his or her current situation and the consequences of his or her behavior and which can be further evaluated by presenting to the patient hypothetical situations that require a choice of a course of action and an explanation of the rationale of that choice
    i. A number of other bedside tests for organic brain disorders, which overlap with the neurologic examination. (Rather than being routine, these tests should be directed by evidence in the patient's history and by the rest of the mental status examination for organic brain syndrome. They include figure copying, dysphasia testing, and describing directions.)

  3. Impulse control data may be available from other parts of the history and the mental status examination; however, the data must be highlighted because of the crucial importance of impulse control in the emergency situation. The patient's history of self-destructive and dangerous behavior as well as current plans and fantasies must be evaluated in detail to assess suicide and homicide potential.

G. Physical examination should be thorough with particular attention paid to evidence of drug intoxication and withdrawal symptoms and to acute and chronic neurologic disease.

H. Laboratory tests should be guided by other findings and by the differential diagnosis. Blood and urine tests for toxic agents may be particularly helpful in the emergency setting.

III. THE SUICIDAL PATIENT

A. Epidemiology

  1. Rate. Suicide is under-reported, but there are about 27,000 deaths by suicide in the United States per year. The rate is 11 to 12/100,000. There are 10 to 20 times as many attempts, however, as successful suicides. Suicide is the tenth leading cause of death in the United States; death by accidents is fourth overall, and this percentage certainly includes some suicides.

  2. Age. Although the age-adjusted suicide rate for individuals under the age of 40 years has doubled in the past 25 years, people over 40 years of age remain at the greatest risk for suicide, with significant rate differences according to sex. The suicide rate in men peaks twice: There is a sharp rise after the age of 12 years and a plateau between the ages of 20 and 30 years; after the age of 45 years, the rate increases again to a higher peak at about the age of 82 years. The suicide rate in women gradually increases to a maximum between the ages of 40 and 60 years and is only slightly lower thereafter. The suicide rate in young men (20 to 30 years old) and elderly men (older than 75 years) is five to seven times greater than the rate in women of comparable ages.

3. **Sex.** Men **commit** suicide three times more often than women. Women **attempt** suicide three times more often than men. Suicide is the seventh leading cause of death in men of all ages, but it is no higher than the eleventh leading cause of death in women overall. Men more often use firearms; women are more likely to ingest drugs.

4. **Marital status.** The rate is higher in single persons than in those married, and it is even higher in those divorced.

5. **Health.** As many as 70% of individuals who commit suicide have some active, usually chronic, illness. Fifty percent of patients who die by suicide have sought medical help within 1 month or less of their deaths, and eighty percent have seen their physicians within 6 months of their deaths.

B. Common presentations

1. **Overt**
   a. **Suicidal behavior.** The patient may have ingested drugs or attempted suicide by wrist-slashing, shooting, jumping, or other means that result in varying degrees of injury. The patient often requires medical or surgical interventions (e.g., gastric lavage or suturing) before complete psychiatric assessment. The patient should be considered acutely suicidal until proven otherwise. Close observation is required to prevent another attempt or to prevent the patient from leaving the emergency department.
   b. **Suicidal ideation.** The patient may be obviously depressed and in considerable pain and distress. The individual may ask for help in controlling his or her suicidal impulses and for relief from depression. He or she may reveal concerns immediately or with little prompting.

2. **Covert**
   a. **Suicidal behavior.** Although the patient may minimize or deny the implications of his or her behavior, he or she may have "accidents," which range from suspiciously to obviously suicidal. The patient may be unconscious of his or her self-destructive impulses but is no less dangerous; in fact, the patient may be more dangerous because the suicidal intent may be missed or ignored. A similar kind of patient is one who appears homicidal or assaultive but whose behavior is primarily an attempt to provoke others, such as the police, to kill him or her.
   b. **Suicidal ideation.** The patient may present for medical evaluation of minor or severe somatic complaints. He or she may appear depressed or may disguise the distress. Empathic questioning may reveal the patient's feelings. The patient may show distress out of proportion to objective findings or may make a series of visits to the emergency department over a short period of time. Although hoping to find help, he or she may take the medication given for somatic complaints in a suicide attempt.

3. **Chronic suicidal ideation and behavior.** The patient repeatedly calls or presents to the emergency room with suicidal ideation and attempts. Self-destructive behavior may be a means to manipulate the environment or to relieve internal discomfort rather than a means to die. These patients evoke tremendous frustration and hostility in caregivers and are at great risk to be ignored or actively rejected. They are also at great risk to kill themselves ultimately by design, miscalculation, or impulsiveness and require careful evaluation.

C. Differential diagnosis.
Patients may become suicidal regardless of or because of preexisting psychopathology. Suicidal ideation is more likely to accompany some diagnoses; conversely, some diagnoses increase the risk of suicide or accidental death in some individuals who are only mildly or not at all suicidal.

1. **Affective disorders.** Both major depression and bipolar disorder, depressed type, carry a high risk of suicide. Some patients may become more actively suicidal as they begin to improve and must be carefully evaluated despite other symptomatic improvement.

2. **Schizophrenic disorders.** Schizophrenic patients may experience a severe depression following resolution of a psychotic episode or may become progressively demoralized by having to cope with a chronic deteriorating disease course. A particularly dangerous situation results from hallucinations or delusions that demand that a patient hurt or kill him- or herself or that motivate the patient to perform dangerous acts, such as trying to fly or stopping traffic on a highway.

3. **Organic mental disorders.** These disorders, whether dementia or delirium, including drug or alcohol intoxication and withdrawal, put a patient at increased risk for suicide because of accompanying impairment of both judgment and impulse control. This is particularly true if the

disorder is superimposed on or concurrent with a depressive disorder. For example, alcoholics have a suicide rate 50 times the normal and account for 25% of all suicides.

4. **Personality disorders** (especially borderline personality disorder). Patients with these disorders are impulsive, provocative, and may be chronically suicidal. Their sensitivity to rejection, tendency to regress and become self-destructive, and propensity to abuse drugs and alcohol put them at risk to kill themselves intentionally or accidentally. They may have a superimposed affective disorder that is missed or ignored because of their tumultuous personality disorder.

D. Assessment of lethality (suicide risk)

1. **Suicidal ideation and behavior is episodic.** Such behavior may remit and relapse both in response to the patient's changing internal emotional and cognitive states and his or her environment. Either the patient, the environment, or both may require intervention to protect the patient.

2. **The suicidal patient is always ambivalent.** The balance between the patient's wish to live and wish to die must be evaluated, and the evaluation must include the factors that tip the balance one way or the other. Eight of ten eventual suicides give prior warning.

3. **Risk factors (predictors).** The patient's ambivalence and the episodic nature of suicidal behavior allow for identification and prevention in many cases. The following predictors may aid the physician in determining both who is at risk and to what extent.

   a. **Demographic indicators.** Unemployed, divorced, Caucasian males over the age of 45 years are at particularly high risk. Any of these factors, occurring singly or in combination, should alert the physician to investigate. [Younger men are also at high risk (see section III A 2).]

   b. **Historic indicators.** A recent loss, real or symbolic, or a change in the status of the affected individual may precipitate a crisis with feelings of anxiety and depression.

   (1) **Present illness.** Reports of hopelessness, helplessness, loneliness, and exhaustion are worrisome. An unexpected change in behavior, such as giving away possessions, or an unexpected change in attitude, such as calm or resignation in the midst of a distressing situation, must be investigated. Overt or indirect talk of death must be followed up with specific questions about fantasies, wishes, plans, and means. In the case of an unsuccessful suicide attempt, the following additional issues are important.

   (a) The patient's perception of the lethality of the attempt, his or her expectations of rescue, and his or her relief or disappointment at being alive are often more important than the objective dangerousness of the attempt, particularly in cases of apparent minimal danger.

   (b) The extent to which the precipitating crisis is resolved or is being resolved may influence the patient's wish to remain alive and his or her attitude towards the future.

   (2) **Past history.** A previous history of suicide attempts increases the risk of suicide, particularly if the attempts have been multiple. The circumstances and lethality of the previous attempts should be determined.

   (3) **Medical history.** A history of chronic illness or an acute change in physical health increases the risk of suicide.

   (4) **Family history.** A family history of suicide is important both in terms of the patient's identification with the individual who died and the possibility of inheritance of an affective disorder. The anniversary date of the death and the patient reaching the same age of the person who died may be particularly stressful times.

   c. **Diagnostic indicators** (see section III C) include conditions of depression, thought disorder, and impairment of impulse control, especially secondary to alcohol or drug abuse.

   d. **Present mental status.** In addition to assessing the severity of depression, any evidence of psychosis, particularly command hallucinations, and the presence of confusion and impairment of impulse control, the physician should be aware of the patient's response to the interview. Does the patient feel understood, experience some relief, and express more hopefulness, or does the patient remain angry, pessimistic, and desperate?

   e. **Resources.** The availability and support of family and friends are crucial. It is essential to get their perceptions of the patient's lethality, and they may need to be interviewed away from the patient to feel comfortable revealing their concerns. Additionally, in planning for disposition and treatment, the physician must be sure of their support and willingness to assume some responsibility for the patient. In particular, the physician must ascertain that there is no collusion with or covert encouragement of the patient's suicidal behavior.

E. Countertransference reactions to suicidal patients.
Countertransference refers to the emotional reactions that the physician has to the patient; these reactions may be unconscious or only

dimly conscious. They may have a powerful influence on the physician's attitude towards the patient, his or her approach to the patient, and even his or her clinical judgment.

1. **The physician** has his or her own particular attitudes towards suicide and death, his or her own set of personal and clinical experiences in these matters, and conflicts about his or her own aggressive or self-destructive impulses. Unless the physician is aware of these reactions, he or she may minimize or distort clinical data from the patient to fit personal feelings or beliefs. The physician may fear being overwhelmed or at loss if the patient admits to suicidal ideation. He or she may even fear (wrongly) that he or she will influence the patient to commit suicide by talking about it.

2. **The patient,** depending on his or her behavior, evokes varying degrees of frustration, anger, and helplessness in most caregivers. At times the patient evokes so much hostility that the physician wishes that the patient was dead. Such a reaction is extremely serious because it is likely that others in the patient's environment feel similarly.

F. **Principles of emergency treatment**

1. The patient must be protected.

2. A psychiatric consultation is necessary if there is any question about the patient's lethality.

3. Treatment options include the following.
   a. **Hospitalization.** A patient should be hospitalized if the lethality of his or her ideation or behavior is high. Lethality might be high because of the persistence of the patient's wish to die, the severity of his or her concurrent psychopathology, or the absence of reliable supports in the patient's social environment.
      (1) A patient can be hospitalized voluntarily if he or she concurs with the need for inpatient treatment.
      (2) A suicidal patient can also be hospitalized involuntarily on a mental health hold if voluntary hospitalization is refused. (The length of time that a patient can be held initially for treatment varies from state to state but is often in the range of 72 hours.) A severely suicidal patient who resists treatment may require one-to-one observation to prevent escape or self-injury.
   b. **Outpatient treatment** is less restrictive than hospitalization and is indicated when there is some crisis resolution, mild concurrent psychopathology, mobilization of environmental resources, and a therapeutic response to the interview. It usually involves a follow-up appointment within 48 hours and intensive crisis treatment thereafter. Somatic treatment can be started on an outpatient basis, but only limited quantities of medication should be dispensed because of the potential for overdose.

IV. **THE VIOLENT PATIENT.** Violent behavior includes, but is not limited to, homicide, assault, child abuse, incest, and rape. Violence is pervasive in our society. Homicide is the twelfth leading cause of death overall; it is the second leading cause of death in men and the third leading cause of death in women between the ages of 15 and 34 years—ahead of suicide for both sexes. Injury and death can be prevented by identifying and managing the potentially violent patient properly.

A. **Common presentations**

1. **Overt**
   a. **Violent behavior.** Overtly violent patients require varying degrees of external controls (see section II). The patient may respond positively and acknowledge his or her capacity for self-control. Once the patient is calmer, the issue becomes one of evaluating ongoing dangerousness.
   b. **Violent ideation.** An individual may present to the emergency department fearing loss of impulse control and asking for help. He or she may be relieved and cooperative at the prospect of forthcoming help, or his or her aggression may escalate during the interview, requiring immediate external control.

2. **Covert violent behavior or ideation.** The affected individual may present with vague somatic complaints or unexplained trauma; although clearly under stress, he or she may be evasive in providing details about his or her illness or injury. The patient may be ashamed of his or her impulses or behavior and yet hope that the physician will see through the initial complaints. The physician should be aware that suicidal ideation may disguise or occur in response to homicidal ideation or violent behavior. The patient may be dangerous both to him- or herself and to others.

3. **Chronic aggressive behavior.** These patients have a violent life-style with frequent episodes of assaultiveness. They may take considerable pleasure in their power and even enjoy the

violence. They show little or no remorse about the pain and injury that they inflict. Their behavior is often chronically impulsive and associated with alcohol or drug abuse. Although they may present with a psychological crisis that requires intervention, more often they present management problems because of their dangerous, threatening behavior. Legal charges and police intervention may be necessary.

B. **Differential diagnosis.** Any individual with any diagnosis may be dangerous in a particular context. As with a suicide risk, an overall assessment of dangerousness overrides the specific clinical diagnosis. However, certain diagnoses are more likely to be associated with violent behavior, and there may be very specific treatment implications with a particular diagnosis.

1. **Alcohol and drug abuse.** Intoxication with alcohol and certain drugs [particularly barbiturates, stimulants, and phencyclidine (PCP)] may impair judgment, distort reality, and lessen impulse control, leading to aggressive behavior. Patients with PCP intoxication and pathologic intoxication triggered by small amounts of alcohol are particularly likely to present with confusion, disorientation, rage, and violent behavior. Such states are commonly seen in emergency departments either as the primary problem or complicating other medical or psychiatric emergencies.

2. **Bipolar disorder, manic type.** Manic patients are pressured, hyperactive, and irritable, with a low frustration tolerance. Euphoric garrulity can quickly change to hostile aggressiveness if a manic experiences interference with his or her immediate wishes, which are often unrealistic and grandiose.

3. **Schizophrenic disorders.** These psychotic disorders may be accompanied by considerable panic and agitation as well as deficient reality testing and impulse control. Although infrequently seen now, a state of catatonic excitement may occur, during which the patient may be extremely dangerous. More commonly seen are patients with paranoid schizophrenia, who are extremely hostile and fearful of attack and who may act aggressively to defend themselves. Schizophrenic patients may experience command hallucinations, ordering them to hurt others.

4. **Paranoid disorders.** Patients with these disorders generally present with stable, well-developed delusions but with better reality testing and impulse control than do those with schizophrenia. However, the overly controlled and often denied hostility may break through as murderous rage if the individual feels particularly threatened or experiences diminished impulse control.

5. **Personality disorders.** Patients with borderline, paranoid, and antisocial personality disorders are especially prone to threatening, assaultive behavior. Their underlying anger and tendency to blame others for their problems lead them to act out rage, particularly when intoxicated with drugs or alcohol.

6. **Post-traumatic stress disorder.** Combat veterans, particularly (now) Vietnam War veterans, with a delayed stress syndrome may show homicidal and assaultive behavior. This may occur in the midst of a flashback to a combat situation, which has been triggered by something in the environment; at these times the patient reexperiences fighting for his life. At other times, in an individual who knows how to fight and kill, there is a breakthrough of chronic frustration and rage, without a dissociative state, but often exacerbated by drugs and alcohol.

7. **Organic mental disorders.** Deliria and dementia of any etiology may present with agitated, aggressive behavior. These disorders may be complicated by paranoid ideation, poor judgment, and impaired impulse control.

8. **Intermittent explosive disorder** results in directed violence and is more common in men. There is a history of violent outbursts with normal behavior between episodes. The disorder is associated with soft neurologic signs, abnormal electroencephalograms (EEGs), and a family history of violence.

9. **Temporal limbic epilepsy.** This diagnosis should be considered, particularly if there are poorly directed episodes of violence with a repetitive pattern, whether or not these episodes are associated with other evidence of a seizure disorder. An abnormal EEG with spikes or slowing over the temporal lobe may be diagnostic of this condition.

10. **Mental retardation.** Mentally retarded patients may have a low frustration tolerance and poor impulse control, resulting in aggressive responses to relatively small environmental changes.

11. **Attention deficit disorder (ADD), residual.** In recent years, an adult-type ADD has been described. It presents with hyperactivity, poor concentration, easy frustration, and poor im-

pulse control continuing from childhood. Affected patients may have a dramatic therapeutic response to treatment with methylphenidate.

C. Assessment of dangerousness. Although making a clinical diagnosis is important, it is only one factor that goes into an overall assessment of imminent and ongoing dangerousness. Future violent behavior is extremely difficult to predict; consideration of the following issues is helpful.

1. Violent behavior is episodic. For most people, violent behavior is an infrequent event; this increases the difficulty in predicting future occurrences. However, there is always a balance between the individual's internal state, including the degree of tension and the controls over expression of aggression, and the environment. Certain combinations of internal and external factors may produce an assaultive crisis. An astute clinician can often identify when a patient is escalating beyond an acceptable expression of anger and frustration towards loss of control and assaultiveness. Appropriate interventions at various points of this cycle may prevent the crisis or minimize the chances of serious injury.

2. All patients have internal controls over the expression of violent impulses. Factors that impair impulse control either transiently or chronically may be crucial in determining whether or not an individual only fears a loss of control or actually acts on his or her impulses. In addition, there are certain contexts in which violence is more likely to occur; the extent to which the current situation recreates a previous one that resulted in a loss of control should be examined. The patient's perception of external danger, whether real or imagined, and the need to protect him- or herself are important factors.

3. Risk factors
   a. Demographic indicators. Young men in the range of 16 to 25 years of age are particularly at high risk for violent behavior. Since domestic violence is so prevalent, parents and spouses are at risk.
   b. Historic indicators
      (1) A recent major life change may place an individual under increasing stress, leading to increasing internal tension and frustration. The patient's feelings of internal pressure, frustration, anger, and potential explosiveness should be carefully explored. Those situations and individuals that increase or decrease the feelings of tension should be identified. The attempts that the patient has made to cope with these feelings and the results achieved should be discussed. Attention should be given to his or her level of optimism or pessimism about prevention of a violent action. The patient's thoughts and fantasies about violence are also extremely important; in particular, there may be certain sadistic fantasies or violent ruminations directed towards a specific individual or individuals. Specific threats require investigation of the patient's relationship with and accessibility to the threatened individual. Specific plans and the availability of and familiarity with weapons increase the danger. The patient's perception of what keeps him or her from carrying out the action is also important. Current use of drugs and alcohol should be explored.
      (2) Past history
         (a) A past history of violent behavior is the most reliable predictor of future violence. This includes fighting, assaults, arrests, and sanctioned violence (e.g., that sanctioned for soldiers and police).
         (b) A past history of impulsive or self-destructive behavior, including accidents, arrests for speeding or reckless driving, and self-mutilation, puts the individual at increased risk.
      (3) Childhood history
         (a) A history of witnessing or experiencing neglect or abuse in childhood increases the likelihood of abuse and brutality directed towards the patient's own children.
         (b) A childhood history of cruelty to animals may be associated with continuing aggressiveness.
   c. Diagnostic indicators (see section IV B). The common diagnostic denominator is the degree to which impulse control and judgment are impaired in the contexts of hostility, irritability, and distorted perceptions of reality.
   d. Present mental status. Fluctuation in the patient's levels of tension and agitation throughout the interview should be noted. The patient's impulse control and judgment during the examination may contradict the content of his or her speech. Command hallucinations to hurt others are particularly worrisome as are escalating delusional perceptions of external danger as these may be accompanied by frantic attempts at self-preservation. Sometimes delusional thinking may place others in danger in the guise of protecting them. For example, a psychotic mother may believe that she must bathe her child in scalding water to purify and cleanse him or her. Any evidence of confusion and organic mental disorders is also crucial as it suggests impairment of impulse control and judgment.

e. Social matrix. The thoughts of family and friends concerning the patient's violence potential should be sought in separate interviews, especially if they are potential victims. The family may provide a reliable history about the patient's access to weapons. The clinician should assess if the potential victim behaves in a challenging or provocative way towards the patient. If the patient appears to be calm enough, an interview with both the patient and the intended victim may be necessary to determine their behavior towards each other and to determine if there has been any resolution of the crisis. Possible use of available community resources beyond those offered by family and friends, such as safe houses, should be assessed.

f. Physician's feelings. Persistent feelings of fear or unease on the part of the physician may be important clues that further investigation and evaluation are necessary.

D. Countertransference reactions to violent patients

1. Physician reaction. An angry, agitated, and threatening patient is likely to frighten and disorganize the physician. The physician's lack of awareness of this fear, previous personal experiences with violence, and conflicts over his or her own aggressive impulses may adversely influence his or her response to the patient.

a. No reaction. The physician may ignore or minimize the patient's concern with loss of control.

b. Anger. The physician may become angry and argue with the patient in response to the fear that he or she experiences. He or she may challenge and humiliate the patient, further escalating a dangerous situation.

c. Counterphobic reaction. The physician may act as though he or she is in control in response to unconscious fear and feelings of lack of control.

d. Overly frightened reaction. The physician may overestimate the patient's violent potential, with the result that the physician is unnecessarily anxious and self-protective.

2. Consequences. Intense, unacknowledged countertransference reactions can interfere with clinical judgment and treatment. The extremes range from being overly concerned with control and even punitive to releasing the patient prematurely or "permitting" him or her to escape in order to avoid dealing with the patient. Either way, the patient may receive an inadequate evaluation and inappropriate treatment. Potential victims may remain in considerable danger.

E. Principles of emergency treatment

1. The patient must be controlled.

2. Although the patient may appear calm, a psychiatric consultation is indicated if there is any question of continuing dangerousness.

3. Treatment options

a. Hospitalization. If the patient remains agitated, is calm but the risk of violence is high, or has not been adequately evaluated, he or she should be hospitalized either voluntarily or involuntarily. Unless the diagnosis is absolutely clear and the patient's treatment history is well-known, he or she should not simply be medicated and released from the emergency department. Medication should generally be given in the inpatient unit or in an observation unit. Haloperidol, administered intramuscularly in 2-mg to 10-mg doses, is probably the safest medication for acute agitation. Diazepam, at intravenous doses of 5 mg to 10 mg over 2 minutes, is also effective, but it may cause respiratory depression. Administration of medication should be delayed until an adequate diagnosis has been made unless:

(1) The patient is so combative even in restraints as to preclude adequate evaluation

(2) The patient's agitation may cause a medical complication (e.g., hyperpyrexia or rhabdomyolysis)

b. Outpatient treatment. The patient's response to the offer of help and willingness to accept treatment, the extent of the patient's psychopathology, the degree of crisis resolution, and the availability of family and community resources all help to determine if the patient is suitable for an outpatient treatment program.

4. Escape. If a patient who is considered to be potentially dangerous does escape from the emergency department, the local police should be notified to help find and pick up the patient. Family and friends who might have contact with the patient should be notified of the severity of the situation and should be instructed as to what to do if they see the patient. Lastly, if the patient has made a credible threat to a specific individual, the potential victim should be notified.

V. THE VICTIMS. Many victims present to the emergency department. Some are obviously victims, and these individuals usually evoke a caring response. Others, particularly subjects of familial vio-

lence, may be less obviously victims; their predicament may be missed, denied, or rationalized such that they return home to face further abuse and trauma. Likewise, the crime of rape may evoke such strong emotional reactions in physicians and the emergency department staff that the woman is victimized further rather than helped. Family violence, which includes child abuse, incest, and spouse abuse, is detected only if there is a high index of suspicion. Often the victim may be of little help because of the attachment to the perpetrator, however ambivalent the relationship may be. The clinician may have to treat the affected individual despite considerable denial. Rape victims may also present with considerable denial because of shame and irrational guilt. Victims may have physical and emotional sequelae to their trauma, which may become apparent immediately or long after the event. If the abuse is repetitive, the sequelae may not appear until long after the abuse has been initiated. Though brutalized, there may be a kind of intrafamilial or intrapsychic equilibrium, through which the victim may resist exposure for fear of unknown consequences.

A. Child abuse. Although child abuse continues to be under-reported in the United States, at least 500,000 children are significantly injured each year. Physical injuries can range from welts or contusions to multiple fractures to death. Concomitant emotional trauma is more difficult to measure but is no less disabling. Physicians may be tempted to rationalize abuse as severe discipline but in the range of normal or to feel that they do not have the right to interfere in family business. This attitude may be particularly prevalent in cases involving middle- and upper-class families, in which abuse is just as prevalent as in families in the lower end of the socioeconomic range.

    1. Clues. There are a number of clues that can guide the physician's exploration of potential abuse despite denials by parents or reluctance to admit to the abuse on the part of the child.

        a. Any **unexplained trauma** should raise the question of abuse, especially if there is evidence of multiple injuries at different stages of healing.

        b. Delay in seeking treatment, especially if poorly explained, may reflect parental fears of detection. Despite being the source of the injury, the parent may be overly concerned, and the child may be clingingly dependent on the parent.

        c. Evidence of **role reversal** between parents and child may be apparent. This may reflect unrealistic expectations on the part of the child to meet parental needs and reflect lack of empathic understanding of the child's needs on the part of the parents.

        d. Pseudomature behavior on the part of the child may be adaptation to the parents' unrealistic expectations.

        e. A child may present with **vague somatic complaints** or **behavioral symptoms,** such as nightmares, phobias, and enuresis, which reflect stress stemming from an abusive home situation.

        f. Any **parent under stress** should be evaluated with regard to child abuse, particularly if there is a history of abuse in the parent's own childhood.

    2. Evaluation. In addition to observing the child and parents together, the clinician should interview the child and parents separately, depending on the age of the child.

        a. Evaluation of the child. The type of examination varies depending on the age of the child and his or her ability to talk about him- or herself and family. After a careful physical examination, x-rays of the long bones and skull to detect old fractures may be indicated for a young child. If the child is able to talk, a description of the family situation may be helpful, particularly of how discipline is carried out on both the affected child and on his or her siblings. A child may be reluctant to talk about this directly, which must be respected; a child may communicate indirectly through expression of wishes, fears, fantasies, and play. Sometimes it is helpful to talk with siblings, especially older ones.

        b. Evaluation of the parents. The parents should be interviewed separately as well as together. Even if only one parent is abusive, there is always collusion (if only out of fear) by the nonabusing partner. Questioning may begin concerning the general stress at home and that caused by the children. How the parents respond to the child's crying and conduct discipline is informative. Description of the pregnancy, labor, and delivery defines the extent to which the child was wanted or unwanted. The current perception of the child and his or her role reveals whether or not the parents have an accurate empathic understanding of the child's needs. An investigation of the quality of the marital relationship and some history of the parents' childhoods, especially their own experiences with discipline and abuse, is helpful. More specific questions about fear of loss of control or actual loss of control, of anger, and of aggression towards the child are necessary.

        c. Assessment of the extent of abuse and potential dangerousness should be made. The specifics should guide the treatment intervention. The clinician should be aware that both parents and children may resist any intervention, no matter how dangerous the situation is.

    3. Emergency treatment. The goal is to protect the child and to initiate treatment that will prevent future abuse.

   a. The child should be given immediate necessary medical treatment.
   b. The child welfare agency and a psychiatric consultant should be called concerning how best to protect this child and other children in the home. Protection may involve:
      (1) Hospitalizing the child
      (2) Placing the child and the siblings out of the home temporarily
      (3) Hospitalizing the abusive parent
   c. The parents should be informed that the abuse has been reported and what this entails. Although initially angry, the parents may also be relieved at the prospect of help.
   d. Under no circumstances should the child be released to the parents, regardless of the intensity of their protests, unless the physician is confident that the child will be safe and unless a treatment alliance has been developed.

B. Sexual abuse (including incest). Sexual molestation of children and adolescents ranges from petting to intercourse. It may involve a single event by a stranger or episodes repeated over a period of years by a family member or friend of the family. There may be little pain, evidence of trauma, or significant injury. Father- (or stepfather-) daughter incest is the most common; it is the example used in the following discussion. Mother-son incest is less common and suggests serious psychopathology, often psychosis, in the mother. Overall, at least 200,000 cases of incest are reported each year, and up to 90% of incidents are not reported.

   1. Clues
      a. If a young daughter appears to have the central role in the family, she may also have replaced the mother as the sexual partner for her father. Overly close and stimulating physical contact between a father and daughter should be discussed, particularly if the mother is absent either physically or emotionally.
      b. Perineal or vaginal trauma at any age requires investigation of sexual abuse. The suspicion of any physical abuse should raise the question of sexual abuse.
      c. Vague somatic complaints or frequent visits to physicians may reflect the child's distress and her search for help.
      d. Antisocial behavior, including sexual promiscuity, truancy, and running away, may be responses to sexual abuse at home. Over 50% of female runaways give sexual molestation as a reason for leaving home.
      e. Any psychiatric symptoms, including suicidal behavior, may stem from sexual abuse. The specific symptom reflects the developmental age of the child or adolescent.
      f. Pregnancy and venereal disease, especially in girls under the age of 12 years, should be evaluated for evidence of sexual abuse.

   2. Evaluation. The age of the child determines the extent to which the child, the parent, or both are the focus of interviews. The child will be more hesitant to talk if she has been molested by a family member rather than a stranger.
      a. Evaluation of the child
         (1) Interview. The physician should talk with the child as well as examine her carefully. Questions must be phrased to match her developmental age. If possible, details of the event, including the identity of the molester, threats made, fear of harm, extent of injury, and feelings, should be obtained. In addition, it is helpful to elicit the child's perception of the reaction of others; children may experience significant shame and guilt and assume responsibility for the situation. In a case of incest, talking about issues of privacy, sleeping arrangements, physical intimacy, and the parental relationship may provide a lead into talking of sexual contact. Also, appreciating the child's fantasies and fears about the consequences of disclosure is important. The child should be reminded that she is not at fault.
         (2) Physical examination should be done carefully and nonintrusively. However, the physician must be aware that he or she is also gathering evidence for what may be a criminal proceeding. As with other cases of abuse and rape, specimens and pictures may be necessary.
      b. Evaluation of the parents
         (1) If a child has been molested by a stranger, the parents may need to ventilate their outrage away from the child so that they can be available to support the child and not confuse, frighten, and overwhelm her with their own feelings.
         (2) In a case of incest, questioning should go from general to specific. Inquiring about sleeping arrangements, privacy, physical contact, and the marital relationship may lead to specific questions about sexual activity. The extent of the sexual activity should be determined, including whether other daughters are involved. The father may deny, minimize, or rationalize his behavior, and it is important to be nonjudgmental. The mother may have colluded with the incest and may have even promoted it; she will not necessarily be an ally early in the treatment process. If both parents deny such activity, they should be confronted with the child's report.

     c. Consequences. There are serious consequences for all family members following disclosure of incest. Disclosure significantly disrupts the existing family equilibrium, however pathologic it may have been. All participants may develop psychiatric symptoms, especially anxiety and depression, and may be at risk for suicide.

  3. Treatment
    a. The indicated medical treatment and follow-up for the victim, including that for venereal disease and pregnancy, must be provided.
    b. The child protection team and a psychiatric consultant must be contacted to plan further intervention. All cases of suspected or actual incest must be reported to the local child welfare agency, which can determine if legal charges and court involvement are indicated.
    c. The child should be protected from further abuse, which may involve hospitalization or placement out of the home. If there are other children at risk, the least disruptive option may be to have the father leave home until treatment is under way.
    d. It may be necessary to hospitalize one or both of the parents, depending on their reaction to the disclosure.
    e. Outpatient treatment is begun by breaking through the denial and conveying the expectation that the problem is treatable if all participate.

C. Spouse abuse. Violence in the home is pervasive, involving all socioeconomic classes. The most frequent pattern is husbands battering wives. At least one-fourth of all homicides occur among family members, and one-half of these involve spouse killing spouse. Husbands and wives kill each other with about equal frequency.

  1. Clues. The physician may be inclined to rationalize the situation as private family business and avoid involvement. As it may be a chronic situation with a certain equilibrium, both partners may resist intervention. Also the distinction between victim and perpetrator may not always be clear. The following are red flags for further investigation.
    a. Unusual or unexplained trauma may point to abuse; this is especially true during pregnancy, which is often a time of particular stress.
    b. Vague somatic complaints may reflect underlying psychological distress in either partner.
    c. Threats of violence from either spouse must be completely investigated.
    d. Evaluation of any psychiatric symptoms, especially those of chronic stress and depression, may result in disclosure of abuse at home.
    e. Overconcern of a spouse or boyfriend, to the extent that the patient is not allowed to be alone or is rushed out of the emergency department, may disguise ongoing abuse and a fear of exposure.
    f. Behavioral problems or psychiatric symptoms in the children may reflect chaos and violence in the home.

  2. Evaluation
    a. Evaluation of the victim. After establishing a supportive relationship, the physician should ask increasingly specific questions about violence, both past and present. The physician should not be put off by evasive answers or initial denial but should appreciate the vulnerable position of the victim (i.e., she may fear abandonment or retaliation if she is candid and may see no alternatives for herself). Some discussion of resources and alternatives, such as safe houses, may be helpful early in the interview if the victim is fearful of cooperating.
    b. Evaluation of the abusive partner. If present, the abusing spouse should be evaluated with respect to dangerousness (see section IV). If he is not present, some assessment of the level of lethality of the situation should still be made. This should include an evaluation of impulse control, the availability of weapons, the provocativeness of the victim, and the homicidal potential of both partners.

  3. Treatment. The goal is to prevent further injury to either partner.
    a. Psychiatric consultation should be requested if there is any question about the lethality of the situation or the psychopathology of the partners.
    b. If lethality or risk of future injury is high, the **wife should not return home.** Options include staying with friends or family, referral to a safe house, or hospitalization. If the victim refuses treatment, the physician should make her aware of resources and options but should not exert further stress by pressuring her to accept help that she does not want unless she is returning to a life-threatening situation.
    c. The physician should support the wife's decision not to return home, although he or she should not make the decision for her, except in the most serious of circumstances. Further treatment is often helpful to the wife during the process of separating from her spouse and establishing herself independently. There may be a tendency on her part to repeat the situation by finding another abusive partner.

d. If the lethality of the present situation is low (i.e., the abusive partner wants help to prevent a recurrence), both husband and wife can be referred for treatment as a couple or individually as indicated. In any case, treatment should be offered to the abusing spouse.

e. The child welfare agency should be notified as there may be concurrent abuse, emotional if not physical, of the children.

D. Rape. Rape is a crime of violence not of sexuality. It is the most common violent crime in America and one of the most under-reported. As many as 70% to 90% of rapes go unreported for a variety of reasons, not the least of which is continued victimization of affected women by police, courts, hospital staff, and even family and friends.

1. **Characteristics of the crime**
   a. Location. Rape can take place anywhere from a deserted city street at night to a supermarket parking lot at midday to a woman's own home.
   b. Violence. In all rapes the woman's life is implicitly threatened. Explicit force is used 85% of the time, and victims are struck or choked 50% of the time. Five percent of women are severely beaten.
   c. The victim. Although rape of males is increasing, women are victims in the majority of cases. In addition, this is the only violent crime, except perhaps spouse abuse, in which the victim's story is suspect unless she fought back. There is frequently the implication and even accusations that the victim invited or encouraged the assault.
   d. The assailant. The rapist is male, usually under 24 years of age, with a prior record. He is often sexually impotent at the time of the rape.

2. **Clinical presentation.** The response of an individual to a rape has much in common with stress response syndromes in general and response to other assaults in particular. However, there are many issues specific to rape, which intensify the conflicts and impair resolution. The following stages can usually be observed, and an accurate diagnosis of where the victim is in the process guides appropriate treatment.
   a. Denial. The first stage is one of shock and disbelief. The woman may describe a feeling of numbness and disbelief, which can last from minutes to hours to days. Though appearing shaken and drained, she may not show much overt emotion. This should not be mistaken for a lack of concern or lack of distress about the assault.
   b. Emotional disorganization. In this stage, the denial alternates with periods of intense feelings of fear, anger, humiliation, and depression. These feelings may be associated with intrusive memories of the event, nightmares, phobias, hypervigilance, and anxiety. This stage may have varying degrees of intensity and continue for months or years.
   c. Resolution. The victim naturally attempts some resolution to her disorganized state, which is distressing in itself and disruptive to normal functioning.
      (1) Maladaptive resolution. The victim's attempts at resolution may be maladaptive, resulting in the establishment of chronic symptoms or creating new problems as bad as or worse than the initial event. Victims may make drastic changes in life-style, which serve to diffuse anxiety about future attacks but which are professionally and socially crippling. There may be loss of relatedness to others and especially a loss of sexual interest. There may be abuse of drugs and alcohol to decrease anxiety and suppress intrusive memories and nightmares. The result may be suicide unless there is active intervention.
      (2) Adaptive resolution. In this case the victim, with or without treatment, gradually integrates the event with a decrease in intrusive recollections and feelings and returns to normal functioning in work and relationships. Future similar situations or particular reminders of the attack may trigger transient reemergence of symptoms but usually with less intensity and distress as time passes.

3. **Evaluation and treatment.** It is particularly difficult to separate evaluation and treatment in cases of rape. Above all, the physician, especially if male, must guard against repeating the humiliation by an intrusive interview and examination. It is helpful if the victim is treated and counseled by a female practitioner.
   a. The rape crisis team or a psychiatric consultant should be called immediately to help assess the patient's current needs and support her through the examination.
   b. The patient's wishes and requests must be respected. If the patient is alone and wants family or friends contacted, she should be helped in doing this. If she prefers not to contact anyone, this must be honored.
   c. If the patient **presents in a stage of denial**, her distress should not be underestimated. With reassurance about her present security, the patient may begin to express the feelings and disorganization of the next stage. If she continues to maintain denial, it should be explained that it is natural to have feelings and thoughts that may cause considerable distress and that talking about these will help her master them.

d. If the patient is **disorganized and upset**, she may feel considerable pressure to review the details of the event and to ventilate feelings, which may include associated feelings of guilt, shame, responsibility, vulnerability, and helplessness.

e. If the patient arrives in the emergency department following a recent rape, an **empathic medical examination** should be done once the patient is prepared. Details of the event are necessary to guide the physical examination. Specimens must be collected should the patient want to press charges immediately or at a later date. There must be discussion, treatment, and follow-up due to the possibility of venereal disease and pregnancy.

f. The patient's resources should be assessed. Meeting with family and friends separately (especially husbands and boyfriends) may help them vent their outrage and conflicting feelings away from the patient and, as a result, be more supportive of her.

g. The patient's own decision about returning home and subsequent treatment should be supported unless it is grossly unreasonable or dangerous. If the patient appears to be placing herself in jeopardy, physically or emotionally, it may be necessary to insist on further crisis intervention immediately.

h. Psychiatric follow-up should be arranged as indicated. If the patient is particularly resistant to treatment, some outreach at a later date by a rape crisis center may be helpful.

VI. TELEPHONE CALLS

A. General issues. People may call the emergency department for a variety of reasons, some of which may be covert or overt requests for help for any of the crises previously described. The physician is quite limited as to what he or she can do over the telephone, but there are general principles of management.

1. The patient's name, telephone number, and address should be obtained as soon as possible in the conversation.

2. The physician should try to develop an alliance with the patient without becoming too involved over the telephone.

3. Acknowledging the limits of the telephone, the physician should encourage the patient to come to the emergency department as the next step in treatment.

4. If the patient refuses to come in, the physician's assessment of potential dangerousness dictates how active he or she must be in getting the patient to the hospital.

B. Covert presentation. Whatever the request by telephone, it may be a subtle clue to a more serious problem. Use of the telephone may reflect the patient's conflict, discomfort, or embarrassment in seeking help. If the underlying reasons for the call are revealed, the patient may feel understood, less alone and isolated, and receptive towards coming to the emergency department or to being referred to the appropriate resources. The physician should follow up his or her referral, both with the patient and the agency or clinic involved, to make sure that they have made contact with each other.

C. Overt presentation

1. The cooperative patient may describe a crisis overtly and simply be requesting help to get into treatment. In other cases the patient's ambivalence may be such that the physician must actively make arrangements with family, friends, or the police to get the patient to the hospital.

2. The uncooperative patient. If the physician is concerned about imminent danger, and the patient refuses to provide information, the physician may be forced to attempt to trace the call and follow up any leads that the patient gives. Although it can be extremely frustrating, the physician should try to build an alliance with that part of the patient desiring help, and he or she should remind the patient of the limitations of telephone contact.

D. Chronic callers. Every emergency department has a contingent of chronic callers. Some of these people are lonely and need reassurance; some are consciously or unconsciously expressing their anger and rage by repeatedly frustrating the staff.

1. Approach. Whatever the motivation for the calls, an attempt should be made to get the caller into the appropriate treatment setting.

2. Plan. Whether or not they go into treatment, a plan for handling them, which identifies these individuals by name, aliases, and content of calls, should be written down. This prevents new staff from becoming tangled in a frustrating situation and minimizes the maladaptive gratification that these individuals receive from making their calls.

STUDY QUESTIONS

Directions: Each question below contains five suggested answers. Choose the **one best** response to each question.

1. In the evaluation of a depressed patient it is most important to

(A) be supportive by accepting his or her history at face value
(B) avoid mentioning suicide so as not to initiate the idea
(C) explore any history of drug and alcohol abuse
(D) honor the patient's request not to get his or her family involved
(E) point out the positive aspects of his or her current situation

2. An individual who unsuccessfully attempts suicide by overdose is most likely

(A) not really serious about dying
(B) a girl younger than 20 years of age
(C) just trying to get attention
(D) a manipulative individual with few friends
(E) without a family history of suicide

3. Which of the following disorders is least likely to present with violent behavior?

(A) Dementia
(B) Schizophrenia
(C) Alcohol withdrawal
(D) Schizoid personality disorder
(E) Borderline personality disorder

4. All of the following are specific clues to potential child abuse EXCEPT

(A) strict religious beliefs in the family
(B) a parent under stress
(C) a child with frequent nightmares
(D) a child with pseudomature behavior
(E) a parent who experienced abuse as a child

5. In the emergency treatment of child abuse it is most important to

(A) keep the family together
(B) avoid offending the parents
(C) educate the parents as to acceptable discipline
(D) encourage the child not to disobey his or her parents
(E) notify the local child protection team

6. What is the suspected percent of cases of sexual abuse of children that are unreported?

(A) 50
(B) 60
(C) 70
(D) 80
(E) 90

Questions 7 and 8

An attractive 32-year-old single woman has come to the emergency department accompanied by a friend. With prompting she reports having been raped at knife point several hours earlier. Although her friend is quite upset, the patient is telling her story with considerable composure and detachment. She is acting as though she is not particularly concerned about the whole matter.

7. The patient's behavior indicates that she

(A) wants to forget about the attack
(B) has put the episode behind her and wants to get on with her life
(C) was not really raped but probably encouraged the man
(D) is in a protective state of numbing and denial
(E) needs to be pushed to reveal her true feelings

Two months later the same patient returns to the emergency department complaining of difficulty in sleeping. She requests medication to help her sleep and fears that she might be going crazy because of repetitive nightmares.

8. The most appropriate treatment at this time would be to

(A) give the patient 1 month's supply of sleeping pills and have her return at the end of the month if she is still having trouble sleeping
(B) encourage the patient to talk about the traumatic experience before she leaves the emergency department
(C) refer the patient for psychological testing to determine if she has evidence of a psychotic depression
(D) reassure the patient that her symptoms are expected and recommend psychotherapy to work through the event
(E) confront the patient about the addictive potential of sleeping medication and encourage her to try to sleep without it

Directions: Each question below contains four suggested answers of which **one or more** is correct. Choose the answer

A   if **1, 2, and 3** are correct
B   if **1 and 3** are correct
C   if **2 and 4** are correct
D   if **4** is correct
E   if **1, 2, 3, and 4** are correct

9.   Complications of sexual abuse include

(1) sexual promiscuity
(2) venereal disease
(3) multiple somatic complaints
(4) ulcerative colitis

Questions 10–13

A 27-year-old man comes to the emergency department in a slightly intoxicated state to have a laceration on his forearm sutured. He becomes increasingly belligerent as he is questioned about the cause of his injury and grabs a pair of scissors from the suture tray.

10. Appropriate responses by the physician include

(1) continuing to suture the laceration and calmly redirecting the patient's attention
(2) insisting that the patient regain self-control and put down the scissors
(3) confronting the patient with his alcohol problem and instructing the nurse to determine the alcohol level in the blood
(4) calling for other staff and security guards

11. Inappropriate responses to this situation reflect various countertransferences to the violent patient. These include

(1) a counterphobic reaction
(2) no reaction
(3) an angry reaction
(4) a limit-setting reaction

12. Further management of this patient requires

(1) inquiring about the details of the injury
(2) searching the patient for weapons
(3) obtaining a past history of violent behavior
(4) performing a mental status examination

13. If the patient escapes from the emergency department, the physician should

(1) pursue the patient
(2) assume that the patient will return when he is ready for treatment
(3) assume that the patient will be all right once he sobers up
(4) notify family and friends about the patient's potential dangerousness

Directions: The group of questions below consists of lettered choices followed by several numbered items. For each numbered item select the **one** lettered choice with which it is **most** closely associated. Each lettered choice may be used once, more than once, or not at all.

Questions 14–17

Match each patient history with the diagnosis with which it is most likely to be associated.

(A) Post-traumatic stress disorder
(B) Schizophrenic disorder
(C) Pathologic intoxication
(D) Intermittent explosive disorder
(E) Bipolar disorder, manic type

14. A 42-year-old man is brought to the emergency department by his family after becoming threatening when they confronted him about his excessive spending. He bought $5000 worth of clothing in the preceding week and then gave it away. He explains that this is part of his presidential campaign, which he has been working on night and day for several weeks.

15. A 23-year-old woman is brought to the emergency department by the police after assaulting her younger sister. She accused the sister of being "a witch" and said that she was ordered by "the voices" to destroy her. She has no friends and has gradually become preoccupied with witchcraft over a period of several years.

16. A 36-year-old Vietnam War veteran is brought into the emergency department in an anxious, tremulous, and diaphoretic state. While coming out of a bar he had attempted to grab a police officer's revolver after hearing a car backfire. He was shouting incoherently about "the enemy."

17. A 20-year-old man is brought to the emergency department after tearing up a restaurant and assaulting his companions. He is confused and agitated. His friends deny any history of violence or prior psychiatric history. They state that he had become violent quite suddenly and that they have been unable to calm him.

ANSWERS AND EXPLANATIONS

1. The answer is C. *(III D, E)* Alcoholics have a suicide rate that is 50 times that of normal and may have a concurrent affective disorder, which also carries an increased risk of suicide. Alcohol and drug intoxication impair judgment and impulse control, which may lead an otherwise mildly depressed patient to be dangerously suicidal. Some patients require detailed questioning and even confrontation before revealing the extent of their depression and their suicidal ideas. Patients experience relief when they are permitted and helped to talk about their suicidal feelings; the physician never puts suicidal ideation in the patient's mind, rather this excuse by the physician may be used to avoid a sensitive subject. History from the family is always important and is crucial if the patient is evasive or minimizes his or her depression. A depressed patient is not able to be optimistic about the present or future and cannot simply be encouraged out of the depression; the patient may not survive at all unless there is an adequate suicide evaluation.

2. The answer is B. *(III A 2, 3, D)* Women **attempt** suicide three times more often than men; men successfully **commit** suicide three times more often than women. The suicide rate in women gradually increases from the teenage years and peaks between 40 and 60 years of age. All suicidal patients are ambivalent; a lack of success does not necessarily suggest a nonlethal intention. An unsuccessful suicide attempt may indeed mobilize support from family and friends, but the self-destructiveness and dangerousness of the behavior must be taken very seriously. Unsuccessful suicide attempts may be a chronic manipulative pattern for some patients with severe character pathology, but for the majority, an attempt reflects a significant crisis of desperate proportions from which the individual can fully recover. A family history of suicide puts an individual at a greater risk both to attempt and actually commit suicide.

3. The answer is D. *(IV B)* Although patients with schizoid personality disorders may have angry outbursts, they have a general style of withdrawal and isolation from others without any psychotic symptoms. The other diagnoses mentioned (i.e., dementia, schizophrenia, alcohol withdrawal, and borderline personality disorder) all can demonstrate varying degrees of agitation, paranoia, impaired reality testing and impulse control, and psychotic thinking. These features singly and especially in combination are associated with an increased possibility of aggressive or assaultive behavior.

4. The answer is A. *(V A 1)* Although many religious groups may emphasize obedience and discipline, this does not in itself suggest an abusive home situation. Parents under stress may take out their hostilities on the children; they may attempt to exercise the absolute control that they do not have elsewhere at the expense of the children. A parent who was abused as a child may see such abuse as acceptable or may be unable to control his or her rage, much as his or her own parent could not. Children may show pseudomature behavior in response to the chaos in the home and their parents' need to be cared for. Any symptomatic behavior in the child, including but not limited to frequent nightmares, may originate from an abusive situation.

5. The answer is E. *(V A 3)* The physician is required by law to notify the local child protection agency of any **suspected** abuse; the agency decides how complete an investigation is indicated. While it is hoped that, with treatment, the abuse can be stopped and the family can stay together, the immediate goal is to protect the child. Although the questioning should be done in an empathic, nonjudgmental way to build a treatment alliance with the parents, an accurate assessment of the dangerousness of the home situation must take precedence over the parents' feelings. Education about alternative ways of discipline may be an important long-range goal, but it is not helpful in the emergency situation. Lastly, although the child's behavior may be problematic and require treatment, the central issue in the emergency situation is the parents' capacity to control aggressive behavior towards the child.

6. The answer is E. *(V B)* At least 200,000 cases of sexual abuse are reported each year, and these reported cases may represent only 10% of all incidents. This includes sexual molestation by strangers and family members. Children experience powerful pressures, both internal and external, to keep the sexual contact hidden. This is particularly so in situations of incest, where exposure may destroy the entire family structure, and children may reveal their distress subtly. Unless the physician has a high index of suspicion, he or she may miss the clues; furthermore, a natural repugnance on the part of the physician and a wish to deny the situation may prevent him or her from making the diagnosis.

7. The answer is D. *(V D 2)* The patient probably does want to forget about the attack, but her apparent composure and detachment reflect the numbing and denial that are often the first stage of a stress-response reaction. The issue for the patient at this moment is survival, not forgetting about the assault or getting on with her life. Her behavior is self-protective and should not be mistaken for a lack of concern about the rape. All victims of life-threatening trauma may wonder if they did something to provoke or cause the assault or accident; this is a reaction to overwhelming helplessness and vulnerability and should not be mistaken for proof that they somehow brought this on themselves. This is particularly true of such a charged issue as rape, in which the male physician may tend to blame the victim for her predicament. While it ultimately is helpful for the woman to discuss her feelings with someone, the physician may repeat the trauma and humiliation of the rape by asking unnecessarily probing questions.

8. The answer is D. *(V D 2, 3)* The patient still may not be able to discuss the details of the assault, of her feelings, or of her symptoms in the emergency department situation; nor is it necessarily therapeutic to pry this open on a one-time visit. Rather, the patient should be reassured that her symptoms, although distressing, are usual following such trauma and are treatable. It probably would be helpful to give the patient a few days' supply of sleeping medication along with a referral for psychotherapy. A 1-month supply of sleeping pills might be used in a suicide attempt, and 1 month is too long to wait for further psychiatric evaluation and treatment. Sleeping medication has some potential for abuse and addiction, but providing this patient with some symptomatic relief at this point is reasonable and humane. Evidence of a psychotic depression would be apparent during the course of treatment, and getting this patient into treatment is the first priority.

9. The answer is A (1, 2, 3). *(V B)* Perineal and vaginal trauma, pregnancy, and venereal disease are all possible medical complications of sexual abuse. Sexual promiscuity, truancy, and running away may be behavioral responses. Multiple somatic complaints, symptoms of anxiety and depression, and other psychiatric symptoms may develop in a young girl experiencing sexual abuse. There is no correlation between ulcerative colitis and sexual abuse.

10. The answer is C (2, 4). *(II A, B, C; IV)* Despite the patient's initial cooperation, he has escalated to overt threatening behavior with minimal provocation. The patient's behavior must be dealt with before anything else. Firm verbal limits that encourage self-control but that do not challenge the patient should be given. If the patient does not respond, the security guards should be called in. If the patient still does not calm down, preparations to disarm him safely must take place. Any discussion with the patient about his alcohol problem must wait until he is sober and in control.

11. The answer is A (1, 2, 3). *(IV D)* A firm limit-setting response on the part of the physician would be appropriate in this situation. A counterphobic reaction, an angry reaction, and no reaction represent countertransference, which can impair clinical judgment and even further increase the danger in dealing with a violent patient. Ignoring the patient's behavior may frighten him because he fears that no one will help him maintain control. An angry response may challenge and humiliate the patient, leading to further escalation. A counterphobic reaction may place the physician in considerable danger since he or she will not take appropriate self-protective measures.

12. The answer is E (all). *(II A, B; IV D)* Once the patient has been controlled (i.e., the scissors have been taken away and he is in restraints if necessary), he should be searched for other weapons and the medical treatment should be completed. At this point he must be evaluated in terms of ongoing dangerousness. The details of the injury and past history of violent behavior are crucial. This data together with a mental status examination will help to determine if the patient requires psychiatric treatment, treatment for alcoholism, or if legal charges for attempted assault should be filed.

13. The answer is D (4). *(IV E)* This patient may be all right once he sobers up, but at present he is volatile and assaultive. To ignore this is a serious countertransference as is pursuing an angry, injured, intoxicated man with a weapon without adequate help. The patient may return, but given his impairment in impulse control and judgment, this seems unlikely. The police and any family or friends who can be reached should be fully apprised of the situation as they too may be in danger if the patient returns home.

14–17. The answers are: 14-E, 15-B, 16-A, 17-C. *(IV B)* The most likely diagnosis of the 42-year-old man is bipolar disorder, manic type. The affected individual's poor judgment and unrealistic behavior motivated by grandiose ideas were sustained over some time, ruling out post-traumatic stress disorder, pathologic intoxication, and intermittent explosive disorder. The specific symptoms of insomnia, hyperactivity, grandiosity, and irritability are consistent with a diagnosis of bipolar disorder rather than schizophrenia

The most likely diagnosis of the 23-year-old woman is schizophrenic disorder. The violent behavior was the culmination of chronically developing delusional beliefs and ultimately the result of command hallucinations. While hallucinations and delusions can occur in bipolar disorder, manic type, there is no evidence of other manic symptoms. In fact, the patient's chronic deteriorating course with poor social relationships suggests schizophrenia.

The most likely diagnosis of the Vietnam War veteran is post-traumatic stress disorder. This patient had a flashback to a combat situation triggered by the sound of a car backfiring. The patient is essentially in a dissociative state and experiences his current situation as though he was back in combat. Despite his appearing anxious and incoherent at the moment, there is nothing else to suggest mania. Although he had been drinking, his violent behavior was not triggered directly by alcohol as occurs with pathologic intoxication.

The most likely diagnosis of the 20-year-old man is pathologic intoxication, which is a dramatic violent behavioral response triggered by a small amount of alcohol and often accompanied by confusion and disorientation. There are no symptoms or previous history in this case to suggest schizophrenia or bipolar disorder, manic type. The diagnosis of intermittent explosive disorder, while more common in men, requires a history of violent behavior and clearly directed violence. There is no history of a traumatic event, post-traumatic symptoms, or a triggering stimulus.

10
Child Psychiatry
William V. Good

I. INTRODUCTION. Child psychiatry is the study and treatment of the mental and behavioral problems of childhood. As such, it overlaps with a variety of pediatric subspecialties. An understanding of standard childhood development is essential to the understanding of childhood psychopathology, since seemingly major difficulties may be normal at certain ages (e.g., negativism is usual at 2 years of age and again at adolescence, but it is problematic during the latency period and in adulthood).

A. Developmental concepts

1. Epigenesis. There is a natural and unalterable sequence in which development must occur (e.g., the anal period must follow the oral stage and cannot be reversed).

2. Developmental continuities. Some childhood personality traits and experiences are continuous with and have ramifications for adulthood; others do not. (For example, a child who is abandoned at the age of 3 years by his or her parents may feel depressed every time someone leaves him or her later in life. Thus, this early childhood experience would be continuous with later experiences.)

3. Critical phases. It is generally accepted that particular phases of development must occur at certain ages. For example, the oedipal period occurs between the ages of 3½ and 6 years. If a child suffers a severe psychological trauma at the age of 4 years, causing a developmental arrest, he or she may not be able to experience a normal oedipal period, even though the trauma is overcome, and development recommences at 7 years of age. The child will have had a distorted oedipal phase. This example is hypothetical; very little is actually known about which developmental phases are critical. In this case, the child might irrationally fear physical or psychological harm in competitive situations. This fear could persist into adulthood.

4. Invulnerability. Certain children are able to negotiate seemingly overwhelming psychological trauma with no apparent effect on their subsequent personality development; however, what makes certain children invulnerable is unknown.

B. Overview of childhood psychopathology

1. All disorders are more common in boys than in girls except thumb sucking. This probably reflects an inherent increased vulnerability of the male to stress and trauma.

2. Isolated traumatic events (e.g., one episode of sexual abuse by a nonfamily member) can cause transient anxiety, anger, and depression. However, they generally do not cause psychopathology unless they generate long-lasting changes in the child's interactions with his or her environment. **Psychopathology is usually the result of chronic, maladaptive interactions** between the child and the environment, often combined with some biologic propensity towards developing a mental illness.

3. Children are usually willing to behave in a way that is consistent with the parents' desires. Their misbehavior may be the result of the parents' conscious or unconscious prompting.

C. Approach to the child patient

1. In child psychiatry **the physician must be an advocate for the child,** not for his or her parents. To do otherwise is to subject the child to the parents' wishes, which may or may not be realistic or appropriate. Nevertheless, the child psychiatrist must develop a working relationship with the child's parents; they often represent a limitation in terms of the child's psychological growth. Parents should be seen frequently, especially at the beginning of psycho-therapy. Preadolescents should be seen alone but usually after the parents have been seen. An attempt to communicate with the child patient by talking should be made. If this is difficult, a small assortment of toys, including a dollhouse, paper and crayons, puppets, checkers, and blocks, can help a child communicate through play. Adolescents should be seen alone and before the parents are seen. Use of unnatural slang to bridge the generation gap should be avoided. An attitude of concern for the adolescent suffices, usually establishing rapport with the patient.

2. The patient interview should reveal:
   a. The child's reaction to separation from the parents
   b. The child's behavior towards the interviewer (e.g., anxious, very open, or shy)
   c. The choice of verbal versus play communication
   d. The child's reaction to rejoining the parents after the interview

3. Gathering information from the child can be facilitated by requesting the child to:
   a. Make three wishes
   b. Draw his or her family
   c. Draw him- or herself
   d. Describe the family
   e. Describe important nonfamily members
   f. Describe the problem that initiated therapy and how the family told him or her of the appointment

II. BONDING AND ATTACHMENT

A. Definition. A **bond** is defined as **an affective relationship of the parent with the child. Attachment describes the child's affective relationship with the parent.** Bonding and attachment develop over time; there appears to be no critical phase of bonding as it is described in the animal literature. Bonding likely commences long before the actual birth of the child and is apparent in the parents' attitudes, fantasies, and wishes for the child.

B. Assessment of bonding

1. The parents should be asked when a name was chosen for the child, which indicates when they began planning for the new arrival. The name can have special meaning; it may indicate how the family perceives the child.

2. What sort of dreams did the parents have about the child during pregnancy?

3. How did the parents' relationship towards each other change during the pregnancy? Usually the husband assumes a maternal role towards his wife. If he begins abusing her, has affairs, or grows uninvolved, a poor relationship between the parents and new baby is likely.

4. Do the parents visit the nursery following delivery or do they seem to avoid it?

5. Is either parent psychotic, depressed, or abusing drugs? These problems can distort the way the parent perceives the child.

6. Special problems are posed if the newborn has had to spend extra time in the nursery due to illness. A family with a child in the critical care unit nursery should be evaluated prior to discharge to assure adequate care for the child.

7. Of whom does the child remind the parents? This question determines transferences and preconceived attitudes about the infant.

C. Disorders of bonding and attachment

1. **Hospitalism** is an extreme example of failure of any affective relationship to develop. Affected infants suffer from susceptibility to infection, apathy, retarded development, and, sometimes, failure to thrive.

2. **Child abuse** may occur if parents have not adequately bonded with the child. This is especially prevalent with premature infants.

3. **Vulnerable child syndrome** was originally described by Green and Solnit. Parents may continue to treat a child who has been ill and recovered as though he or she is still vulnerable. Such children can later show a variety of psychological traits, including:
   a. Those resulting from parental overprotectiveness
   b. Hypochondriasis
   c. Hyperactivity

        d. Separation anxiety
        e. Learning difficulties
   4. Children who are separated from their parents in infancy probably also suffer a range of reactions later in life.

D. Treatment

   1. Parents should be counseled to spend time with the newborn. In situations in which the parents have not visited a sick infant or have been reluctant to see a newborn, **a structured plan to facilitate parent-child interactions should be implemented.** There should be a mandatory visitation of at least 24 consecutive hours. Nursing support should be available when parents' questions arise. Grief over a child's prematurity and illness may require psychiatric intervention when the grief is thought to contribute to the lack of parental involvement.

   2. Follow-up in a special clinic for premature infants is indicated.

   3. When parents cannot demonstrate a bond to their child and an understanding of the child's needs and when these problems may contribute to the development of either hospitalism or child abuse, the child should be placed in a foster home.

   4. Psychopathology in either parent should be evaluated and treated.

   5. Vulnerable child syndrome is managed by informing the parents that the child has recovered and is doing well. Surprisingly, parents may not realize this, and their attitude towards the child may change with this reassurance. However, if reassurance fails, psychotherapy for the parents is indicated.

III. CHILDHOOD PSYCHOSES

A. Infantile autism

   1. Clinical data. Infantile autism is an illness commencing early in childhood (before the age of 30 months) in which the child is relatively unresponsive to other human beings, demonstrates bizarre responses to his or her environment, and has unusual language development.
      a. Autistic children treat other individuals indifferently, almost as though they are inanimate objects.
      b. Language abnormalities include echolalia, pronoun reversals (e.g., use of the pronoun "you" when "I" is correct), mutism, and delays.
      c. Autistic children have a great need for consistency in their environment and may decompensate if, for example, furniture is rearranged. The etiology of this need for sameness is unknown.
      d. Social development is usually abnormal.

   2. Epidemiology. Although the disorder has an even socioeconomic distribution, it occurs more commonly in boys.

   3. Etiologic theories
      a. A cold, distant mother figure was thought to be responsible for the development of coldness and aloofness in the child (i.e., growing up in an emotional vacuum leads to unrelatedness in the child). However, this theory is old and has been replaced by the abnormal sensory integration theory.
      b. Abnormal sensory integration theory. An increased threshold to sensory stimuli or delayed integration of communicative stimuli could place the child out of synchrony with the environment.

   4. Associated findings
      a. Abnormal auditory-evoked potentials (which are tracings of the transmission of sound stimuli from the brain stem to the cerebral cortex)
      b. Decreased nystagmus in response to vestibular stimulation

   5. Differential diagnosis
      a. Hearing deficits
      b. Mental retardation—global developmental delays, not simply social delays as in autism, are evident
      c. Organic brain disorders, such as hepatic encephalopathy and congenital cytomegalovirus, which can mimic autism

   6. Treatment
      a. A highly structured classroom setting is important to help autistic children focus their atten-

tion on learning and communication tasks. Precautions should be taken to insure that the environment remains stable.

b. Psychotherapy for both the child and parents may be of value in cases in which parental factors are considered to be partly etiologic. It may also be indicated when the family is having trouble coping with the stress of having an autistic child.

c. Medication is rarely of value unless agitation is pronounced, in which case thioridazine at an oral dose of 0.5 to 1.0 mg/kg daily may be necessary.

d. Language therapy may be beneficial.

7. **Prognosis.** Many autistic children develop grand mal seizures prior to adolescence. However, the prognosis for infantile autism is better the higher the IQ of the child. It is also better with reasonable language development.

B. Childhood schizophrenia

1. **Clinical data.** Pervasive developmental disorder* and borderline psychosis of childhood are sometimes used synonymously with the term childhood schizophrenia. However, there are differences. Childhood schizophrenia is a regression to a psychotic state after previous attainment of better mental functioning. Borderline psychosis of childhood is similar to the borderline personality disorder of adults. Pervasive developmental disorder begins after 30 months of age and includes:

a. Preoccupation with gory or grotesque fantasies

b. Hallucinations (usually not prominent and not a criterion in the *DSM III*)

c. Propensity to digress with poor attention span

d. Responsiveness to individuals in the environment without demonstration of sociability or empathy

e. Possible abnormal motor movements

f. Unusual mannerisms

2. **Etiology.** A genetic cause for childhood schizophrenia has not been well delineated as it has for adult schizophrenia. A **grossly chaotic upbringing** with constant exposure to aggressive and sexual themes (e.g., chronic violence in the family) could be causative. A failure of repression is also considered to be active in the disorder. For example, a child who is repeatedly exposed to violence may be unable to repress sexual and aggressive fantasies, which normally occurs by the age of 6 years.

3. **Treatment**

a. Psychotherapy is very helpful. Family therapy may be indicated when disruption of the family is evident.

b. Antipsychotic medication, especially thioridazine at an orally administered dose of 1 mg/kg daily, is often necessary.

C. Symbiotic psychosis

1. **Clinical data.** Symbiotic psychosis is a disorder in which a parent misperceives herself as her child. The reciprocal is usually true also. Although this disorder usually occurs in mothers and their children, fathers occasionally are affected.

a. A loss of ego boundaries (i.e., the inability to distinguish oneself from others) is apparent.

b. Great anxiety at the threat of separation of the child from the parent is seen in both. Upon reuniting, the anxiety clears.

c. The overlap between parent and child can be manifested in almost any area (e.g., if the parent diets, she assumes the child needs to diet too).

2. **Etiology.** A parent who has poor object relations may see her child as an extension of herself. Borderline psychopathology may predispose to the disorder. Although the parent is the cause of the problem, the child usually manifests the symptoms (e.g., severe separation anxiety).

3. **Treatment.** Psychotherapy aimed at separating the child from the parent is needed. Sometimes the parent may require support to help her permit the separation and development of autonomy in the child.

4. **Prognosis** is good; symbiotic psychosis carries the best prognosis of all the childhood psychoses.

IV. CHILDHOOD AFFECTIVE DISORDERS

A. Depressive illness presents at all developmental stages.

---

*This is the nomenclature of the *Diagnostic and Statistical Manual of Mental Disorders*, third edition (*DSM III*). See the bibliography at the end of the chapter.

1. **Anaclitic depression** occurs between the ages of 7 months and 30 months. The cause is a lengthy separation (more than 1 week) from caregivers. Symptoms include listlessness, anorexia, psychomotor retardation, and sad facial expressions. The treatment is restitution of the relationship.

2. When depressed, **preschool children** show more behavioral symptoms than older children (e.g., hyperactivity and aggressiveness). These symptoms are called **depressive equivalents.** Separation from caregivers or a sense of poor mastery over developmental tasks (e.g., toilet training) may be etiologic. Treatment should be aimed at changing the child's environment. Psychotherapy may help.

3. **School-aged children** may manifest the usual signs and symptoms of depression (e.g., vegetative signs and a depressed mood). Biologic vulnerabilities and a sense of helplessness or incompetence may play an etiologic role at this age. Treatment is psychotherapy aimed at helping the child feel a sense of competence vis à vis his or her environment.

4. **Adolescents** also show usual signs of depression. The incidence of affective disorders increases in adolescence, with girls affected more than boys.

B. **Manic-depressive illness** rarely presents in childhood. Hyperactivity can be mistaken for mania.

C. **Biologic markers** are even less valuable in identifying childhood affective disorders than in identifying adult disorders. They remain under investigation.

D. **Childhood suicide** may be a complication of affective illness. The incidence of suicide is probably increasing in preadolescence. Depressed children should be carefully evaluated for suicidal ideation.

V. **TOURETTE'S SYNDROME** is recurrent, involuntary, purposeless motor movements accompanied by vocal tics (e.g., coprolalia and involuntary swearing). Other findings include the voluntary suppression of tics for minutes or hours. Motor tics may precede or follow the development of coprolalia. Psychological stress exacerbates the symptoms, but the cause, although unknown, is probably organic.

A. **Epidemiology**

1. The disorder is more common in boys and is usually noticed at the age of 5 to 7 years.

2. There may be a familial pattern.

3. It occurs in all socioeconomic classes.

B. **Treatment**

1. **Psychotherapy** is indicated when the tics are causing psychological problems.

2. **Medical treatment** includes the use of haloperidol, which suppresses tics. The use of pimozide for Tourette's syndrome is under investigation, and the drug appears to be effective. However, pimozide can cause cardiac arrhythmias.

VI. **SLEEP DISORDERS**

A. **Parasomnias** usually affect stages 3 and 4 of sleep, which predominate early in the sleep cycle. Thus, these disorders usually occur early in the night.

1. **Somnambulism (sleep walking)** is exacerbated by psychological stress in some cases. It is normal much of the time. Alcoholism unmasks somnambulism in adults.

2. **Night terrors** are very common between the ages of 2½ and 5 years, affecting 30% of children in this age bracket. Terrors are sometimes exacerbated by stress. There is usually no treatment unless immobilization is required, in which case administration of chloral hydrate should suppress the deep stages of sleep.

3. **Nocturnal enuresis** (see section VII A 1) is due generally to stress or slow central nervous system maturation. The disorder dissipates with increasing age and is, therefore, self-limited.

B. **Narcolepsy** is a sleep disorder that is characterized by sleep-onset rapid eye movement (REM). REM sleep normally occurs after sleep stages 1 to 4.

1. **Manifestations**
   a. The entire sleep cycle is affected, resulting in **excessive daytime drowsiness**.
   b. **Cataplexy** is the loss of motor tone in response to an emotion (e.g., anger and excitement).

c. On awakening, the patient may be transiently completely **paralyzed**.

d. **Hypnagogic hallucinations** are vivid hallucinations occurring at sleep onset.

2. **Treatment.** Administration of amphetamines and tricyclic antidepressants helps.

VII. ENURESIS

A. **Clinical data.** The child with enuresis continues to urinate at inappropriate times and places after the time when he or she normally should have been toilet trained (i.e., between the ages of 2 and 4 years). The disorder is much more common in boys.

1. **Primary enuresis** is that which has never been interrupted by a period of good bladder control.

   a. **Nocturnal enuresis** is a parasomnia occurring during stages 3 and 4 of sleep.

   b. **Daytime enuresis** occurs during the waking hours.

2. **Secondary enuresis** is that which develops after a period of at least 1 year of good bladder control. As in primary enuresis, the disorder may occur both during the sleeping and waking hours.

B. **Etiology**

1. **Organic disorders** may cause enuresis. These include:

   a. **Systemic illness**, including:

      (1) Juvenile-onset diabetes mellitus

      (2) Sickle cell anemia or sickle cell trait

      (3) Diabetes insipidus

   b. **Central nervous system disorders**

      (1) Frontal lobe tumor

      (2) Spinal cord lesion (e.g., spina bifida or spina bifida occulta)

      (3) Peripheral nerve damage

   c. **Anatomic disorders**

      (1) Posterior urethral valvular dysfunction

      (2) Proximal genitourinary malformations

   d. **Urinary tract infections**

   e. **Delayed central nervous system maturation** (after the age of 4½ years, as many as 10% of boys remain enuretic, frequently due to delayed maturation.

2. **Psychological factors** account for the majority of cases of enuresis.

   a. Acute stress can cause enuresis (e.g., the birth of a sibling or starting kindergarten).

   b. Enuresis sometimes occurs in very ambitious boys. Strength and quality of the urine stream may become equated with physical prowess. Micturition can then become conflicted, resulting in urination at inappropriate times.

   c. Hostility can be expressed through the symptom of enuresis. Such an expression of hostility is nearly always unconscious; the child does not deliberately void at inappropriate times.

   d. Family reaction to the enuresis sometimes causes more psychopathology than the psychological causes of the enuresis per se.

   e. The family may encourage enuresis unconsciously. A possible vicarious pleasure for the parents in the child's enuresis may exist.

   f. Some children wet their pants because they are too busy or preoccupied to use the bathroom.

C. **Treatment** may be only sporadically helpful, with the exception of tricyclic antidepressant therapy. Since enuresis is a self-limited disorder, sometimes no treatment is the best.

1. Probing diagnostic procedures to search for an organic etiology, unless the preponderance of evidence points to such, should be avoided.

2. The parents should be assured that the child is not purposefully wetting (enuresis is usually beyond the child's control). Reduction of fluid intake after dinner, awakening the child to urinate after 1 to 2 hours of sleep, bladder exercises (having the child try to hold urine during the daytime), and the use of special feedback devices that set off an alarm upon urination in bed may all be remedial.

3. Tricyclic antidepressant therapy can be effective. Imipramine should be administered in a 10- to 25-mg dose after school. The medicine should be kept out of reach in a child-proof bottle since overdoses can cause serious problems. Enuresis is a self-limited condition; therefore, the use of antidepressants is discouraged except in refractory or unusual cases (e.g., the parents are completely intolerant of the condition).

4. The child should be treated for any psychological stress. In refractory cases, long-term psychotherapy may be indicated.

VIII. ENCOPRESIS

A. Clinical data. Encopresis is fecal incontinence beyond the period when bowel control should normally have developed. Most encopresis is unconscious and involuntary; only occasionally does it occur deliberately.

   1. Primary encopresis is that which has occurred continuously throughout the child's life.

   2. Secondary encopresis develops following a period of at least 1 year of good bowel control.

B. Etiology

   1. Organic disorders. Hirschsprung's disease rarely presents in older children as encopresis.

   2. Psychological factors
   a. Unresolved anger at a parent sometimes is expressed unconsciously through fecal incontinence. The child consciously and unconsciously perceives that his or her stool has a negative impact on the family.
   b. Fecal smearing may be a psychotic symptom, especially if the child is older than 4 or 5 years.
   c. As is true with enuresis, parents can get vicarious pleasure from their child's symptoms.
   d. When autonomy and control battles focus on toilet training at the age of 2 to 3 years and when parents are too punitive and unyielding in their approach to the toilet training, conflicts over bowel evacuation develop in the child.

C. Treatment

   1. Correcting fecal impaction is necessary. Some pediatricians recommend a bowel regimen that consists of periodic cathartic administration to insure that no impaction develops and to help regulate bowel control [e.g., administration of a bisacodyl (Dulcolax) suppository daily at the same time, immediately followed by placing the child on the toilet].

   2. Behavior modification that reinforces continence is effective in some children (e.g., rewarding a child after a day of good bowel control or after evacuation in the toilet).

   3. Long-term psychotherapy is indicated in refractory cases. Occasionally encopresis is a symptom of psychosis. The underlying disease should then be treated.

IX. MASTURBATION

A. Definition. Childhood masturbation involves genital manipulation and fondling. It definitely is not a disease, but many parents complain to the physician about this behavior in their children. An open attitude on the part of the physician is important in allowing the parents to express concern. Any notions that masturbation may cause growth retardation or mental retardation should be dispelled.

B. Incidence. Masturbation occurs in 100% of children. It can develop before the age of 1 year. During the oedipal period (i.e., between the ages of 3½ and 6 years), there is heightened focus on the genitalia.

C. Continuous masturbation may be a sign of severe understimulation or environmental deprivation.

   1. Other signs of self-stimulation (e.g., rocking, head banging, and hair pulling) should be sought. The child should be enrolled in a stimulation program, and the situation should be followed up fully.

   2. Signs of child abuse should also be sought.

X. THUMB SUCKING

A. Thumb sucking is more common in girls and is normal at transitional periods in the child's life (e.g., at bedtime and at times of separation from the parents).

B. Treatment is not usually needed. If thumb sucking is chronic and occurs after the age of 3½ years, it can cause changes in dentition. An in-depth exploration of the child's relationship with the parents is indicated as is, usually, psychotherapy. Thumb sucking in the older child can be a sign that the child is insecure or withdrawn. Behavior modification can be useful.

XI. SCHOOL PHOBIAS

A. Definition. School phobias are a phobic attitude towards and avoidance of school. In adolescence, they can herald schizophrenia.

B. Incidence. School phobias most commonly occur when a child is first introduced to school (at age 4 or 5 years) and in early adolescence when children are required to shower at school after gym. They occur throughout childhood, however.

C. Etiology. School phobia is best considered as a symptom. It is caused by a variety of conditions, including:

1. Vulnerable child syndrome

2. Extreme separation anxiety suffered by the parent (as opposed to that suffered by the child)

3. Malingering (e.g., the child has not completed a homework assignment)

4. A legitimate cause of fear to the child at school (e.g., gangs or a cruel teacher)

5. Homosexual panic in an older child

6. Separation anxiety suffered by the child

D. Treatment

1. Legitimate causes of fear should be eliminated, and the child should usually be sent back to school immediately. Thus, school avoidance is not reinforced by staying home.

2. Psychotherapy to treat the underlying disorder may be needed.

3. Some cases are exceedingly refractory to treatment interventions and may even require psychiatric hospitalization.

XII. HYPERACTIVITY

A. Definition. Hyperactivity is defined subjectively as an increase in motor activity to a level that interferes with the child's functioning either at school or at home. The *DSM III* term for this problem is **attention deficit disorder**, with or without the symptom of hyperactivity.

B. Etiology

1. Medication (paradoxically, sedatives frequently cause hyperactivity in children)

2. Depression (depression is poorly tolerated by some children, who express their sad feelings by means of increased activity)

3. Anxiety

4. Vulnerable child syndrome

5. Severe central nervous system disease (e.g., a grossly abnormal central nervous system or a history of significant head trauma)

6. Constitutional hyperactivity (some children have a hyperactive temperament, which is present from birth)

7. An intolerant parent, teacher, or supervisor (i.e., factitious hyperactivity—the child is not truly suffering from increased motor activity)

8. Specific learning disabilities, which may be associated with hyperactivity

C. Treatment

1. Any underlying disorder should be treated (e.g., depression should be treated by means of psychotherapy).

2. Medication
a. Methylphenidate administered in divided doses of 5 mg to 50 mg per day is effective.
b. Tricyclic antidepressants, phenytoin, and thioridazine have all proved to be valuable in certain refractory cases.

3. Although studies have not proven any beneficial dietary effects as yet, **an alteration in the child's diet** may be helpful, presumably because the emphasis on food alters a parent's relationship with a child in some meaningful way. Many parents of hyperactive children report that reducing the child's sugar intake reduces the hyperactivity. These parents may pay more attention to their child, feel more in control of the problem, and spend more time with the child at mealtime as a result of changing the child's diet. All of the secondary effects can be beneficial.

XIII. LEARNING DISORDERS

A. There are a wide range of disorders that interfere with the child's ability to perform certain intellectual functions. Children may suffer from specific reading, processing, writing, mathematical, and language disabilities, which can be diagnosed with IQ testing and other specialized learning examinations. In this paper, the focus is on psychiatric conditions that can interfere with learning.

1. **Depression** develops in childhood and manifests itself differently at varying ages.
   a. In infancy anaclitic depression occurs between 7 and 30 months of age in response to prolonged separation from the primary caretaker.
   b. In toddlers, depression may present as heightened aggression or clinging.
   c. Latency-aged children may be hyperactive, aggressive, frankly depressed, or withdrawn.
   d. Adolescents may act out as a depressive equivalent.

2. **Hyperactivity** can be either primary or secondary to the learning disorder. This distinction is important since treatment differs with the etiology of the hyperactivity.

3. **School phobias** of any etiology can lead to learning disorders.

4. An **interaction problem with the teacher** (specific transference reactions) can prove causative.

5. **Homosexual panic** (in older children) may interfere with learning.

6. **Childhood psychosis,** with its attendant developmental delays, may be at the root of a learning disability.

B. **Treatment** is aimed at the underlying disorder.

XIV. PROBLEMS OF ADOLESCENTS. A variety of disorders increase in incidence during adolescence (e.g., anorexia nervosa, adult schizophrenia, and depression). Specific problems of adolescent development are discussed below.

A. **Identity disturbances.** Adolescents struggle to achieve a stable identity. Certain problems result when this aspect of development breaks down.

1. **Identity diffusion.** An adolescent has a poor sense of him- or herself and is easily swayed by the opinions of others.

2. **Peer-related disorders.** Some adolescents can be persuaded to do dangerous things (e.g., take drugs and drive recklessly) to meet the identity of their peer groups.

B. **Adult sexual development.** In adolescence, adult sexual functioning is achieved and sexual preferences are solidified.

1. **Homosexuality** can be normal in early adolescence, but when it occurs consistently throughout adolescence, it usually represents a true homosexual preference.

2. **Sexual perversions.** Disorders such as transvestism, voyeurism, and exhibitionism usually become full-blown in adolescence.

3. **Pregnancy** may be the outcome of increased sexual promiscuity or may manifest emancipation difficulties. For example, an adolescent who is struggling with separating from her family may become pregnant and turn the baby over to the parents for care. The baby thus replaces her and makes her emancipation easier.

C. **Separation.** In adolescence, the individual negotiates leaving his or her family.

1. Difficulty with emancipation can be etiologic in a variety of clinical disorders. For example, psychosis becomes evident in many schizophrenics when they first leave home. The battle over food is really a struggle for autonomy and independence in anorectics. Separation and loss can trigger depressive feelings.

2. Difficult emancipation can lead to **mobilization of aggression** on the part of the adolescent, and intrafamily fighting ensues.

3. **Incest** can develop to prevent a child from emancipating, and inappropriate sexual contact within a family sometimes signifies separation problems.

D. **Treatment.** Special problems develop in the psychotherapy of adolescents.

1. **Labile allegiances.** Adolescents love the therapist one day and hate him or her the next day. They have trouble forming an alliance to work on problems.

2. **Labile moods.** Because adolescents are in great endocrine and psychological turbulence, unstable moods frequently result.

3. **Communication difficulties.** Adolescents may not be comfortable with verbal communication but are too old for communication through play. Some adolescents communicate by means of their behavior (e.g., reckless driving may signify anger or depression). Obstinancy may signify an emancipation problem because the child refuses to take responsibility for him- or herself.

4. **Overprotective parents** may meddle in an adolescent's treatment. An adolescent should be seen by a physician for evaluation even if he or she asks that the parents not be made aware of the request for treatment. However, parents should be notified under these circumstances:
   a. If the patient is a danger to him- or herself
   b. If the patient is a danger to others
   c. If the patient is gravely disabled

XV. **CHILD ABUSE** occurs when the individuals in a child's environment retard his or her development by hurting the child.

A. **Epidemiology**

1. Approximately 15% of children who come to the emergency room with obvious trauma have been physically abused.

2. Parents who were abused as children are at greater risk for abusing their own children.

3. Premature infants are abused more often than full-gestation infants, which is probably due to poor bonding.

4. Reasons for the abuse of infants probably differ from those for the abuse of older children. Abuse of the latter is often associated with psychosexual development (e.g., a 3-year-old soils her pants and is beaten). The former are abused because their parents are emotionally needy and feel that the infant is taking attention away from them. Problems with feeding may result in abuse of infants. It is unusual for child abuse to begin after the age of 6 years.

5. Abuse occurs in all socioeconomic groups.

B. **Effects on the child**

1. Occasionally, development may be precocious. The expectation that a child function as "a parent" causes some children to develop quickly. Fear of being abused for mistakes can also lead to precocious development.

2. Development may be retarded if the abuse is severe.

3. There may be a role reversal with the parents. Abusive parents may expect their children to function as adults and care for them.

4. Physical injuries are constantly a risk.

5. There is a risk of abusing future offspring when the abused child grows up and identifies with his or her parents.

6. Exposure to chronic violence can increase aggression and antisocial behavior in the abused child.

C. **Treatment**

1. Suspected abuse must be reported to the county protective services. If the child's health or life is in jeopardy, he or she should be removed from the abusive environment. If there is no improvement at 1 to 2 years postdiagnosis, severance of parental rights should be considered.

2. Most abused children need psychotherapy.

3. Parents almost always need long-term psychotherapy and occasionally parenting classes.

BIBLIOGRAPHY

American Psychiatric Association: *Diagnostic and Statistical Manual of Mental Disorders*, 3rd ed. Washington, D.C., American Psychiatric Association, 1980

Emde RN, Harmon RJ, Good WV: Depressive feelings in children: a transactional model for research. In *Depression in Childhood: Developmental Perspectives.* Edited by Rutter M, Izard D, Reed P. New York, Gilford Press. In press, 1985

Green M, Solnit AJ: Reactions to the threatened loss of a child. A vulnerable child syndrome. *Pediatrics* 34:58–65, 1964

Klaus MH, Kendall JH: *Parent-Infant Bonding.* St. Louis, CV Mosby, 1982

Spitz RA: Hospitalism: an inquiry into the genesis of psychiatric conditions in early childhood. *Psychoanal Study Child* 1:53–74, 1945

Steele BF, Pollock CB: A psychiatric study of parents who abuse infants and small children. In *The Battered Child.* Edited by Helfer RE, Kempe CH. Chicago, University of Chicago Press, 1968, pp 103–145

STUDY QUESTIONS

Directions: Each question below contains five suggested answers. Choose the **one best** response to each question.

1. Which of the following statements about childhood psychopathology is true?

(A) Childhood psychiatric disorders are more common in boys than in girls
(B) Childhood disorders are more common in latency-aged children (i.e., those 6 to 12 years of age)
(C) Childhood psychopathology is always transient
(D) It is impossible to evaluate children alone; their families must also be evaluated
(E) None of the above

2. Which of the following statements concerning the sequence of oral-anal-genital psychosexual stages is true?

(A) It starts when a child is 2 years old
(B) It must be negotiated in this order
(C) It does not really exist
(D) It is based on Jungian theory
(E) None of the above

3. What statement is true concerning the issue of confidentiality in treating a child?

(A) It does not apply because parents have a right to know what their children are thinking and talking about
(B) It does not apply because children think that their parents know and understand most things
(C) It applies except when a child is a danger to him- or herself or others
(D) It applies to children over the age of 15 years
(E) None of the above

4. The first measure that should be taken in the treatment of encopresis is to

(A) determine if the child has an impaction
(B) help the child understand his or her anger
(C) perform a rectal examination to rule out Hirschsprung's disease
(D) assure the parents that the child is not soiling deliberately
(E) recommend negative reinforcement for soiling behavior

5. Which statement is most accurate concerning the syndrome of infantile autism?

(A) The prognosis is good if the onset of the illness is at birth
(B) The prognosis is good if the child has normal auditory-evoked potentials
(C) The prognosis is determined by language development
(D) The prognosis is bad if either of the child's parents has manic-depressive illness
(E) None of the above

Directions: Each question below contains four suggested answers of which **one or more** is correct. Choose the answer

A if **1, 2, and 3** are correct
B if **1 and 3** are correct
C if **2 and 4** are correct
D if **4** is correct
E if **1, 2, 3, and 4** are correct

6. True statements concerning the use of toys in child psychiatry include

(1) toys should be available for the child's enjoyment
(2) toys facilitate communication between the child and the therapist
(3) toys may be used by a child to avoid thinking or talking about his or her problem
(4) toys are used symbolically by the age of 3 years

7. Causes of enuresis include

(1) juvenile-onset diabetes mellitus
(2) a urinary tract infection
(3) psychological factors
(4) spina bifida occulta

8. Methods of treating infantile autism include

(1) electroconvulsive therapy (ECT)
(2) behavior modification
(3) imipramine administration
(4) psychotherapy

9. Phases of the life cycle during which the bonding process occurs include

(1) the mother's childhood
(2) pregnancy
(3) the immediate postnatal period
(4) the toddler stage

10. Signs and symptoms that are found in the syndrome of hospitalism include

(1) severe inanition in infancy
(2) bad bonding
(3) susceptibility to infection
(4) jaundice

11. Of the following conditions, parasomnias include

(1) night terrors
(2) enuresis
(3) somnambulism
(4) narcolepsy

Directions: The group of questions below consists of lettered choices followed by several numbered items. For each numbered item select the **one** lettered choice with which it is **most** closely associated. Each lettered choice may be used once, more than once, or not at all.

Questions 12–16

Match the conditions listed below with the most appropriate medication.

(A) Thioridazine
(B) Imipramine
(C) Methylphenidate
(D) Phenobarbital
(E) No medication

12. Childhood schizophrenia

13. Hyperactivity

14. Enuresis

15. Infantile autism

16. Idiopathic grand mal epilepsy

ANSWERS AND EXPLANATIONS

1. The answer is A. (*I B 1, C 1, 2; X; XIII*) The incidence of almost all childhood psychiatric conditions is higher in boys; only anorexia nervosa and thumb sucking occur more frequently in girls. Boys are more vulnerable for a number of reasons. They may be raised differently, and they probably have a genetic vulnerability. The incidence of many psychiatric conditions such as anorexia nervosa, depression, and schizophrenia increases at puberty. Childhood psychopathology is more likely to be transient when it follows a clear psychological stressor. When a child has been raised in a chronically damaging way, he or she may have lasting psychological problems. Although family history and evaluation are helpful, a child can be evaluated alone.

2. The answer is B. (*I A 1, 2*) Epigenesis is a principle that states that development must occur in a sequential fashion. Although some children may become arrested at certain points of development, they still progress through these psychosexual stages in the correct order. When a child is psychologically traumatized at one of these levels, he or she may continue to show characteristics of that level. For example, the child might have anal traits of compulsions, stinginess, and extreme orderliness if hospitalized for 6 months at the age of 2 years; however, he or she would still continue through all phases. These psychosexual stages begin in the first year of life; they were discovered by Freud.

3. The answer is C. (*I C 1; XIV D 4*) A child should be assured that the information that he or she provides the therapist is confidential. When a child is at risk of harming him- or herself or others, it is appropriate and necessary to inform the family. Although children assume that parents know a great deal, the ability to understand and keep a secret probably develops before 3 years of age, and the child's sense of confidentiality allows him or her to discuss feelings without fear of reprisal or loss of love.

4. The answer is A. (*VIII C 1*) A significant percentage of children with encopresis have an impaction, and before psychiatric treatment is initiated, the presence of an impaction must be determined. A rectal examination might be appropriate in cases of encopresis but should probably be performed by a pediatrician. Because children with this disorder are not usually consciously aware of angry feelings, too early an interpretation of these feelings may cause problems in therapy. Children rarely soil deliberately, and negative reinforcement does not eliminate this behavior.

5. The answer is C. (*III A 4, 7*) Although the prognosis of infantile autism is better with good language development and relatively high intelligence, in general, the prognosis for the syndrome is very guarded. There probably are some associated neurologic deficits (e.g., development of grand mal seizures prior to adolescence and possible vestibular dysfunction). Most autistic children have abnormal auditory-evoked potentials; however, this finding does not correlate with the prognosis. A manic-depressive parent would not affect the prognosis; there is no association of manic-depressive illness (bipolar affective disorder) with infantile autism.

6. The answer is E (all). (*I C 1, 3*) As with all forms of communication, play and the use of toys inform the therapist of conflict and can be used defensively. For example, a child may insist on playing checkers for the entire session to avoid talking or playing out his or her problems. If he or she has problems with competition and throws the checkerboard after losing, the game is probably being used to express a conflict. Symbolic play—using toys to express an idea—develops very early in childhood.

7. The answer is E (all). (*IV B*) A variety of organic and psychological factors cause enuresis. Metabolic conditions (e.g., diabetes), infections (e.g., those of the urinary tract), anatomical problems (e.g., those of the posterior urethral valves), neurologic conditions (e.g., spina bifida or spina bifida occulta), and psychological problems can all cause enuresis. Because psychological problems are most frequently causative, painful invasive procedures should be avoided unless they are absolutely indicated. Psychological causes include repressed anger on the part of the child, psychological stress (e.g., birth of a sibling), and ambition expressed through enuresis (boys may express pride and ambition with the strength and quality of their urine stream; when ambition is conflicted, enuresis can develop).

8. The answer is C (2, 4). (*III A 6*) Neither electroconvulsive therapy (ECT) nor administration of imipramine is effective in treating infantile autism. Behavior modification is most suitable, and psychotherapy is a useful adjunct. Behavior modification aims to promote social behavior and to eliminate autistic or idiosyncratic behavior. A structured educational setting with a low student-to-teacher ratio, a constant environment, and specific language therapy is helpful. Psychotherapy may be needed when the family is having trouble coping with an autistic child or when environmental factors have played a role in the genesis of the illness.

9. The answer is E (all). (*II A*) Bonding occurs throughout an individual's life span. There is no critical phase. Bonding is defined as the affective relationship that develops between a parent and child. Bonding to a child can develop before the child is born. A 3-year-old girl, for example, plays with dolls and imagines her attitudes towards her future children. When she is pregnant, these vague attitudes about children become focused on the fetus and child to be. After the child is born, the affective relationship grows and changes. It probably persists throughout the child's life span and is passed on to the next generation.

10. The answer is A (1, 2, 3). (*II C 1*) Hospitalism is the result of no bond between a parent and child. Although it can cause severe inanition and susceptibility to infection, it is not associated with jaundice. The syndrome develops in infants and is associated with a high mortality rate. Treatment consists of providing the infant with a bonding (i.e., nurturing) experience. If parents are unavailable, surrogate parents should be provided.

11. The answer is A (1, 2, 3). (*VI A, B*) Night terrors and somnambulism (sleepwalking) are parasomnias. Although enuresis is not necessarily a parasomnia, when it occurs nocturnally, it usually is associated with the deep stages of sleep. Narcolepsy is a disorder characterized by sleep-onset rapid eye movement (REM), cataplexy, daytime drowsiness, hypnagogic hallucinations (hallucinations at sleep onset), and sleep paralysis. It is not a parasomnia. Parasomnias are common, can be aggravated by daytime stress, and seldom require treatment.

12–16. The answers are: 12-A, 13-C, 14-B, 15-E, 16-D. (*III A 6, B 3; VII C 3; XII C 2*) Childhood schizophrenia is now termed pervasive developmental disorder (see the *DSM III*). Low doses of thioridazine can help. It should be kept in mind, however, that neuroleptics cause serious side effects (e.g., tardive dyskinesia).

Imipramine is used for the treatment of enuresis. It has anticholinergic properties, and it affects the central nervous system, both of which are therapeutic in this condition. Side effects can be serious, the lethal dose ratio is low, and cardiac arrhythmias can develop with an overdose. The drug should be prescribed with caution.

Methylphenidate treats hyperactivity. Side effects include growth retardation, tics, anorexia, and excitation. It, too, should be prescribed cautiously.

Phenobarbital treats grand mal seizures. This drug can cause hyperactivity, necessitating a change of anticonvulsants.

There is no medication that treats infantile autism. However, infantile autism is probably an organic condition, and studies of nonmethylphenidate stimulants are showing modest, but promising, results.

11
Personality Disorders
James H. Scully

I. DEFINITION. Each of us has a repertoire of coping devices or defenses that allows us to maintain an equilibrium between our internal drives and the world around us. This repertoire is **personality—the set of characteristics that define the behavior, thoughts, and emotions of an individual**. The characteristics become ingrained and dictate our life-styles.

A. Personality traits are generally viewed as a result of development that has been influenced by culture and society as well as by the child-rearing practices of the individual family. In addition, recent studies in child development suggest that there may be genetically determined temperamental factors involved in the course of personality development. Certain genetic characteristics may make a specific behavioral response more likely to occur, thus leading to a specific personality style. When this stable pattern of response leads to problems, a personality disorder may be present. The *Diagnostic and Statistical Manual of Mental Disorders*, third edition, (*DSM III*) defines a personality disorder as present when personality traits are inflexible and maladaptive and cause either significant impairment in social or occupational functioning or subjective distress. Manifestations of a personality disorder are generally recognized by adolescence or earlier and continue throughout most of adult life; they often become less obvious in middle or old age.

B. Personality disorders are the most common emotional disorders seen in psychiatric practice, particularly in the outpatient clinic. The patient's perception of the problem and the expression of symptoms, however, are different than those demonstrated in other psychiatric illnesses and make treatment difficult. Patients with personality disorders may complain of mood disturbances, particularly depression or anxiety. However, they do not see the cause of this disturbance as coming from themselves. It results from the rest of the world being out of step with them. This kind of symptom is called **ego-syntonic**, that is, patients do not see anything wrong with themselves that needs to be changed. Sometimes patients with personality disorders have ego-dystonic or internally distressing symptoms but, nevertheless, are unable to alter their behavior.

C. Symptoms of personality disorders almost always affect other individuals. The symptoms involve work and play and relationships of all sorts. People with personality disorders have trouble in their work settings; they have often had many jobs and work below their capacities. Social relationships are disrupted or absent altogether. Often the reactions to personality disorders are more pronounced in the individuals surrounding an affected person than in that person. Those with personality disorders can be irritating and infuriating to those involved with them, and among the people with whom they come into contact are physicians and other health professionals. These patients may seek help as a result of a concurrent medical or surgical problem or because of a primary emotional distress; in any case, these patients have the ability to elicit strong negative reactions in those who take care of them. In general, these patients tolerate stress poorly, and they do not seek help to change their characters but to alleviate the outside stress. If stress is great, as it can be in physical illness, patients may regress even more and can develop transient psychotic reactions, in which they lose touch with reality and become unable to function for brief periods of time.

D. Diagnosis of a personality disorder should be made with care in someone who is reacting to a major environmental or social stress. For example, some young men develop maladaptive coping mechanisms in the military that they do not otherwise employ. On the other hand, some environments are compatible with certain personality traits and even reward them: The histrionic and narcissistic personality types may function well in the entertainment field, while schizoid and avoidant types might do better isolated in laboratories.

II. CLASSES OF PERSONALITY DISORDERS

A. Eleven specific personality disorders are defined in the *DSM III* and can be grouped into three classes.

    1. The dramatic, emotional, and erratic class includes histrionic, narcissistic, antisocial, and borderline personality disorders.

    2. The odd and eccentric class includes paranoid, schizoid, and schizotypal personality disorders.

    3. The anxious and fearful class includes avoidant, dependent, compulsive, and passive-aggressive personality disorders.

B. The dramatic, emotional, and erratic group of personality disorders are the most problematic to treat because of the reactions that they stir up in the therapist. Affected individuals tend to use certain **defense mechanisms** such as dissociation, denial, splitting, and acting out.

    1. Dissociation involves the "forgetting" of unpleasant feelings and associations. It is the unconscious splitting off of some mental processes and behavior from the normal or conscious awareness of the individual. When extreme, this can lead to multiple personalities.

    2. Denial is closely associated with dissociation. In denial the patient disavows a thought, feeling, or wish but is unaware of doing so.

    3. In **splitting**, often seen in borderline personalities, the patient divides individuals into all good and all bad and cannot experience an ambivalent relationship. The patient cannot even be ambivalent in regard to his or her own self-image.

    4. Acting out involves the actual motoric expression of a thought or feeling that is intolerable to the patient; this can involve both aggressive and sexual behavior. Patients with these types of personality disorders may be **biologically vulnerable to stress because of a tendency to low cortical arousal and disinhibited autonomic and motoric activity**. Thus, a psychobiologic pattern may develop, which increases the potential for acting out and which is not associated with any particular anxiety.

C. Odd and eccentric group of personality disorders. Affected individuals use the **defense mechanisms** of projection and fantasy and may have a tendency towards psychotic thinking. Biologically, patients with this group of personality disorders may have a **vulnerability to cognitive disorganization when stressed**. Schizotypal patients have been found to have some of the same biologic markers that are seen in schizophrenic individuals, which include low levels of monoamine oxidase (MAO) activity in platelets and disorders of smooth pursuit eye movements. It is speculated that not everyone who has a genetic vulnerability to schizophrenia becomes psychotic, and some of these individuals may be diagnosed as having a schizotypal personality disorder.

    1. Projection involves attributing to another thoughts or feelings of one's own that are unacceptable; this can take the form of prejudice, excessive fault finding, and a tendency towards paranoia.

    2. Fantasy is the creation of an imaginary life with which the patient deals with loneliness. A fantasy can be quite elaborate and extensive.

D. Anxious and fearful personality disorders. Individuals with avoidant, dependent, compulsive, and passive-aggressive personality disorders use **defenses** of isolation, passive aggression, and hypochondriasis.

    1. In **isolation**, an unacceptable feeling, act, or idea is separated from the associated emotion. Patients are orderly and controlled and can speak of events of their lives without feeling.

    2. In **passive aggression**, resistance is indirect and often is turned against the self. Thus, failing examinations, clownish conduct, and procrastinating are aspects of passive-aggressive behavior.

    3. Hypochondriasis (see Chapter 6, "Somatoform Disorders") is often present in patients with personality disorders, particularly in dependent, passive-aggressive patients. **Biologically, these patients may have a tendency towards higher levels of cortical arousal and an increase in motor inhibition**. Thus, stressful stimuli may lead to greater anxiety or affective arousal.

III. SPECIFIC PERSONALITY DISORDERS

A. Borderline personality disorder

1. Definition (*DSM III*).* Previously referred to as borderline schizophrenia, pseudoneurotic schizophrenia, or ambulatory schizophrenia, borderline personality disorder is now felt to have little relationship to schizophrenia and is a distinct disorder itself. **The most important feature of this disorder is instability in a variety of areas**, including interpersonal behavior, mood, and self-image. However, no single area is always a problem.

2. Symptoms
   a. Relationships with others are often intense and unstable, with marked shifts of attitudes. Other individuals are idealized and then devalued. Manipulation of others is common.
   b. Impulsive and unpredictable behavior is frequent and potentially physically self-damaging. This behavior includes suicidal gestures, self-mutilation, recurrent accidents, and fighting.
   c. Mood is often unstable, shifting from normal to dysphoric. Intense and inappropriate anger is seen. Patients easily lose their tempers.
   d. Symptoms of a profound identity disturbance include uncertainty about self-image, gender, and long-term goals.
   e. There is an inability to tolerate being alone; the affected individual becomes frantic when faced with the prospect. At the same time there are chronic feelings of emptiness and boredom.

3. Epidemiology. The results of epidemiologic studies are unclear, but borderline personality disorder is an increasingly common and probably overused diagnosis in psychiatric settings.

4. Etiology. Almost all theories related to the cause of the borderline personality have postulated problems in early development. It is speculated that there is failure of the child to separate and individuate, and, therefore, a symbiotic relationship with the parental figures persists.

5. Medical-surgical setting. When an individual with a borderline personality becomes ill, there is an increase of stress and the potential for an exacerbation of symptoms related to the personality. The illness can mean a threat to any emotional homeostasis that the patient has developed. **Splitting** is seen. The hospital staff may unconsciously take sides and, with the patient, see things as all good or all bad. This split often occurs between the physicians and the nurses. The intensity of the feelings stirred up by the patient may make medical treatment difficult.

6. Treatment
   a. Psychological. There are two general approaches to the psychological treatment of the borderline patient.
      (1) The **psychodynamic approach** aims to understand the underlying psychopathology. In general, standard long-term psychotherapy is difficult because the patient tends to regress and therapist reaction is intense.
      (2) **Treatment oriented towards supportive reality** is confrontational rather than interpretational. The therapist helps the patient recognize the feelings that are being stirred up and their connection with behavior. The therapist sets limits and provides structure. This approach is more appropriate in the general hospital setting.
   b. Pharmacologic treatment. Leibowitz and Klein have described a group of patients who meet the criteria of borderline personality disorder and who they see as suffering from "**hysteroid dysphoria.**" This represents a subtype of **atypical depression**, characterized by overeating and oversleeping, affective instability, poor self-esteem, which is particularly dependent upon external approval, and intolerance of personal rejection. These patients respond to **monoamine oxidase inhibitors (MAOIs)** better than to tricyclic antidepressants. While there is some controversy over the diagnosis of atypical affective disorder, certainly any patient with borderline personality disorder should be evaluated for an affective illness.

B. Antisocial personality disorder

1. Definition (*DSM III*). Individuals with this disorder have a **history of continuous and chronic antisocial behavior** by which the rights of others are violated. The essential defect is one of character structure in which affected individuals are seemingly unable to control their im-

---

*Terms in this chapter followed by the designation *DSM III* are defined as they are in the current formal psychiatric nomenclature of the *Diagnostic and Statistical Manual of Mental Disorders*, third edition.

pulses and postpone immediate gratification. There is a lack of sensitivity to the feelings of others. They are egocentric, selfish, and excessively demanding. They are usually free of anxiety, remorse, and guilt. Antisocial personalities have been termed as sociopathic and psychopathic. They persist in lifelong habits of violating the laws and customs of the communities in which they live.

   a. The antisocial behavior, which begins before the age of 15 years and persists into adult life, is **not due to manic episodes, schizophrenia, or mental retardation**.
   b. An inability to maintain adequate job performance over a period of several years is evident. (Some individuals, such as housewives, students, and the self-employed may not demonstrate this particular feature of the disorder.)

2. Symptoms
   a. For diagnosis, the individual must be at least 18 years old but have had personality problems beginning before the age of 15 years, including at least three of the following symptoms:
     (1) Truancy
     (2) Expulsion or suspension from school for misbehavior
     (3) Delinquency
     (4) Running away
     (5) Persistent lying
     (6) Repeated sexual intercourse in casual relationships
     (7) Repeated drunkenness or substance abuse
     (8) Vandalism
     (9) School grades markedly below expectations
     (10) Chronic violation of rules at home or at school
     (11) Initiation of fights
   b. Problem behavior occurs after the age of 18 in at least four of the following areas:
     (1) Frequent job changes, significant unemployment, serious absenteeism, and walking off the job
     (2) Inability to function as a responsible parent
     (3) Failure to accept social norms with respect to lawful behavior as indicated by repeated thefts, an illegal occupation (e.g., pimping, prostitution, and drug selling), multiple arrests or felony convictions
     (4) Inability to maintain an enduring attachment to a sexual partner as indicated by two or more divorces, separations, or both as well as desertion and promiscuity
     (5) Irritability and aggressiveness as indicated by repeated physical fights or assaults, including spouse and child abuse
     (6) Failure to honor financial obligations and debts, failure to provide child support, and failure to support other dependents on a regular basis
     (7) Failure to plan ahead or impulsiveness as indicated by moving about without a prearranged job or clear goal or the lack of a fixed address for 1 month or more
     (8) Disregard for the truth as indicated by repeated lying or conning others for personal profit
     (9) Recklessness as indicated by driving while intoxicated or recurrent speeding

3. Prevalence. It is estimated that 3% of American men and 1% of American women have an antisocial personality disorder. The disorder is more common among individuals of lower socioeconomic groups, and individuals with this disorder tend to do poorly economically and leave their families destitute. Illiteracy and substance use disorders are frequent complications.

4. The etiology is not clear. There is a history of antisocial personality disorder often found in both men and women in the family. Some antisocial behavior is precipitated by brain damage secondary to closed head trauma or encephalitis. In these cases, the proper diagnosis is organic personality syndrome rather than antisocial personality disorder. The causative factors are generally felt to be psychosocial. A sociopathic or alcoholic father is a powerful predictor of an antisocial personality whether or not the child is reared in the presence of the father. Other studies show that inconsistent and impulsive parenting is more damaging than the loss of a parent.

5. Medical-surgical setting. Patients with antisocial personality disorder may be superficially charming when under stress and not cause any particular problems initially. However, they tend to be manipulative if given a chance and will chafe against the rules of the hospital. Younger patients with antisocial personality have particular difficulty with the authority of physicians and tend to be noncompliant with treatment. They are likely to bolt the hospital against medical advice when threatened and generally disrupt the hospital setting.

6. Treatment
  a. The setting of firm limits is crucial, and, in general, inpatient settings are the only places where behavior can be controlled.
  b. Group therapy is more helpful than individual therapy because the patient sees it as less authoritative. Inpatient groups can confront antisocial behavior since the group is made up of experts at recognizing this behavior. Group treatment may involve therapeutic communities as well.
  c. Outpatient treatment usually is totally unsatisfactory because the patient flees treatment as soon as unpleasant affects are elicited.

C. Narcissistic personality disorder

1. Definition (*DSM III*). Individuals with narcissistic personality disorder **constantly seek admiration and attention**; however, they are more concerned about appearance than substance. Their self-esteem is often fragile, and these individuals respond to criticism with cool indifference and emptiness or rage and shame.

2. Symptoms. Narcissistic individuals are significantly impaired by the following:
  a. A **grandiose sense of self-importance** or uniqueness, which may be manifested as extreme self-centeredness and self-absorption
  b. An **exhibitionistic need for constant attention** and admiration
  c. A **sense of entitlement**, with the expectation of special favors without the assumption of reciprocal responsibilities
  d. Interpersonal exploitation; advantage is taken of others for self-aggrandizement and to indulge personal desires
  e. Relationships with others that alternate between the extremes of **overidealization** and **devaluation**, with lack of empathy; **splitting**
  f. Excessive and unrealistic fantasies involving unlimited success, ability, power, wealth, brilliance, beauty, and ideal love, which substitute for realistic activity

3. The prevalence of this disorder is unknown. The diagnosis is being made more often in recent years; however, this may be due to greater interest in the disorder rather than an increased prevalence.

4. Associated features often include a depressed mood.

5. Medical-surgical setting. An individual with a narcissistic personality reacts to illness as a threat to his or her sense of grandiosity and self-perfection. There is usually intensification of characteristic behavior and either overidealization or devaluation of the physician. The patient expects special treatment.

6. Treatment. Individual psychotherapy is the treatment of choice with an attempt at understanding the pain suffered by the patient with this disorder. The therapist must deal with transitions from being overidealized to being devalued. These transitions can be stormy, and they occur when the therapist has misunderstood the patient or has not been perfectly empathic. It is important that the therapist is not defensive about his or her mistakes.

D. Histrionic personality disorder

1. Definition (*DSM III*). This disorder formerly was called **hysterical personality**, but that term has been dropped because of the many meanings of hysterical. Over the years the word hysterical has been described as a personality type, a conversion reaction, a psychoneurotic disorder characterized by phobias and anxiety, and generally has been a pejorative term usually applied to women. A histrionic personality disorder can occur in men as well as women. It is sometimes associated with homosexual arousal patterns in men.

2. Symptoms
  a. Individuals with histrionic personality disorder are prone to **self-dramatization**, exaggerated expression of emotions, excessive drawing of attention to themselves, craving for activity and excitement, **overreaction to minor events**, and irrational angry outbursts.
  b. They need constant stimulation with what is new and exciting and become bored with the routine.
  c. The **interpersonal relationships** of histrionic individuals show characteristic disturbances.
    (1) They are often perceived by others as being **shallow** and lacking genuineness even if they are superficially warm and charming.
    (2) They are **egocentrics**, often self-indulgent and inconsiderate of others.
    (3) They are **vain and demanding**.
    (4) They **constantly seek reassurance** from others and present themselves as being dependent and helpless on the one hand.

(5) On the other hand, **they tend to manipulate** others with suicide threats and gestures.

d. They are often attractive and even seductive. Their sex lives tend to involve romantic fantasies rather than real relationships. While some individuals may be promiscuous, others are naive and sexually unresponsive.

3. **Prevalence.** Histrionic personality disorder is apparently not uncommon; however, the prevalence is not known with certainty.

4. **Associated features** include depression and dysphoric moods. There are general complaints of poor health and somatic symptoms.

5. **Medical-surgical setting**
   a. Patients may be seen as charming and fascinating by the physician, especially when they are of the opposite sex.
   b. The illness is often seen as a threat by patients to their physical attractiveness. It may be seen as a punishment for their thoughts or feelings, and in men it may be seen as a threat of castration.
   c. Men may behave in an inappropriate sexual manner with nurses and physicians who are women. The sexual behavior may be a cover for deeper concerns about dependency. These patients learn that they can be taken care of by being cute or sexually attractive, and this behavior is accentuated under the stress of illness. The physician should approach the patient as a professional and remind him or her that the roles are set; at the same time, it is important to remain warm and noncritical.

6. **Treatment. Psychotherapy**, either as an individual or in a group, is generally the treatment of choice for this disorder. In general, the therapist helps the patient become aware of the real feelings underneath the histrionic behavior.

E. **Paranoid personality disorder**

1. **Definition** (*DSM III*). The central features of paranoid personality disorder are a **pervasive and unwarranted suspicion and mistrust of people**, hypersensitivity to others, and an inability to deal with feelings. Individuals with this disorder are neither psychotic nor schizophrenic.

2. **Symptoms**
   a. Paranoid individuals are hypervigilant.
      (1) They continually scan the environment for signs of a threat.
      (2) They expect to be tricked or harmed.
      (3) They are guarded and secretive.
      (4) They avoid accepting blame when it is deserved.
      (5) They question the loyalty of others.
      (6) They search continuously and intensely for confirmation of their biases with loss of appreciation of the larger context.
      (7) They exhibit overconcern for hidden motives and special meanings.
      (8) They exhibit pathologic jealousy.
      (9) They have difficulty relaxing and are ready to counterattack when any threat is perceived.
      (10) They make mountains out of mole hills.
      (11) They are quick to take offense.
   b. Paranoid individuals are often litigious.
   c. The affectivity of paranoid individuals is restricted.
      (1) They appear cold to others.
      (2) They have no sense of humor.
      (3) They lack passive, soft, tender, and sentimental feelings.
      (4) They pride themselves on being objective and rational.

3. **The prevalence** of paranoid personality disorder is unknown, and it should be noted that these patients rarely come to treatment. They tend to group themselves in esoteric religions and pseudoscientific and quasipolitical groups. Groups of paranoid individuals who set themselves apart and see others as ''the enemy'' tend to provoke negative reactions from the outside, thus reinforcing their paranoid views.

4. **Medical-surgical setting.** Illness tends to exacerbate the personality style of paranoid patients. They tend to become more guarded, suspicious, and quarrelsome. They are frequently overly sensitive to slights and project their concerns onto others. They complain and are suspicious. Physicians should be courteous, honest, and respect the defenses of paranoid patients. There is a need to be straightforward and explain everything. Physicians should not ex-

pect to be trusted and should not impose closeness upon these patients but remain professional and even a little aloof.

5. **Treatment.** Individuals with schizoid, paranoid, and schizotypal personality disorders do not usually seek treatment. If treatment is sought, the physician should be respectful but scrupulously honest in dealing with the patient. Individual psychotherapy is usually the only possible way to begin, but, if the patient can tolerate it, **group therapy** can be more successful.

F. Schizoid personality disorder

1. **Definition and symptoms** (*DSM III*)
   a. **Schizoid individuals have defects in their capacity to form social relationships.** They lack warm, tender feelings and are indifferent to praise, criticism, and the feelings of others.
   b. **These individuals are characterized by emotional coldness and aloofness.** Their close friendships are limited to no more than one or two people, including family members. They are not psychotic, and they do not have the eccentric thoughts, speech, and behavior seen in individuals with schizotypal personality disorder.
   c. These people are loners; they tend to be humorless and dull. They are self-absorbed and absentminded and seem to be unrelated to their surroundings.
   d. Men with this disorder are very unlikely to marry because they lack social skills. Women may passively accept a relationship and marriage.

2. **The prevalence** of schizoid personality disorder is unknown as these patients rarely come to treatment.

3. **Medical-surgical setting.** Illness brings these patients into close contact with caregivers, which is often seen as a threat to their equilibrium. Patients may intensify their aloofness and are likely to leave the hospital against medical advice if intruded upon too much. Physicians should respect the patients' distance and intrude as little as possible. They should expect the development of trust to take a long time and not demand emotional reactions from their patients.

4. **Treatment** is the same as that for paranoid personality disorder (see section III E 4).

G. Schizotypal personality disorder

1. **Definition** (*DSM III*). **Individuals with a schizotypal personality disorder are "strange" in that their speech, behavior, and thoughts are odd**; however, the symptoms of these patients are not so severe that they can be termed schizophrenic. There are no histories of psychotic episodes.

2. **Symptoms.** No single feature of the disorder is invariably present. In order for a diagnosis to be made, at least four of the following characteristics of the disorder must be found:
   a. Magical thinking (e.g., superstitiousness, clairvoyance, and telepathy)
   b. Ideas of reference
   c. Social isolation (i.e., there are no close friends or confidants, with social contacts limited to the essential)
   d. Paranoid ideation
   e. Recurrent illusions sensing a force or individual not actually present
   f. Odd speech, without loosening of associations or incoherence (i.e., speech that is digressive, overelaborate, circumstantial, and metaphoric)
   g. Inadequate rapport in face-to-face interactions due to constricted or inappropriate affect
   h. Undue anxiety about social situations and hypersensitivity to real or imagined criticism

3. **The prevalence** of schizotypal personality disorder is unknown.

4. **Medical-surgical setting.** The problems in treating illness are similar to those encountered with schizoid patients. Schizotypal individuals tend to put off caregivers. Illness threatens their isolation.

5. **Treatment.** If treatment is sought, the physician should be very honest in dealing with the patient. The odd behavior of these patients can cause uneasiness in the physician, who must avoid all ridicule of his or her patient. If the patient is able to tolerate **group therapy**, there is more chance of success than with individual psychotherapy.

H. Avoidant personality disorder

1. **Definition and symptoms** (*DSM III*). **Avoidant individuals are exceptionally sensitive to the possibility of rejection, humiliation, and shame.** They are unwilling to become friends unless given unusual reassurance that they will be accepted without criticism. Despite their

wish for friendship and closeness, they withdraw from social situations. They have poor self-esteem and are self-critical.

2. **The prevalence** is unknown, but the disorder is thought to be common.

3. **Medical-surgical setting.** Unlike schizoid patients, patients who are avoidant may do well in the hospital. These patients are undemanding and generally cooperative; their illness can allow them to be taken care of and to establish relationships with the staff. They are sensitive to criticism and may misinterpret equivocal statements as being derogatory or ridiculing and withdraw emotionally.

4. **Treatment. Psychotherapy**, either individual or group, can be useful. **Assertiveness training** may give these patients new social skills and be very useful. These patients respond to genuine caring and support.

I. **Compulsive personality disorder**

1. **Definition** (*DSM III*). **Compulsive individuals are impaired in their ability to express warm and tender feelings.**

2. **Symptoms**
   a. These individuals are perfectionists in a way that they "miss the forest for the trees." They are obsessed with minutiae such as rules, lists, procedures, and so forth.
   b. They insist that things be done their way, and they are insensitive about how others may be affected.
   c. They avoid or postpone pleasure by devoting all of their time and energy to work. At the same time, they are inefficient because they cannot make decisions due to their fears of making a mistake.
   d. Individuals with this disorder rarely give compliments or gifts. They are stingy with their emotions and material possessions.
   e. They are always aware of their status in relationship to authority. They do well at work as subordinates.
   f. In Freudian terminology, they are seen as anal characters who are rigid, orderly, and constricted. They are inflexible in dealing with others.
   g. Relationships are generally stable.
   h. Depressed mood is common. When compulsive individuals become angry, they do not generally express it directly, but ruminate about the details.

3. **Prevalence.** This disorder is more common in men, although the prevalence is not known with certainty.

4. **Medical-surgical setting**
   a. Illness may be perceived by compulsive individuals as a threat to their control over impulses. Generally stress increases compulsive behavior with an intensification of self-restraint and obstinacy. Patients become more inflexible than before, which may lead to complaints about the sloppiness of the hospital and imprecision of the care being given. When these patients are critical of failure to meet their standards, physicians should avoid defensive, authoritarian rebuttal. There is a fear of losing control of a situation on the part of these patients, and this may lead to a struggle for control with their physicians.
   b. Control should be shared with the patient in as many ways as possible. The patient should be allowed active participation in the decisions and details of his or her actual medical care. This may include charting medication times, carefully calculating caloric intake, and monitoring fluid intake and output.

5. **Treatment.** In general, individuals with compulsive personalities recognize that they have problems, unlike those with the other personality disorders. These patients know that they suffer from their inability to be flexible and realize that they do not permit themselves to have good feelings. **Individual psychotherapy** can be helpful, but treatment is difficult because these patients use the defense of isolation of affect. Group therapy may be more useful. Therapy should focus on current feelings and situations, and excessive time should not be spent on examining the psychological etiology of the condition. Struggles for control should be avoided. Depression, when present, should be treated.

J. **Dependent personality disorder**

1. **Definition and symptoms** (*DSM III*)
   a. Individuals with dependent personality disorder are **passive**. They allow others to direct their lives because they are unable to do so themselves. Other people, such as a spouse or parents, make all of the major decisions of their lives, including where to live and what type of employment to obtain. Their own needs are placed secondary to those of the peo-

ple upon whom they depend to avoid any possibility of having to be self-reliant. They lack self-confidence and see themselves as helpless or stupid.

  b. Commonly, there is another personality disorder present, such as histrionic, schizotypal, narcissistic, or avoidant.

  c. In psychoanalytic terminology, dependent individuals exhibit oral characteristics such as concern with oral satisfaction, pessimism, passivity, and self-doubt.

  d. Authorities believe that the presence of this disorder depends, to a large extent, upon cultural roles (i.e., certain groups are expected to assume dependent roles on the basis of criteria such as gender and ethnic background).

2. The prevalence is unknown, but the disorder is apparently common. The diagnosis is more frequently given to women.

3. Medical-surgical setting

  a. Being sick usually means being taken care of, and one might expect that dependent individuals would be good patients. However, illness may stir up intolerable feelings of fear of abandonment and helplessness for these patients. There is a pull to regress to an earlier state of dependency, which may frighten the patients because of its intensity. Feelings of dependency increase. Generally these patients become demanding and complaining when sick.

  b. Physicians need to set limits. It is important for the physicians, nurses, and other staff to get together to plan with the patient what kind of care is going to be given. For instance, it should be clear to the patient how often the nurses will come by to check on him or her. If this is not done early, the negative reactions that these patients stir up can lead to punitive behavior on the part of the caregivers.

4. Treatment. Psychotherapy can be very useful in the treatment of dependent patients. Focus is on the current behavior and its consequences. Behavioral therapies, including **assertiveness training**, can be helpful. The therapist should be careful when there is a challenge to a pathologic but dependent relationship. The patient may leave therapy rather than give up such a relationship.

K. Passive-aggressive personality disorder

1. Definition and symptoms (*DSM III*)

  a. Passive-aggressive individuals refuse to perform adequately at work or in social situations. This refusal is expressed indirectly. Such individuals are assumed to be expressing hidden aggression passively, which is expressed indirectly through at least two of the following:

  (1) Procrastination
  (2) Dawdling
  (3) Stubbornness
  (4) Intentional inefficiency
  (5) Forgetfulness

  b. The result of this behavior is long-standing impairment in work and social situations. These patients are often dependent and lack self-confidence. They may be aware of some conscious resentment towards authority figures but do not connect this with their behavior.

2. The prevalence is unknown.

3. Medical-surgical setting

  a. Some illnesses require patients to take an active role in the treatment. When this situation occurs with passive-aggressive patients, they tend to be noncompliant and develop new symptoms when discharge is pending. Staff reactions generally are anger and frustration in dealing with these patients. This may be the first clue to the personality diagnosis.

  b. The physician should support the positive aspects of the behavior (e.g., encouraging the patient to walk rather than to be pushed in a wheelchair). Early confrontation of the passive-aggressive behavior is preferable before angry feelings become too strong and the wish to punish the patient interferes with care. It is sometimes important for physicians to recognize that these patients cannot be cured and that it is not the physician's responsibility if the patient continues to smoke or abuse alcohol in the face of multiple warnings.

4. Treatment. In general, **supportive psychotherapy** is indicated for those patients who seek therapy. The therapist should calmly confront the patient's behavior and its consequences. The goal is to help the patient see that his or her behavior causes certain reactions in the environment that then cause pain in the patient.

L. Atypical, mixed, and other personality disorders. A patient may often have features of one or

more personality disorders. A specific personality disorder should be diagnosed even if there are mild features of another, coexisting, personality disorder.

1. The diagnosis of **atypical personality disorder** can be used when it is clear that a personality disorder is present but there is insufficient information as to a more specific diagnosis.

2. **Mixed personality disorder** can be used when the individual has features of several personality disorders but does not meet the criteria for any specific personality disorder.

3. **Other personality disorders** may include:
   a. **Masochistic personality disorder.** Many clinicians feel that masochistic personality disorder can be distinguished from sexual masochism, and that it is a common disorder seen more often in women than in men. This disorder involves long-standing, self-induced suffering and martyrdom. The patient sacrifices herself over and over again in relationships. There is a concomitant angry feeling of being exploited and a sense of righteous indignation. This disorder should be distinguished from altruistic behavior in which a sacrifice is also made for others but the attendant feelings of being put upon are not present.
   b. Other disorders that are sometimes considered by clinicians include **impulsive and immature personality disorders**.

BIBLIOGRAPHY

American Psychiatric Association: *Diagnostic and Statistical Manual of Mental Disorders*, 3rd ed. Washington, D.C., American Psychiatric Association, 1980

Leibowitz M, Klein D: Interrelationship of hysteroid dysphoria and borderline personality disorder. *Psychiatr Clin North Am* 4(1):67–87, April, 1981

STUDY QUESTIONS

Directions: Each question below contains five suggested answers. Choose the **one best** response to each question.

1. A personality trait is defined as a personality disorder when

(A) there is no genetic predisposition to the behavior
(B) problems are manifested by adolescence or earlier
(C) there is an unstable pattern of response to stress
(D) the behavior patterns become worse in middle age
(E) social impairment is less significant than occupational impairment

2. The difference between individuals with personality disorders and those with other mental disorders is most obvious in that

(A) these patients may have fewer symptoms than those around them
(B) these patients have often come into contact with health care professionals
(C) these patients do not handle stress very well
(D) social relationships with others tend to be absent or problematic
(E) these patients often work below their capacities

3. An individual who commonly uses projection as a way of dealing with stress may have a tendency towards

(A) schizoid behavior
(B) passive-aggressive behavior
(C) dependent behavior
(D) obsessive behavior
(E) paranoid behavior

4. Schizotypal patients have been found to have some of the same biologic markers that are seen in schizophrenics. These include

(A) low levels of monoamine oxidase (MAO) activity in platelets
(B) low cortical arousal
(C) electroencephalographic (EEG) abnormalities
(D) retinal disorders
(E) a tendency towards affective instability

5. Patients who are orderly and controlled and can speak of the events of their lives with no feelings are using the defense of

(A) denial
(B) splitting
(C) dissociation
(D) repression
(E) isolation

6. What personality disorder was previously referred to as pseudoneurotic schizophrenia?

(A) Schizoid
(B) Schizotypal
(C) Borderline
(D) Passive-aggressive
(E) Paranoid

7. Patients with atypical depression who also meet the criteria for borderline personality disorder seem to respond best to

(A) tricyclic antidepressants
(B) monoamine oxidase inhibitors (MAOIs)
(C) benzodiazepines
(D) neuroleptics
(E) none of the above

8. Characteristics of individuals with antisocial personality disorder include all of the following EXCEPT

(A) sexual promiscuity
(B) repeated drunkenness
(C) below normal intelligence
(D) poor work record
(E) a tendency towards running away

9. While the etiology of antisocial personality disorder is not known with certainty, it is known that a major contributing factor is

(A) a head injury in childhood
(B) encephalitis
(C) alcoholism
(D) loss of a parent
(E) inconsistent, impulsive parenting

10. All of the following are features of narcissistic personality disorder EXCEPT

(A) exaggerated concern about the motives of others
(B) exploitation of others
(C) lack of empathy
(D) a sense of entitlement
(E) feelings of emptiness

11. What is the best treatment approach for the patient with a narcissistic personality disorder?

(A) Administration of monoamine oxidase inhibitors (MAOIs)
(B) Group psychotherapy
(C) Individual psychotherapy
(D) Administration of tricyclic antidepressants
(E) Hospitalization

12. Characteristics of the histrionic personality disorder include all of the following EXCEPT

(A) self-indulgence
(B) suicidal gestures
(C) sexual promiscuity
(D) sexual naiveté
(E) pathologic jealousy

13. What is the best approach that a physician can take with a hostile, paranoid patient who is hospitalized?

(A) Offer straightforward explanations of procedures
(B) Be sympathetic about the patient's fears
(C) Set firm limits on the patient's behavior
(D) Avoid isolating the patient
(E) Let the patient share in the treatment decisions

Directions: Each question below contains four suggested answers of which **one or more** is correct. Choose the answer

A   if **1, 2, and 3** are correct
B   if **1 and 3** are correct
C   if **2 and 4** are correct
D   if **4** is correct
E   if **1, 2, 3, and 4** are correct

14. Features that an individual with a compulsive personality disorder is likely to exhibit include

(1) explosive behavior when angry
(2) constant awareness of status in relation to authority
(3) impulsive decisions when stressed
(4) generally stable relationships

15. The physician can best manage a hospitalized individual with a compulsive personality disorder by

(1) carefully explaining the roles of physician and patient
(2) allowing the patient the emotional distance that he or she needs
(3) setting limits on the patient's regressive behavior
(4) allowing the patient participation in decisions concerning his or her medical care

16. Characteristics essential to the diagnosis of passive-aggressive personality disorder include

(1) forgetfulness
(2) ideas of reference
(3) stubbornness
(4) aloofness

17. Individuals with the anxious, fearful personality disorders, a group that includes avoidant, dependent, compulsive, and passive-aggressive disorders, are most likely to use psychological defenses including

(1) projection
(2) isolation
(3) splitting
(4) hypochondriasis

ANSWERS AND EXPLANATIONS

1. The answer is B. (*I A*) Most personality disorders are manifested by adolescence or even earlier. In fact, there may be a genetically determined factor involved in the development of a personality disorder. A pattern in response to stress becomes stable and involves certain defenses. This behavior pattern often becomes less obvious in middle and old age. While occupational impairment is common in many of the personality disorders, it is not always present. Compulsive individuals may do well at work, but impairment in their relationships is almost always present.

2. The answer is A. (*I C*) People in contact with individuals affected by some of the severe personality disorders can become irritable and infuriated with the individuals with those disorders. These patients may view themselves as not having any problems but only reacting to environmental stresses, which, of course, their personalities stir up. With most other mental disorders, the patients suffer the most. Almost all patients with mental disorders come into contact with physicians at one point or another. It is uniformly true of mental disorders that stress is not handled well, but this may be more of a problem with schizophrenia and other disorders than with personality disorders. Relationships with others are problematic in patients with the psychoses as well as other mental disorders. Patients with schizophrenia and bipolar illness tend to have poor work histories as well.

3. The answer is E. (*II C 1*) Projection involves attributing unacceptable thoughts and feelings of one's own to another. This can take the form of defenses such as prejudice, excessive fault finding, and a tendency towards paranoid thinking and behavior. Projection is the hallmark of paranoid thinking. Schizoid patients tend to use fantasy as a defense mechanism. Passive-aggressive patients tend to use action. The passive-aggressive, dependent, and obsessive personalities tend to use the defenses of isolation and hypochondriasis along with aggression more than defenses such as projection.

4. The answer is A. (*II C*) In searching for biologic markers in schizophrenia, researchers have found a number of phenomena that are present in schizophrenic patients and not generally present in others. These include low levels of monamine oxidase (MAO) activity in platelets as well as disorders of smooth pursuit eye movements. Speculation is that not everyone who has a genetic vulnerability towards schizophrenia develops the illness and that some of these individuals may be diagnosed as having a schizotypal personality disorder. Low cortical arousal is seen in patients who exhibit a lot of acting out, and this group includes more of the patients with histrionic and narcissistic personality disorders. Electroencephalographic (EEG) abnormalities have not been useful in distinguishing character disorders, although there is an increase in EEG abnormalities in a number of psychiatric illnesses. Retinal disturbances are not an issue. There is a tendency towards affective instability in patients who are diagnosed as having the dramatic and emotional personality disorders, including borderline and antisocial disorders.

5. The answer is E. (*II D 1*) Avoidant, dependent, compulsive, as well as passive-aggressive patients use defenses of isolation, passive aggression, and hypochondriasis. In isolation, the unacceptable feeling, act, or idea is separated from the emotional charge associated with it. A patient can talk about it without feeling anything, and some of the anxiety is handled in this way. Denial can sometimes be seen in these patients, but it is more likely to be seen in dramatic, emotional individuals, in whom it is associated with dissociation. In dissociation the patient "forgets" unpleasant feelings and associations rather than isolating the affective charge. Splitting, in which ambivalence is never experienced, is more likely to be seen in the dramatic, erratic group of personality disorders. Repression is unconscious forgetting of events, and although similar to dissociation in some ways, it is seen in individuals with all kinds of personality disorders as well as in normal people.

6. The answer is C. (*III A*) Initially, patients with borderline personality disorder were thought to be borderline psychotic, and borderline psychosis was thought to be a kind of schizophrenic process. The patients would have transient psychotic episodes along with other symptoms of intense and unstable relationships and would demonstrate impulsive and unpredictable behavior. The diagnosis that they carried included borderline schizophrenia and ambulatory schizophrenia. Schizotypal patients were often previously referred to as schizophrenics and occasionally as chronic schizophrenics because of their bizarre behavior and thinking, but they were not included in the diagnosis of pseudoneurotic schizophrenia. The same is true of individuals with schizoid personality disorder, who do not have the intense affect that was seen as somehow neurotic. In the same way, individuals with paranoid personalities were sometimes thought to have schizophrenia but rarely pseudoneurotic schizophrenia. Passive-aggressive patients occasionally have been seen as neurotic but rarely as schizophrenic.

7. The answer is B. (*III A 6 b*) Borderline patients who have a subtype of atypical depression, which is characterized by overeating, oversleeping, affective instability, and poor self-esteem, seem to respond better to treatment with monoamine oxidase inhibitors (MAOIs) than they do to tricyclic antidepressants. Benzodiazepines and neuroleptics are not particularly helpful in the management of atypical depression.

8. The answer is C. (*III B 2*) Individuals with antisocial personality disorder may have normal or above normal intelligence. Occasionally, antisocial behavior is seen in mentally retarded patients; however, antisocial personality disorder should not be diagnosed when mental retardation is present as the mental retardation is felt to be partly responsible for the aberrant behavior. Sexual promiscuity is seen more often in women than in men with this diagnosis. Substance abuse, particularly repeated drunkenness, is a common feature. Symptoms must be present before the age of 15 years for diagnosis. Running away from home is among the more common symptoms. After the age of 18 years, the inability to sustain consistent work behavior, such as changing jobs too frequently, significant unemployment, serious absenteeism, and walking off the job, are common features of this disorder.

9. The answer is E. (*III B 4*) Although the studies are not conclusive, the intermittent presence of inconsistent and impulsive parents may be more damaging than the loss of a parent. Having a sociopathic or alcoholic father is a powerful predictor of antisocial personality disorder, whether or not the father is present, but it is unclear what the etiologic significance of this is. Some antisocial behavior can be precipitated by brain damage secondary to either a head injury or encephalitis. In these cases the disorder is called organic personality syndrome rather than antisocial personality disorder. Alcoholism can also be associated with antisocial behavior, but the personality disorder is not necessarily present.

10. The answer is A. (*III C 1, 2*) To be overly concerned about the motives of others is characteristic of paranoid personality disorder; it is not a primary feature of narcissistic personality disorder. Disordered relationships with others involving interpersonal exploitation and lack of empathy are features of narcissistic personality disorder. A sense of entitlement along with the expectation of special favors without assuming any reciprocal responsibilities is seen. These individuals may respond to criticism with feelings of emptiness, cruelty, and indifference as well as with rage and shame.

11. The answer is C. (*III C 6*) The best initial treatment approach for the patient with narcissistic personality disorder is individual psychotherapy. Group psychotherapy would be difficult because of the patient's sense of entitlement. The therapist must try to understand the pain that this disorder causes the patient. A problem of therapy is a tendency for the narcissistic patient to overidealize and then devalue the therapist. Monoamine oxidase inhibitors (MAOIs) and tricyclic antidepressants are indicated only if there is an associated affective illness; however, they are not the primary treatment for narcissistic personality disorder. In general, inpatient treatment is not necessary, and an affected individual can do well as an outpatient.

12. The answer is E. (*III D 1*) Pathologic jealousy is a feature of the paranoid personality, who has difficulty trusting and is threatened by others. The histrionic individual is overly dramatic and egocentric but is not particularly concerned with others except as they relate to him- or herself. Self-indulgence and inconsideration of others is typical of the histrionic individual. These people often tend to manipulate others by suicidal gestures and threats. While some are sexually promiscuous, others may be naive and sexually unresponsive; these are not mutually exclusive aspects of the disorder.

13. The answer is A. (*III E 4*) In general, paranoid patients are suspicious and look for a hidden motive and special meaning in the behavior of others. They are often litigious. When a paranoid individual is ill in the hospital, it is important for the physician to explain everything in a courteous, straightforward manner. The physician should not expect to be trusted and should not impose closeness upon the patient but should remain professional and even a bit aloof. Setting firm limits on the patient's behavior is not usually necessary. Isolating the patient may be more helpful than trying to place him or her in close contact with other people. While it is sometimes useful to let the patient share in some decisions concerning his or her care, it is not usually the most important aspect of the management.

14. The answer is C (2, 4). (*III I 2*) Compulsive individuals are restricted and are perfectionists. They are exquisitely sensitive to the status of authority figures and try to please them. They are excessively devoted to work and productivity and therefore do well at work. Individuals with this personality type generally have stable relationships when compared to those of individuals with the other personality disorders. They do not explode angrily when stressed but tend to ruminate about the details of an insult. They are not impulsive decision makers but tend to be indecisive and obsessive about all of the possibilities.

15. The answer is D (4). (*III I 4*) An individual with a compulsive personality perceives illness as a threat to his or her control over impulses, and this leads to an intensification of self-restraint and obstinacy. In the management of this type of patient, it generally is not helpful for the physician to retreat to a position of authority. The patient is not seeking emotional distance but control. Setting limits is not necessary with this kind of patient. It is more helpful to allow the patient active participation in the decisions and details of his or her actual medical care. This includes charting medication times, carefully calculating caloric intake, and so forth.

16. The answer is B (1, 3). (*III K 1 a*) The essential feature of passive-aggressive personality disorder is a resistance to demands for adequate performance in both occupational and social functioning, which is expressed indirectly rather than directly. This kind of covert aggression is expressed in terms of stubbornness, intentional forgetfulness, inefficiency, and procrastination. Ideas of reference in which the patient feels that events have special personal meaning are more often seen in paranoid and schizotypal personality disorders. Aloofness also is seen in the group of disorders that include schizoid, schizotypal, and paranoid personality disorders.

17. The answer is C (2, 4). (*II D*) Individuals with the anxious and fearful personality disorders use defenses to help them deal with their anxiety. These defenses include isolation, in which the unacceptable feeling, act, or idea is separated from the emotion that is associated with the idea. These patients can speak of events in their lives with no feelings. They are also hypochondriacal and complain of multiple somatic problems. Projection is more likely to be seen in the odd or eccentric group of personality disorders, such as schizoid and paranoid, and involves attributing to another unacceptable thoughts and feelings of one's own. Splitting is seen in the dramatic, emotional group and involves dividing people into all good and all bad.

Post-test

QUESTIONS

Directions: Each question below contains five suggested answers. Choose the **one best** response to each question.

1. A patient with endogenous anxiety can become phobic if

(A) the phobic trait is inherited along with the anxiety trait
(B) the patient becomes frightened of situations in which anxiety attacks were experienced
(C) the patient has experienced some sort of environmental stress resulting in phobia
(D) the anxiety attacks symbolize deep-seated conflicts that frighten the patient
(E) the phobias are side effects of drug therapy for endogenous anxiety

2. All of the following statements about electroconvulsive therapy (ECT) are true EXCEPT

(A) the success rate is greater than 90%
(B) it is indicated in manic patients who have not responded to other modes of therapy
(C) temporary memory loss is a common side effect
(D) the therapeutic effect results from seizure activity in the limbic area of the brain
(E) it is associated with low morbidity and mortality when properly administered

3. All of the following personality types are grouped into the anxious and fearful personality disorders EXCEPT

(A) dependent
(B) avoidant
(C) paranoid
(D) compulsive
(E) passive-aggressive

4. Why is developmental testing in infancy important?

(A) It can provide parents with a prediction of their child's future intelligence
(B) It accurately predicts a child's future development
(C) It can begin to prepare a child for future development and IQ tests
(D) It can screen for phenylketonuria
(E) None of the above

Questions 5–7

A 38-year-old woman has a 10-year history of pelvic pain, which is partially relieved by narcotics. Extensive workup, including laparotomy, has not revealed organic pathology. The patient denies feelings of depression and other psychiatric problems but expresses anger at physicians for being unable to cure her.

5. The most likely diagnosis for this disorder is

(A) depressive disorder
(B) somatization disorder
(C) malingering
(D) factitious disorder
(E) psychogenic pain disorder

6. All of the following disorders should be considered in the differential diagnosis of this case EXCEPT

(A) malingering
(B) schizophrenia
(C) bipolar illness
(D) organic illness
(E) conversion disorder

7. Although the psychological mechanisms of this disorder are not fully known, all of the following etiologic theories concerning this case are possible EXCEPT

(A) the pain may enable the patient to avoid an untenable situation
(B) the patient did not learn to verbalize her emotions as a child
(C) the patient had a painful illness as a child
(D) the patient needs to deceive her physicians in order to feel better about herself
(E) the pain may arise from a central nervous system response to stress

8. In evaluating potentially violent patients, all of the following are important EXCEPT

(A) obtaining a complete history of drug and alcohol abuse
(B) assessing the patient's capacity for impulse control
(C) determining which situations result in violent behavior
(D) feeling relaxed and comfortable with the patient
(E) contacting family and friends for further information

9. In contrast to most hallucinogens, phencyclidine (PCP) is more likely to cause

(A) hallucinations
(B) mydriasis
(C) dangerous behavior
(D) depersonalization
(E) anxiety

10. A patient with endogenous anxiety is most likely to respond to which of the following drugs?

(A) Diazepam
(B) Diphenhydramine
(C) Trifluoperazine
(D) Imipramine
(E) Secobarbital

11. Which syndrome is associated with anorexia nervosa?

(A) Klinefelter's syndrome
(B) Turner's syndrome
(C) Fragile X syndrome
(D) Down's syndrome (trisomy 21)
(E) None of the above

12. What percentage of patients show a social recovery from schizophrenia after 5 years of illness?

(A) 15%
(B) 30%
(C) 45%
(D) 70%
(E) 90%

13. All of the following statements about organic mental conditions due to vascular disease are true EXCEPT

(A) early signs of vascular disease include memory loss, irritability, and mental fatigue
(B) these conditions usually occur in individuals between 50 and 65 years of age
(C) insomnia is treated through sedating medications
(D) men are affected more often than women
(E) signs and symptoms of these disorders result from cellular hypoxia and disrupted metabolism

14. Which of the following statements is most characteristic of paraphilias?

(A) Patients feel little shame or guilt
(B) These disorders occur with equal frequency in men and women
(C) The etiology is thought to be genetic
(D) Depression is a common finding
(E) Patients see themselves as "sick"

15. The most important feature that differentiates the avoidant personality from the schizoid personality is

(A) hypersensitivity to criticism
(B) a wish for acceptance
(C) social isolation
(D) no sense of humor
(E) magical thinking

16. Most authorities believe that the lifelong risk for major depression is approximately

(A) 5%
(B) 10%
(C) 20%
(D) 40%
(E) 50%

17. What percentage of patients who commit suicide had a concurrent medical illness?

(A) 20%
(B) 45%
(C) 50%
(D) 70%
(E) 85%

18. Which of the following syndromes is associated with poor bonding and attachment?

(A) Enuresis
(B) Encopresis
(C) Child abuse
(D) Night terrors
(E) Sleepwalking

19. The percentage of United States Army enlisted men who became dependent on narcotics while in Vietnam was roughly

(A) 10%
(B) 20%
(C) 30%
(D) 40%
(E) 50%

20. The unconscious detachment of certain behavior from the normal conscious feelings associated with it is called

(A) denial
(B) splitting
(C) projection
(D) dissociation
(E) acting out

21. All of the following statements about bipolar disorder are true EXCEPT

(A) some patients have inherited an abnormality of membrane lithium transport in red blood cells
(B) depression follows each manic episode
(C) bipolar disorder is equally common in men and women
(D) bipolar disorder is usually clinically evident before 30 years of age
(E) levels of norepinephrine and its metabolites are often elevated in mania

22. Essential elements of a psychiatric emergency include all of the following EXCEPT

(A) internal or external stress
(B) a maladaptive solution by the affected individual
(C) increased tension between the individual and the environment
(D) a preexisting psychiatric history
(E) a tendency towards increasing disorganization

23. The mortality rate associated with anorexia nervosa is

(A) less than 1%
(B) 5% to 15%
(C) 20% to 30%
(D) 35%
(E) 50%

24. A 26-year-old woman presents to the emergency room with shortness of breath, dizziness, and tingling in her fingers for which no organic cause can be found. The psychiatric diagnosis that would most immediately explain her symptoms is

(A) situational reaction
(B) endogenous anxiety
(C) caffeinism
(D) hyperventilation syndrome
(E) post-traumatic stress disorder

Directions: Each question below contains four suggested answers of which **one or more** is correct. Choose the answer

- **A** if **1, 2, and 3** are correct
- **B** if **1 and 3** are correct
- **C** if **2 and 4** are correct
- **D** if **4** is correct
- **E** if **1, 2, 3, and 4** are correct

25. Bereavement is characterized by

(1) thoughts of dying
(2) weight loss
(3) sleeping difficulties
(4) a duration of 2 to 6 months

26. True statements concerning encopresis include

(1) soiling is rarely deliberate
(2) the symptom may signify severe psychopathology
(3) the illness is usually self-limited
(4) soiling is an expression of ambition

27. The differential diagnosis of anorexia nervosa includes

(1) Addison's disease
(2) Turner's syndrome
(3) panhypopituitarism
(4) tracheoesophageal fistula

28. Features of delirium include

(1) emotional lability
(2) disorientation
(3) rapid onset
(4) depression

29. Anaclitic depression can be described as occurring

(1) after 4 months of life
(2) after 6 months of life
(3) anytime in the life span
(4) prior to 24 months of life

30. A 28-year-old schizophrenic man lives at home with his parents. His mother is critical of his appearance, and his father considers him lazy for not getting a job and moving out. The patient has had three hospitalizations in 8 months with florid psychotic symptoms, which respond well to treatment with trifluoperazine. Treatment interventions at this point might include

(1) measuring the blood levels of trifluoperazine
(2) switching to fluphenazine decanoate injections
(3) beginning a daily activities program at the clinic
(4) encouraging the patient to get a job and find his own place to live

31. The gender identity disorder, transsexualism, can be described as

(1) usually beginning after puberty
(2) involving males dressing in female clothing
(3) caused in part by a sex-linked chromosome
(4) more common in males than in females

32. A 30-year-old chronic schizophrenic individual who is maintained on antipsychotic drugs develops anxiety and increased psychotic symptoms. Approaches to management might include

(1) reality testing
(2) support of defenses
(3) advice
(4) insight therapy

33. Medical illnesses that are misdiagnosed as somatoform disorders, particularly early in the disease course, include

(1) multiple sclerosis (MS)
(2) systemic lupus erythematosus
(3) thyrotoxicosis
(4) rheumatoid arthritis

34. An agitated 24-year-old man is brought to the emergency room in handcuffs by the police after he was found wandering along the highway in a confused state. The patient becomes mute and appears to be calm. The first steps in managing this patient include

(1) taking a history from the police
(2) removing the handcuffs to make the patient comfortable
(3) talking with the patient about his impulse control
(4) administering a 5-mg dose of haloperidol intramuscularly

35. A 68-year-old woman with chronic obstructive pulmonary disease is brought to the hospital by her husband. Four times in the last month he has found her wandering about their yard at 2 A.M. in her bedclothes. Which of the following etiologic factors should be considered?

(1) Hypoxia
(2) Aminophylline toxicity
(3) Senile dementia
(4) Cerebral vascular disease

36. Medical diseases that are known to produce a full depressive syndrome include

(1) pancreatic cancer
(2) hypertension
(3) hypothyroidism
(4) peptic ulcer disease

37. The most important features of the dependent personality disorder include

(1) a lack of self-confidence
(2) subordination of one's own needs
(3) failure to take responsibility
(4) the presence of other personality disorders

Directions: The groups of questions below consist of lettered choices followed by several numbered items. For each numbered item select the **one** lettered choice with which it is **most** closely associated. Each lettered choice may be used once, more than once, or not at all.

Questions 38–43

Match each case history with the most appropriate diagnosis.

(A) Acute phencyclidine (PCP) intoxication
(B) Alcohol hallucinosis
(C) Schizophrenia
(D) Bipolar disorder, manic
(E) Paranoid disorder

38. A successful 52-year-old businessman is admitted to an orthopedic ward with a femur severely factured in a skiing accident. After 2 days, the patient becomes agitated, complaining that people are making derogatory comments about him from the hallway, despite the fact that no one is there. Within 1 week, the patient has returned to normal.

39. A 30-year-old woman has not slept in 3 days following the delivery of her first child. She speaks continuously in a pressured, intrusive fashion of needing to prepare the world for the Son of God. She has no previous psychiatric history, but her father, who becomes quite agitated and pressured when given antidepressants, has a history of recurrent depressions.

40. A 19-year-old woman, who had dropped out of college to join a religious commune, is brought to the emergency department for bizarre behavior. During the 18 months that she has lived at the commune, she has been frequently observed talking to herself, and she often speaks of the devil trying to enter her head through her left ear. She has become uncontrollably agitated following an acute ingestion of an unknown substance; she is visibly responding to threatening voices. These symptoms continue for several weeks. Physical and neurologic examinations are unremarkable.

41. A 32-year-old man with three previous psychiatric hospitalizations is admitted to the hospital for harassing two young boys in front of a store. He insists that he is a special agent for the FBI and wants to report their misbehavior to the police. He lives alone in a cheap hotel room and spends his days talking to people on television. He is isolated and shows little affective response, regardless of the situation.

42. A 48-year-old mechanical engineer is referred for evaluation by his attorney because of his insistence that his employer's request to change his job is part of a communist conspiracy against him. He has no previous psychiatric history and appears to be normal except when talking about his employer and communists.

43. A 20-year-old man without a previous psychiatric history is brought in for evaluation after violently attacking his best friend. He has auditory and visual hallucinations and screams about being attacked when anyone approaches him. He has slurred speech and moves in an unsteady fashion. He is noted to have vertical and horizontal nystagmus.

Questions 44–47

Match each sign or symptom below with the alcohol-related syndrome with which it is most commonly associated.

(A) Delirium tremens
(B) Intoxication
(C) Hallucinosis
(D) Korsakoff's psychosis
(E) Wernicke's encephalopathy

44. Visual and tactile hallucinations

45. Blackouts

46. Confabulation

47. Dehydration

Questions 48–51

For each disorder listed below, select the clinical observation with which it is most likely to be associated.

(A) Bipolar disorder
(B) Major depression
(C) Dysthymic disorder
(D) Cyclothymic disorder
(E) Atypical depression

48. A change in personality in adolescence

49. Uninhibited spending

50. A tendency to experience more health problems than most people

51. Delusions of grandeur

Questions 52–57

Match each description of personality disorders with the appropriate disorder.

(A) Schizoid
(B) Borderline
(C) Antisocial
(D) Schizotypal
(E) Narcissistic

52. Splitting occurs. The affected patient divides people into all good or all bad and is unable to experience an ambivalent relationship.

53. The affected patient may have low levels of monoamine oxidase (MAO) activity in platelets and disorders of smooth pursuit eye movements.

54. Previously referred to as pseudoneurotic or ambulatory schizophrenia, the disorder is now felt to be a distinct diagnosis.

55. While this disorder should not be diagnosed until after the age of 18 years, the symptoms must be present before the age of 15 years.

56. The interpersonal relationships of individuals affected by this disorder alternate between the extremes of overidealization and devaluation.

57. The speech of affected individuals is often circumstantial, overelaborate, or metaphoric.

Questions 58–60

For the investigators listed below, select the theory concerning schizophrenia with which each is associated.

(A) Bateson
(B) Burnham and Gladstone
(C) Mahler
(D) Winnicott
(E) Leff and Vaughan

58. In the absence of "good-enough" mothering, the preschizophrenic individual develops a pathologic false self.

59. Psychosis develops as an attempt to deal with repeated double-bind communications.

60. Patients returning to families that rate high in critical comments and emotional overinvolvement have an increased rate of relapse.

ANSWERS AND EXPLANATIONS

1. The answer is B. (*Chapter 5 I A 1*) A patient with endogenous anxiety becomes progressively more phobic of situations in which he or she experienced spontaneous anxiety attacks. Although biologic factors seem to be strongly implicated in spontaneous anxiety attacks and some phobias, there is no evidence that these conditions are inherited together. Phobias that develop after exposure to a frightening situation are called exogenous phobias and are not associated with endogenous anxiety. Patients may become phobic of benign situations that stimulate unconscious conflicts; however, the symbolism of the phobia is usually apparent, and exogenous rather than endogenous anxiety occurs. While psychological therapies are generally ineffective in endogenous anxiety and many phobias, drug treatment often is effective for both of these conditions.

2. The answer is D. (*Chapter 2 VIII A 4*) Electroconvulsive therapy (ECT) has been a very effective treatment when judiciously used with patients for whom it is indicated. However, it is not known how it works. The limbic area of the brain is associated with emotional control and expression, but it is not known if ECT affects functioning in this area. Properly administered, ECT is associated with very low morbidity and mortality, and its success rate is higher than 90%.

3. The answer is C. (*Chapter 11 II D*) Paranoid individuals may appear occasionally fearful to outsiders, but their symptoms go beyond this to the odd and eccentric. The results can be avoidance of others, but this is primarily due to the inability to trust others and to suspiciousness. The dependent individual is fearful of abandonment. The avoidant personality is frightened of being humiliated. The compulsive personality is anxious about everything being perfect, and the passive individual is too frightened to express his or her anger openly.

4. The answer is E. (*Chapter 10 I A*) Developmental testing in infancy does not correlate with the future functioning of the child. Developmental testing only provides an accurate measure of the child's current level of functioning, and results can point to interventions to help the child at that point in time. For example, if a child is found to have developmental delays in motor milestones, physical therapy or special exercises might be recommended. Childhood IQ tests differ substantially from infant development tests. Developmental testing is not used to screen for phenylketonuria; however, phenylketonuria can cause developmental delays.

5. The answer is E. (*Chapter 6 II C 1*) The primary issue in this case seems to be one of a psychogenic pain disorder since pain is the major complaint of the patient. Depression may be present, but it is not the fundamental problem. Also, the physician should be wary of malingering to obtain narcotics, but there is, with the information given, no strong evidence of this. The diagnosis of somatization disorder requires the existence of multiple symptoms, and diagnosis of factitious illness is determined by the patient's awareness that the symptoms are not real.

6. The answer is B. (*Chapter 6 II C, E*) The least likely diagnosis in this case is schizophrenia, the diagnosis of which requires that the patient exhibit some disorders in thinking beyond that in the information given. In malingering the patient would be faking an illness for a clear gain, which is possible in this case. A bipolar illness involving somatic symptoms is also possible as is conversion disorder, which involves pseudoneurologic symptoms. The question of an undiagnosed organic illness must always be raised in patients with somatoform disorders.

7. The answer is D. (*Chapter 6 II C 3*) The psychological mechanisms are not fully understood in any of the somatoform disorders. Some researchers speculate that children who do not learn how to express their emotions verbally are more at risk for developing somatoform disorders. Also, patients with somatoform disorders tend to have a history of illness in childhood. Part of the mechanism may also be that they simply have a different kind of central nervous system response to stressful stimuli. In Munchausen syndrome (factitious disorder), patients seem to have a need to fool the physician and fake an illness to that end.

8. The answer is D. (*Chapter 9 IV D, E*) While it is essential to insure one's safety when evaluating a potentially violent patient, it is unlikely that the physician will feel relaxed and comfortable. Some degree of anxiety and tension is to be expected, and its absence suggests a countertransference denial of the patient's dangerousness. The patient's capacity to control his or her aggressive impulses is central to the evaluation; both drug and alcohol intoxication may significantly impair this capacity. The patient may be unable or unwilling to provide the necessary information; family and friends may be able to describe more accurately the patient's behavior and the precipitants for violence. Not only is the patient's impulse control important, determination of the likelihood of his or her returning to a situation that previously produced violent behavior is also crucial.

9. The answer is C. (*Chapter 4 II D 1, 2*) Hallucinogens produce autonomic arousal, increased temperature, illusions, hallucinations, anxiety, depersonalization, and paranoia without clouding the sensorium. In addition to these effects, phencyclidine (PCP) intoxication causes violent behavior and neurologic signs.

10. The answer is D. (*Chapter 5 VII C*) Benzodiazepines with the exception of alprazolam and antihistamines such as diphenhydramine may be useful to a patient with exogenous anxiety or with anticipatory anxiety with endogenous panic attacks. Antidepressants such as imipramine may ameliorate endogenous anxiety or endogenous phobias. Because of the danger of addiction and abstinence syndromes, barbiturates such as secobarbital and related compounds should not be prescribed for any form of anxiety or insomnia. Neuroleptics such as trifluoperazine may help some anxiety patients who are bothered by sedation; however, they are not specifically useful in endogenous anxiety.

11. The answer is B. (*Chapter 8 I B 5*) Turner's syndrome is associated with anorexia nervosa; however, this association does not mean that Turner's syndrome causes anorexia nervosa. Turner's syndrome patients often have short stature, a webbed neck, and learning difficulties, which could be screened for when examining a patient with anorexia nervosa.

12. The answer is D. (*Chapter 1 V D 1 a*) With the diagnostic criteria for schizophrenia requiring a deteriorating course and a duration of at least 6 months, the likelihood of a complete recovery from the disease is quite small, with some clinicians placing it at less than 4%. Approximately 60% to 70% of patients are socially recovered, which means that, despite varying degrees of impairment and continuing symptoms, they are able to function within society. Approximately 10% of patients require chronic hospitalization; another 20% have such marked impairment as to require custodial placement, nursing homes, and boarding homes.

13. The answer is C. (*Chapter 3 IV E 1–7*) Confusion is one of the more problematic symptoms of cerebral vascular insufficiency, and sedating medications exacerbate confusion. Although nocturnal restlessness often must be treated, a sedative is not indicated. More appropriate treatment is low-dose neuroleptic medication (e.g., 1 mg to 2 mg of haloperidol).

14. The answer is D. (*Chapter 7 IV A*) Depression is a common finding in the paraphilias, especially when a patient's interpersonal relationships suffer because of the sexual problem. Patients often feel shame and guilt about their impulses to act in deviant ways. Most of these disorders are seen only in men, with the exception of masochism. The etiology is thought to be psychological rather than biologic in nature, although it is not known for certain. Despite the distress that the disorders cause, patients do not always see themselves as "sick" and often come to medical attention only after they have been legally apprehended.

15. The answer is B. (*Chapter 11 III H 1*) Patients with avoidant personality disorder have a great wish for acceptance and affection, unlike individuals with schizoid personality disorder. Both personality types are hypersensitive to criticism and potential rejection, which leads to social isolation and few friends. Schizoid patients may have less of a sense of humor than avoidant patients. Magical thinking is a feature of schizotypal personality.

16. The answer is B. (*Chapter 2 III A 1 b*) Although the figure is controversial, most authorities agree that 10% to 15% of the population will suffer a major depression sometime during their lifetimes. The effects of the disease are widespread, and all physicians must be alert for it, especially since it does not always present in a classic manner (e.g., depression in men may present as substance abuse or be otherwise masked).

17. The answer is D. (*Chapter 9 III A 5*) Not only are many medical illnesses, especially those with chronic courses, associated with significant pain and disability, they represent a loss to be grieved and require the patient to make a shift in his or her self-image and expectations for future professional and social functioning. The patient's future may appear bleak and hopeless in the context of the plans and aspirations of a once healthy and younger person. Chronic medical illness can put severe strain on families and not only diminish their potential to support the patient but create further pressure on the patient, who may experience increased feelings of personal failure and isolation.

18. The answer is C. (*Chapter 10 II C 2*) Follow-up studies of premature infants suggest that they are at higher risk of being abused, probably because parents have not adequately bonded with them. Premature infants can exert other effects on parents. Parents may respond to the premature child by being overly protective. Over-protectiveness (which can last well into childhood) can cause a child to have hypochondriacal complaints, separation anxiety, hyperactivity, and learning problems at school. Parents may react to the birth of a premature child with grief, marital discord, substance abuse, or psychological growth.

19. The answer is B. (*Chapter 4 V A 3 a*) Forty percent of enlisted men tried narcotics while they were in Vietnam, and about one-half of these individuals became dependent. The finding that only a minority of men continued to use drugs upon return to the United States suggests that easy availability of drugs and the encouragement of a peer group that supports abuse are necessary for drug abuse to continue.

20. The answer is D. (*Chapter 11 II B 1*) Dissociation involves the "forgetting" of the unpleasant feelings that are associated with some behavior. When those feelings are too unpleasant, the patient has an ability to dissociate them unconsciously from the action. This is associated with denial, in which the patient totally disavows the feelings and thoughts that he or she has. In splitting, the patient sees others as either all good or all bad and cannot be ambivalent about anyone. The patient attributes his or her own feelings to others in projection. Acting out involves the motoric expression of the thoughts and feelings rather than a dissociation of them.

21. The answer is B. (*Chapter 2 IV A 1; V A 3; VI A 1, 2*) The clinical course of bipolar disorder varies. Many patients have manic episodes without any interceding depressive episodes. Others have many more depressive episodes than manic episodes. Unlike major depression, bipolar disorder is equally common in men and women. Symptoms are usually evident before 30 years of age. Investigators have discovered an inherited abnormality of membrane lithium transport in red blood cells, which suggests an autosomal dominant pattern of transmission. In mania, levels of norepinephrine and its metabolites are often elevated.

22. The answer is D. (*Chapter 9 I A*) Patients with preexisting psychopathology are often vulnerable to making maladaptive responses to stressors, but even healthy individuals may decompensate in the face of overwhelming stress or inadequate environmental support. Although some kind of stress, internal or external, initiates the process of increasing tension and disorganization, maladaptive responses, such as violence, alcohol abuse, and depression, continue the destructive spiral leading to a psychiatric emergency. Sometimes a formal psychiatric diagnosis, where none was present initially, is a sequela of an individual's response to stress.

23. The answer is B. (*Chapter 8 I D 2, G 3*) The usual causes of death in anorexia nervosa are serum electrolyte abnormalities and suicide. The workup of a patient with anorexia nervosa should include the following: careful physical examination, determination of the serum electrolyte count, electrocardiogram (ECG), and a blood chemistry profile (i.e., serum protein and liver and renal function studies). A mental status examination should be performed. This screens for suicidal ideation and other psychiatric conditions that cause weight loss (e.g., depression and schizophrenia).

24. The answer is D. (*Chapter 5 IV*) Hyperventilation, which may be caused by any type of anxiety, often results in shortness of breath, dizziness, paresthesia, headache, weakness, and, occasionally, carpopedal spasm. Situational anxiety, endogenous anxiety, and caffeinism all can cause hyperventilation if the patient becomes sufficiently anxious. Post-traumatic stress disorder more typically causes anxiety and other signs of distress and occurs as a reaction to a traumatic event that had taken place more than 3 months previous to the onset of the psychological disorder. However, hyperventilation could conceivably be caused by anxiety due to post-traumatic stress syndrome.

25. The answer is E (all). (*Chapter 2 VII C*) A full depressive syndrome is a normal reaction to loss. Preoccupation with the loss leads to a decrease in appetite, weight loss, ruminations, troubled sleep, distractibility, thoughts about dying, and impaired concentration. Family and cultural expectations play a role in the duration of bereavement. The typical duration is 2 to 6 months. Severe, disabling symptoms marked by feelings of hopelessness and worthlessness signal the presence of a major depression.

26. The answer is A (1, 2, 3). (*Chapter 10 VIII B 2*) Soiling is rarely deliberate and is usually self-limited. Sometimes encopresis does signify severe psychopathology, but not necessarily. The symptom may be associated with harsh or punitive toilet training. It is often an expression of anger but not ambition. With no treatment, an encopretic child could be expected to stop soiling by adolescence. Underlying psychopathology would probably remain, however.

27. The answer is B (1, 3). (*Chapter 8 I D 1 a–f*) Addison's disease can cause vomiting and weight loss. It is characterized by dark pigmentation, low sodium and high potassium concentrations, and low serum cortisol levels. Turner's syndrome is associated with anorexia nervosa; however, it is not part of the differential diagnosis. Panhypopituitarism mimes anorexia nervosa by causing amenorrhea, weight loss, and delayed puberty. Tracheoesophageal fistulas usually are congenital anomalies, and anorexia nervosa is usually a disorder of early adolescence.

28. The answer is A (1, 2, 3). (*Chapter 3 III A 1, 2*) Delirium is an acute process in which brain functioning is severely compromised. Widespread deficits result from delirium, which is defined as a global disorder. Emotional expression fluctuates rapidly. If an individual cannot remember or think clearly, maintaining orientation becomes difficult or impossible. Delirium arises suddenly and must be addressed quickly as a true medical emergency. Emotions typical of delirium are fear and anxiety; depression is not a feature. Depression is commonly seen in dementia, however.

29. The answer is C (2, 4). (*Chapter 10 IV A 1*) Anaclitic depression occurs after 6 months of life and before 24 months of life. During this phase of development children are aware of who their primary caretaker is but do not yet have object constancy, that is, they lack the ability to maintain an image of their caretaker in the caretaker's absence. Therefore, they are vulnerable to lengthy separations (i.e., more than 1 week). Such separations from caretakers can result in a depressive syndrome that includes sad facial expressions, anorexia, apathy, and withdrawal from other individuals. The best treatment is to avoid prolonged separations. If that is not possible, a familiar individual or surrogate caretaker should be available to the child.

30. The answer is A (1, 2, 3). [*Chapter 1 VII G 6; VIII C, H 1 d, e (3)*] Maintenance neuroleptics and a supportive family can have powerful effects on preventing a relapse of schizophrenia. A patient who responds well to neuroleptics should be evaluated with respect to compliance and adequate blood levels of the drugs. If oral compliance is a problem, fluphenazine decanoate administered every 2 to 3 weeks may be a successful alternative. While education and therapy can improve the quality of family interactions, some families are not willing to change. If a patient must live in a family with a high expressed emotion (EE), his or her likelihood of relapse can be decreased by reducing face-to-face contact with the family. It is not reasonable to expect a patient with frequent psychotic relapses to become independent and self-supporting immediately, although this might be a reasonable long-term goal.

31. The answer is C (2, 4). (*Chapter 7 III A*) Transsexualism, as defined, involves males dressing in female clothing; transsexuals crossdress because they are more comfortable living as females. In comparison are transvestites, who crossdress in order to obtain sexual gratification. Transsexualism is more common in males, as are most sexual disorders. The disorder almost always begins in childhood; 75% of males with this disorder have a history of crossdressing before the age of 4 years. The etiology is unknown.

32. The answer is A (1, 2, 3). (*Chapter 5 VII A 1*) Psychotherapy that is primarily supportive is useful to a patient with limited psychosocial resources, such as a schizophrenic. Techniques such as reality testing, support of adaptive defenses, and advice may help to suppress psychotic anxiety, while patient insight into deeper conflicts may increase the symptoms.

33. The answer is A (1, 2, 3). (*Chapter 6 II E*) Multiple sclerosis (MS), systemic lupus erythematosus, and thyrotoxicosis are illnesses that present in their early stages with vague symptoms and often are associated with psychiatric complaints such as anxiety, mood disorders, and occasionally psychotic episodes. Because of these vague, transient symptoms and the associated psychiatric complaints, patients are often misdiagnosed. Rheumatoid arthritis, while associated with psychiatric complaints, is less commonly misdiagnosed due to the physical findings of swollen and painful joints.

34. The answer is B (1, 3). (*Chapter 9 II A, B; IV D*) Although the patient appears to be calm, his muteness prevents taking the initial history from him, but it should still be attempted. The observations of the police are crucial to the diagnostic process; the patient's confusion and muteness suggest serious psychopathology. The patient's calmness may be the result of the external control exerted by the police and the handcuffs. Removal of the handcuffs without adequate precautions may lead to a reescalation of agitated behavior. Although external control may be necessary, administration of haloperidol at this point without a diagnosis might confuse the picture and even make the patient worse [e.g., neuroleptics are contraindicated in cases of phencyclidine (PCP) intoxication]. This patient might be best managed with 2- or 4-point leather restraints until he cooperates with history taking, physical examination, and mental status examination.

35. The answer is E (all). [*Chapter 3 IV D 1, 2, E 1–7, F 2 g (1), J 5*] Oxygenation of the blood is compromised by impaired alveolar gas exchange in chronic obstructive pulmonary disease. At her best, this patient may barely get enough oxygen to her brain; at night, most individuals hypoventilate. She has no margin of safety; if she hypoventilates, she no longer delivers enough oxygen to her brain. Hypoxia produces confusion, impairment of judgment, erratic behavior, and irrational thinking. Aminophylline is an analeptic agent chemically related to sympathomimetic amines. Intoxication with aminophylline can produce a delirious, confused state. Senile dementia presents in a variety of ways: A change in behavior in an elderly woman may be the first sign of the dementing process. A demented individual may suffer acute disturbances in behavior if an acute insult such as hypoxia is present. Cerebral vascular disease is common in the elderly, and an early sign is confusion. Nocturnal confusion may be particularly prominent. Judgment is impaired, and erratic behavior occurs.

36. The answer is B (1, 3). (*Chapter 2 VII A 2*) Hypertension is not known to lead to major depression, although antihypertensive medications such as reserpine have been implicated in the illness. Pancreatic cancer presents as depression in as many as 40% of cases, but the mechanism of disturbance is not known. Hypothyroidism leads to fatigue, apathy, and disinterest; affected individuals feel slowed down and become discouraged. Although it is known that thyroid hormone is necessary for normal functioning of the central nervous system, the mechanism by which depression is produced is not known.

37. The answer is E (all). (*Chapter 11 III J 1*) Individuals with dependent personality disorder allow others to assume responsibility for the major areas of their lives because they lack the self-confidence to function independently. They subordinate their own needs to those upon whom they feel dependent in order to avoid any possibility of having to be self-reliant. There is commonly another personality disorder present, such as histrionic, schizotypal, narcissistic, or avoidant.

38–43. The answers are: 38-B, 39-D, 40-C, 41-C, 42-E, 43-A. [*Chapter 1 IV; V; VI A 1 a (2), b (2), B 1, 2*]
The only symptoms described in question 38 are agitation and auditory hallucinations in an otherwise successfully functioning 52-year-old man. Acute phencyclidine (PCP) intoxication, alcohol hallucinosis, schizophrenia, bipolar disorder, manic, and paranoid disorder all may present with auditory hallucinations, except for paranoid disorder, which is characterized by persistent delusions, not hallucinations. Schizophrenia may present with auditory hallucinations, but this patient is too old for a first schizophrenic episode and functions on a high occupational level, and there is no description of prodromal or residual symptoms. In the manic phase of a bipolar disorder, auditory hallucinations, even if mood-incongruent, should occur secondary to a prominent mood disturbance; there are no affective symptoms described. The rapid onset and resolution of this man's symptoms suggest an organic mental disorder, such as an intoxication or a withdrawal state. PCP intoxication would have been present from the outset and would have been accompanied by numerous physical symptoms, including nystagmus and dysarthria. The patient, his symptoms, and the time course of his condition are most consistent with alcohol hallucinosis induced by forced abstinence during the hospitalization.

While the acute onset and lack of a previous psychiatric history suggest an intoxication withdrawal state in the patient in question 39, the other symptoms are not consistent with PCP intoxication or alcohol hallucinosis. Although paranoid and schizophrenic disorders may present initially in the postpartum period, this woman has a family history of an affective disorder and clinical symptoms consistent with mania. Furthermore, the observation that her father displayed some manic symptoms when treated with antidepressants suggests that he too may have a bipolar disorder, although he has not had a clear-cut manic episode.

Although the patient in question 40 has had an acute decompensation following ingestion of a substance, there are no physical symptoms consistent with PCP intoxication nor is there a history of chronic alcohol abuse. What is most striking is the chronicity of her symptoms in the absence of a mood disturbance prior to the ingestion. Not only was she delusional about the devil but probably chronically responded to auditory hallucinations when talking to herself; this latter symptom would exclude even a chronic paranoid disorder. What is most likely is that some substance triggered an acute psychotic decompensation in a chronic schizophrenic woman who has found some acceptance and comfort in a religious communal situation where her bizarre beliefs and behavior have been tolerated.

The man in question 41 has a chronic psychiatric history without acute evidence of intoxication or withdrawal. His delusional belief about his association with the FBI could be observed in a bipolar disorder, in a paranoid disorder, as well as in schizophrenia. However, the significant chronic impairment of his social and occupational functioning is more consistent with schizophrenia, as is his blunted affective responsiveness.

In question 42, the chronicity of the patient's beliefs in the absence of other symptoms, physical or psychiatric, rules out a state of intoxication or withdrawal. The lack of a psychiatric history prior to age 48, the preservation of good occupational functioning despite his belief, and the absence of other psychiatric symptoms make schizophrenia unlikely. There is no evidence of a mood disturbance or vegetative symptoms consistent with an affective disorder. Rather the patient's symptoms are most consistent with a paranoid disorder, including his extreme sensitivity to the humiliation implied in his job being changed and his litigiousness.

Acute PCP intoxication, alcohol hallucinosis, schizophrenia, bipolar illness, manic, and paranoid disorder all might present with violent behavior, as occurs in question 43. The lack of a prior psychiatric history in a 20-year-old is not as helpful as that in a 50-year-old in narrowing the diagnostic possibilities. The visual hallucinations and young age would exclude a paranoid disorder and alcohol hallucinosis. The acute onset makes schizophrenia and bipolar disorder less likely but does not exclude them; the particular symptoms do not discriminate among these disorders and PCP intoxication. In this case, the physical findings of dysarthria, ataxia, and nystagmus suggest an acute intoxication consistent with PCP. A history of drug ingestion and a drug screen showing evidence of PCP would substantiate the diagnosis.

44–47. The answers are: 44-A, 45-B, 46-D, 47-A. (*Chapter 3 IV F 2 x*) Hallucinations occur in both delirium tremens and alcohol hallucinosis. The sensory modality is critical. Typically, auditory hallucinations are present in hallucinosis. Visual and tactile hallucinations, such as spiders crawling over the skin, are much more likely to occur in delirium tremens.

Blackouts refer to transient periods of amnesia that result from intoxication. They stand out because the individual has no trouble with memory when he or she is not drinking. The individual has a memory gap of a few hours and may be painfully aware of it. Amnestic periods of different types appear in delirium tremens, Wernicke's encephalopathy, and Korsakoff's psychosis.

Memory is grossly impaired in Korsakoff's psychosis. Amnesia is severe and persistent. Confabulation is common. Stories are told with an air of certainty, even though no memory of events is present. This typically occurs without the confabulator being aware of the process. It is an attempt to adapt in the face of overwhelming deficits.

Delirium tremens is a condition in which an individual is often febrile and agitated. Loss of water may be enormous. Furthermore, the delirium interferes with the capacity for appropriate response to thirst and dehydration. Careful monitoring and replenishment of fluids is crucial in this disorder.

48–51. The answers are: 48-D, 49-A, 50-C, 51-A. (*Chapter 2 IV A 1, 2 d, B 1; VI B 2*) The cyclothymic individual experiences marked shifts in mood, level of energy, enthusiasm, and sociability. These symptoms typically begin in adolescence. An individual who was relatively consistent in interactions with others becomes erratic as these shifts in mood occur. The personality is changed.

The exuberant, enthusiastic manic individual is usually hyperactive. Judgment is often impaired. Money is spent freely, even if money is not there to spend. The financial consequences may be severe.

Chronic depression interferes with health care. An individual may not seek care when indicated because he or she does not have the motivation to do so and may feel unworthy of being helped. Some investigators believe that depression hampers the body's immune system. Symptoms in the chronically depressed may be interpreted as signs of depression instead of signs of physical disease.

Psychotic symptoms occur in both bipolar disorder and major depression. The expansive, exuberant mood of bipolar disorder leads to ideas that reflect that mood. The individual believes that he or she is as important as he or she feels, and delusions of grandeur result. Delusions in depression are usually focused on decay, guilt, and death.

52–57. The answers are: 52-B, 53-D, 54-B, 55-C, 56-E, 57-D. (*Chapter 11 II B 3, C 2; III A 1, B 1, 2, C 1, 2, G 1, 2*) Individuals with borderline personality disorder have profound identity disturbances, including disturbances in gender identity. Previously, these patients were felt to be affected by a type of schizophrenia on the borderline between schizophrenia and neurosis. This was called pseudoneurotic or ambulatory schizophrenia. Borderline personality disorder is now considered to be a distinct entity.

Splitting is a hallmark of the borderline personality disorder along with the intense and unstable relationships experienced by these patients. It can occur, however, in some of the other dramatic and emotional disorders such as narcissistic, histrionic, and antisocial personality disorders.

The essential features of schizotypal personality disorder are oddities of thought, perception, speech, and behavior, which are not severe enough to be called schizophrenia. Among these oddities is speech that is digressively overelaborate, circumstantial, or metaphoric.

Schizotypal patients have some of the same biologic markers that are seen in schizophrenic patients, including low levels of monoamine oxidase (MAO) activity in platelets and disorders of smooth pursuit eye movement. The speculation is that not everyone who has a genetic predisposition to schizophrenia becomes psychotic and may, in fact, be diagnosed as schizotypal.

Antisocial personality disorder should not be diagnosed before the age of 18 years because often juvenile distress is expressed as delinquent behavior and will dissipate in time. However, the symptoms must be present before the age of 15 years and include school problems and misbehavior as well as running away and vandalism. Age requirements are less strict for the diagnosis of other personality disorders.

An individual with narcissistic personality disorder has feelings of entitlement and exploits interpersonal relationships. Similar to splitting, but not as severe, are the patient's tendencies towards overidealization and devaluation.

58–60. The answers are: 58-D, 59-A, 60-E. (*Chapter 1 VII F 5 c, G 3, 6*) Winnicott focused on the importance of "good-enough" mothering, that is, empathic responses to the infant's needs without excessive gratification or undue frustration. Such mothering permits the infant to differentiate between him- or herself and others and maintain a stable sense of self. Without this type of mothering, the child may develop a vulnerable and pathologic false self to meet the mother's narcissistic needs; a breakdown in this system produces psychosis.

Bateson and associates studied the psychotogenic potential of double-bind situations. In double-bind communications, the child is presented simultaneously with conflicting messages on different levels; he or she can neither escape the situation nor comment on the conflicting messages. Therefore, whatever he or she says or does is wrong; however, a confusing, ambiguous response may be self-protective in this context. In this way, a schizophrenic thought disorder is viewed as an adaptive response to an untenable situation.

Leff and Vaughan identified family situations associated with high and low rates of relapse of schizophrenic symptoms. Families that show a hostile and overinvolved attitude are rated as having a high expressed emotion (EE). Patients living in such families have a relapse rate of 92%, which can be reduced by maintaining them on neuroleptics and by reducing the total time of face-to-face contact with the family. Some families can change from high to low levels of EE with education about schizophrenia and treatment of the disruptive communication patterns.

Index

Note: Page numbers in *italics* denote illustrations; those followed by (t) denote tables.